AMERICAN ACADEMY™
OF OPHTHALMOLOGY

9

Intraocular Inflammation and Uveitis

Last major revision 2015–2016

2016–2017
BCSC
Basic and Clinical Science Course™

Protecting Sight. Empowering Lives.™

EB

Published after collaborative review with the European Board of Ophthalmology subcommittee

The American Academy of Ophthalmology is accredited by the Accreditation Council for Continuing Medical Education to provide continuing medical education for physicians.

The American Academy of Ophthalmology designates this enduring material for a maximum of 10 *AMA PRA Category 1 Credits*™. Physicians should claim only the credit commensurate with the extent of their participation in the activity.

CME expiration date: June 1, 2018. *AMA PRA Category 1 Credits*™ may be claimed only once between June 1, 2015, and the expiration date.

BCSC® volumes are designed to increase the physician's ophthalmic knowledge through study and review. Users of this activity are encouraged to read the text and then answer the study questions provided at the back of the book.

To claim *AMA PRA Category 1 Credits*™ upon completion of this activity, learners must demonstrate appropriate knowledge and participation in the activity by taking the posttest for Section 9 and achieving a score of 80% or higher. For further details, please see the instructions for requesting CME credit at the back of the book.

The Academy provides this material for educational purposes only. It is not intended to represent the only or best method or procedure in every case, nor to replace a physician's own judgment or give specific advice for case management. Including all indications, contraindications, side effects, and alternative agents for each drug or treatment is beyond the scope of this material. All information and recommendations should be verified, prior to use, with current information included in the manufacturers' package inserts or other independent sources, and considered in light of the patient's condition and history. Reference to certain drugs, instruments, and other products in this course is made for illustrative purposes only and is not intended to constitute an endorsement of such. Some material may include information on applications that are not considered community standard, that reflect indications not included in approved FDA labeling, or that are approved for use only in restricted research settings. **The FDA has stated that it is the responsibility of the physician to determine the FDA status of each drug or device he or she wishes to use, and to use them with appropriate, informed patient consent in compliance with applicable law.** The Academy specifically disclaims any and all liability for injury or other damages of any kind, from negligence or otherwise, for any and all claims that may arise from the use of any recommendations or other information contained herein.

Cover image: From BCSC Section 10, *Glaucoma.* Typical gonioscopic appearance of angle recession. *Courtesy of Steven T. Simmons, MD.*

FSC www.fsc.org MIX Paper from responsible sources FSC® C103061

Basic and Clinical Science Course

Louis B. Cantor, MD, Indianapolis, Indiana, *Senior Secretary for Clinical Education*
Christopher J. Rapuano, MD, Philadelphia, Pennsylvania, *Secretary for Ophthalmic Knowledge*
George A. Cioffi, MD, New York, New York, *BCSC Course Chair*

Section 9

Faculty

Russell W. Read, MD, PhD, *Chair,* Birmingham, Alabama
Nisha Acharya, MD, San Francisco, California
Ralph D. Levinson, MD, Los Angeles, California
P. Kumar Rao, MD, St Louis, Missouri
H. Nida Sen, MD, MHS, Bethesda, Maryland
Jonathan D. Walker, MD, Fort Wayne, Indiana
Daniel V. Vasconcelos-Santos, MD, *Consultant,* Belo Horizonte, Brazil

The Academy wishes to acknowledge the American Uveitis Society (AUS) for recommending faculty members to the BCSC Section 9 committee.

The Academy also wishes to acknowledge the following committees for review of this edition:

Committee on Aging: Kelly L. Larkin, MD, Houston, Texas

Vision Rehabilitation Committee: Paul I. Homer, MD, Boca Raton, Florida

Practicing Ophthalmologists Advisory Committee for Education: Dasa V. Gangadhar, MD, *Primary Reviewer,* Wichita, Kansas; Edward K. Isbey III, MD, *Chair,* Asheville, North Carolina; Alice L. Bashinsky, MD, Asheville, North Carolina; David J. Browning, MD, PhD, Charlotte, North Carolina; Robert G. Fante, MD, Denver, Colorado; Bradley D. Fouraker, MD, Tampa, Florida; Steven J. Grosser, MD, Golden Valley, Minnesota; James A. Savage, MD, Memphis, Tennessee

EB

European Board of Ophthalmology: Carlos E. Pavesio, MD, *EBO Chair,* London, United Kingdom; Talin Barisani-Asenbauer, MD, FEBO, *EBO Liaison,* Vienna, Austria; Bahram Bodaghi, MD, PhD, Paris, France; Marc D. de Smet, MD, PhD, Lausanne, Switzerland; Arnd Heiligenhaus, MD, PhD, Münster, Germany; Richard W. J. Lee, PhD, Bristol, United Kingdom; Elisabetta Miserocchi, MD, Milan, Italy; Philip I. Murray, MBBS, DO (RCS), PhD, Birmingham, United Kingdom; Piergiorgio Neri, MD, PhD, FEBO, Ancona, Italy; Miles Stanford, MD, London, United Kingdom

Financial Disclosures

Academy staff members who contributed to the development of this product state that within the past 12 months, they have had no financial interest in or other relationship with any entity discussed in this course that produces, markets, resells, or distributes ophthalmic health care goods or services consumed by or used in patients, or with any competing commercial product or service.

The authors and reviewers state that within the past 12 months, they have had the following financial relationships:*

Dr Acharya: Santen (C), Xoma (C)

Dr Barisani-Asenbauer: Askin Austria (L), Croma Pharma (S), Laboratoires Thea Austria (L), Novartis Pharmaceuticals (S), Teva Pharmaceutical Industries (C)

Dr Bodaghi: Abbott Medical Optics (C), Allergan (C, S), Bausch + Lomb Surgical (C), Novartis Pharmaceuticals (S), Santen (C), Xoma (C)

Dr Browning: Aerpio Therapeutics (S), Alimera Sciences (C), Diabetic Retinopathy Clinical Research (S), Genentech (S), Novartis Pharmaceuticals (S), Pfizer (S), Regeneron Pharmaceuticals (S)

Dr de Smet: Allergan (C, L, S), Arnhem Ophthalmic Research (O, P), Bayer Pharmaceuticals (C), Centocor Pharmaceuticals (C, S), GlaxoSmithKline (C), Regeneron Pharmaceuticals (C), Sanofi (C), Santen (C), Thrombogenics (C, L, P, S)

Dr Fante: Ophthalmic Mutual Insurance Company (C)

Dr Fouraker: Addition Technology (C), Alcon Laboratories (C), Keravision (C), Ophthalmic Mutual Insurance Company (C)

Dr Grosser: Ivantis (O)

Dr Isbey: Alcon Laboratories (S), Allscripts (C), Bausch + Lomb (S), Medflow (C)

Dr Larkin: AbbVie Humira (C), Xoma Eyeguard Study (C)

Dr Lee: EMD Serono (C), Genentech (C), UK National Institute for Health Research (S), US Patent Application No. 61/919,404 (P)

Dr Miserocchi: Abbott Immunology (C), Allergan (C), Santen (C)

Dr Neri: AbbVie (L), Bausch + Lomb (C, L), Santen Pharma (C)

Dr Pavesio: Alcon (C), Alimera Sciences (C), Bausch + Lomb (C)

Dr Rao: National Eye Institute (S), Regeneron Pharmaceuticals (S), Servier Laboratories (C)

Dr Read: EyeSight Foundation of Alabama (S), Matthew Family Foundation (S), Research to Prevent Blindness (S)

Dr Savage: Allergan (L)

The other authors and reviewers state that within the past 12 months, they have had no financial interest in or other relationship with any entity discussed in this course that produces, markets, resells, or distributes ophthalmic health care goods or services consumed by or used in patients, or with any competing commercial product or service.

*C = consultant fees, paid advisory boards, or fees for attending a meeting; L = lecture fees (honoraria), travel fees, or reimbursements when speaking at the invitation of a commercial sponsor; O = equity ownership/stock options of publicly or privately traded firms (excluding mutual funds) with manufacturers of commercial ophthalmic products or commercial ophthalmic services; P = patents and/or royalties that might be viewed as creating a potential conflict of interest; S = grant support for the past year (all sources) and all sources used for a specific talk or manuscript with no time limitation

Recent Past Faculty

Bahram Bodaghi, MD, PhD
Ramana S. Moorthy, MD
Russell N. Van Gelder, MD, PhD
Albert T. Vitale, MD

In addition, the Academy gratefully acknowledges the contributions of numerous past faculty and advisory committee members who have played an important role in the development of previous editions of the Basic and Clinical Science Course.

American Academy of Ophthalmology Staff

Dale E. Fajardo, *Vice President, Education*
Beth Wilson, *Director, Continuing Professional Development*
Ann McGuire, *Acquisitions and Development Manager*
Stephanie Tanaka, *Publications Manager*
D. Jean Ray, *Production Manager*
Beth Collins, *Medical Editor*
Naomi Ruiz, *Editorial Assistant*

American Academy of Ophthalmology
655 Beach Street
Box 7424
San Francisco, CA 94120-7424

Contents

General Introduction

The Basic and Clinical Science Course (BCSC) is designed to meet the needs of residents and practitioners for a comprehensive yet concise curriculum of the field of ophthalmology. The BCSC has developed from its original brief outline format, which relied heavily on outside readings, to a more convenient and educationally useful self-contained text. The Academy updates and revises the course annually, with the goals of integrating the basic science and clinical practice of ophthalmology and of keeping ophthalmologists current with new developments in the various subspecialties.

The BCSC incorporates the effort and expertise of more than 80 ophthalmologists, organized into 13 Section faculties, working with Academy editorial staff. In addition, the course continues to benefit from many lasting contributions made by the faculties of previous editions. Members of the Academy's Practicing Ophthalmologists Advisory Committee for Education, Committee on Aging, and Vision Rehabilitation Committee review every volume before major revisions. Members of the European Board of Ophthalmology, organized into Section faculties, also review each volume before major revisions, focusing primarily on differences between American and European ophthalmology practice.

Organization of the Course

The Basic and Clinical Science Course comprises 13 volumes, incorporating fundamental ophthalmic knowledge, subspecialty areas, and special topics:

1 Update on General Medicine
2 Fundamentals and Principles of Ophthalmology
3 Clinical Optics
4 Ophthalmic Pathology and Intraocular Tumors
5 Neuro-Ophthalmology
6 Pediatric Ophthalmology and Strabismus
7 Orbit, Eyelids, and Lacrimal System
8 External Disease and Cornea
9 Intraocular Inflammation and Uveitis
10 Glaucoma
11 Lens and Cataract
12 Retina and Vitreous
13 Refractive Surgery

In addition, a comprehensive Master Index allows the reader to easily locate subjects throughout the entire series.

References

Readers who wish to explore specific topics in greater detail may consult the references cited within each chapter and listed in the Basic Texts section at the back of the book.

These references are intended to be selective rather than exhaustive, chosen by the BCSC faculty as being important, current, and readily available to residents and practitioners.

Videos

This edition of Section 9, *Intraocular Inflammation and Uveitis,* includes videos related to topics covered in the book. The videos were selected by members of the BCSC faculty and are available to readers of the print and electronic versions of Section 9 (www.aao.org/bcscvideo_section09). Mobile-device users can scan the QR code below (a QR-code reader must already be installed on the device) to access the video content.

Study Questions and CME Credit

Each volume of the BCSC is designed as an independent study activity for ophthalmology residents and practitioners. The learning objectives for this volume are given on page 1. The text, illustrations, and references provide the information necessary to achieve the objectives; the study questions allow readers to test their understanding of the material and their mastery of the objectives. Physicians who wish to claim CME credit for this educational activity may do so by following the instructions given at the end of the book.

Conclusion

The Basic and Clinical Science Course has expanded greatly over the years, with the addition of much new text and numerous illustrations. Recent editions have sought to place a greater emphasis on clinical applicability while maintaining a solid foundation in basic science. As with any educational program, it reflects the experience of its authors. As its faculties change and as medicine progresses, new viewpoints are always emerging on controversial subjects and techniques. Not all alternate approaches can be included in this series; as with any educational endeavor, the learner should seek additional sources, including such carefully balanced opinions as the Academy's Preferred Practice Patterns.

The BCSC faculty and staff are continually striving to improve the educational usefulness of the course; you, the reader, can contribute to this ongoing process. If you have any suggestions or questions about the series, please do not hesitate to contact the faculty or the editors.

The authors, editors, and reviewers hope that your study of the BCSC will be of lasting value and that each Section will serve as a practical resource for quality patient care.

Objectives

Upon completion of BCSC Section 9, *Intraocular Inflammation and Uveitis,* the reader should be able to

- describe the immunologic and infectious mechanisms involved in the development of and complications from uveitis and related inflammatory conditions, including acquired immunodeficiency syndrome
- identify general and specific pathophysiologic processes in acute and chronic intraocular inflammation that affect the structure and function of the uvea, lens, intraocular spaces, retina, and other tissues
- differentiate infectious from noninfectious uveitic entities
- formulate appropriate differential diagnoses for ocular inflammatory disorders
- based on the differential diagnosis, choose examination techniques and appropriate ancillary studies to differentiate infectious from noninfectious causes
- describe the principles of medical and surgical management of infectious and noninfectious uveitis and related intraocular inflammation, including indications for, adverse effects of, and monitoring of immunosuppressive drugs
- describe the structural complications of uveitis, their prevention, and their treatment
- describe the main principles for differentiating masquerade syndromes from true uveitis and increasing clinical suspicion for these syndromes

Introduction

This section of the BCSC is divided into 2 parts. The information in Part I, Ocular Immunology, has evolved from progress in studies of the basic and regional immunology of the eye, which has translated into major advances in our understanding of uveitis. This advancement has allowed clinicians to better define uveitic entities and develop treatments directed at specific immune processes. The section on immunology describes basic aspects of the human immune response, including ocular-specific ones; the effector mechanisms of immunity, including antibody-mediated and lymphocyte-generated mechanisms; and the various pro- and anti-inflammatory cytokines and other effector molecules, including reactive oxygen species and nitric oxide products. Clinical examples are interspersed, discussing issues of clinical relevance. A clear understanding of the involved immune mechanisms should enhance the clinician's approach to the management of uveitis.

Part II, Intraocular Inflammation and Uveitis, introduces a clinical approach to uveitis, divided into chapters focusing on infectious uveitis, noninfectious uveitis, endophthalmitis, masquerade syndromes, and complications of uveitis; it concludes with a section on ocular involvement in human immunodeficiency virus infection. Because most clinicians approach noninfectious uveitis from an anatomical perspective, the chapter discussing it is organized topographically. The chapter on infectious uveitis, which can occur in any anatomical location, is organized by causative agent.

PART I

Ocular Immunology

Introduction to Ocular Immunology and Immune-Mediated Eye Disease

Immune-mediated eye diseases are a leading cause of visual disability and blindness worldwide. Understanding the pathogenesis, diagnosis, and treatment of this class of diseases requires familiarity with basic concepts of immunology, as well as an understanding of the unique aspects of ocular immune function. The introduction provided over the ensuing 4 chapters is not a substitute for a full immunology course, and the reader unfamiliar with current concepts in immunology is directed to several excellent texts covering this material.

Abbas AK, Lichtman AH, Pillai S. *Basic Immunology: Functions and Disorders of the Immune System.* 4th ed. Philadelphia, PA: Elsevier Saunders; 2012.

Abbas AK, Lichtman AH, Pillai S. *Cellular and Molecular Immunology.* 7th ed. Philadelphia, PA: Elsevier Saunders; 2011.

Murphy KM. *Janeway's Immunobiology.* 8th ed. London: Garland Science; 2011.

CHAPTER 1

Basic Concepts in Immunology: Effector Cells and the Innate Immune Response

Definitions

An immune response is a sequence of molecular and cellular events intended to rid the host of a threat: offending pathogenic organisms, toxic substances, cellular debris, or neoplastic cells. There are 2 broad categories of immune responses, *adaptive* and *innate.*

Adaptive (or *acquired*) responses are higher-order specific responses directed against unique antigens and will be discussed in detail in Chapter 2. Innate immune responses, or *natural immunity,* require no prior contact with or "education" about the stimulus against which they are directed. This chapter introduces the crucial cells of the immune system and discusses their functions in innate immunity.

Components of the Immune System

Leukocytes

White blood cells, or *leukocytes,* comprise several kinds of nucleated cells that can be distinguished by the shape of their nuclei and the presence or absence of cytoplasmic granules as well as by their uptake of various histologic stains.

Neutrophils

Neutrophils possess a multilobed nucleus of varying shapes; hence, they are also called *polymorphonuclear leukocytes* (PMNs). Neutrophils feature cytoplasmic granules and lysosomes and are the most abundant granulocytes in the blood. They are efficient phagocytes that readily clear tissues and degrade ingested material and act as important effector cells through the release of granule products and cytokines.

Neutrophils dominate the infiltrate in experimental models and clinical examples of active bacterial infections of the conjunctiva, sclera (scleritis), cornea (keratitis), and vitreous (endophthalmitis). They are also dominant in many types of active viral infections of the cornea (eg, herpes simplex virus keratitis) and retina (eg, herpes simplex virus retinitis). Neutrophils constitute the principal cell type in ocular inflammation induced by lipopolysaccharides (discussed later) and after direct injection of most cytokines into ocular tissues.

Eosinophils

Eosinophils, a second type of polymorphonuclear leukocyte, also contain abundant cytoplasmic granules and lysosomes, but the biochemical nature of eosinophilic granules consists of more basic protein (thus acidic dyes, such as eosin, will bind to these proteins). Eosinophils have receptors for, and become activated by, many mediators; interleukin-5 (IL-5) is especially important. Eosinophilic granule products such as major basic protein and ribonucleases destroy parasites efficiently; thus, these cells accumulate at sites of parasitic infection. Eosinophils are also important in allergic immune reactions.

Eosinophils are abundant in the conjunctiva and tears in many forms of atopic conjunctivitis, especially vernal and allergic conjunctivitis. They are not considered major effectors for intraocular inflammation, with the notable exception of helminthic infections of the eye, especially uveitis caused by toxocariasis.

Basophils and mast cells

Basophils are the blood-borne equivalent of the tissue-bound mast cell. Mast cells exist in 2 major subtypes—connective tissue and mucosal—both of which can release preformed granules and synthesize certain mediators de novo that differ from those of neutrophils and eosinophils. *Connective tissue mast cells* contain abundant granules with histamine and heparin, and they synthesize prostaglandin D_2 upon stimulation. In contrast, *mucosal mast cells* require T-lymphocyte cytokine help for granule formation, and they normally contain low levels of histamine. Mucosal mast cells primarily synthesize leukotrienes after stimulation. Tissue location can alter the granule type and functional activity, but regulation of these differences is not well understood.

Mast cells act as major effector cells in IgE-mediated, immune-triggered inflammatory reactions, especially allergic or immediate hypersensitivity reactions. They perform this function through their expression of high-affinity Fc receptors for immunoglobulin E (IgE). *Fc* (from "*f*ragment, *c*rystallizable") refers to the constant region of immunoglobulin that binds cell surface receptors (see Chapter 2). Mast cells may also participate in the induction of cell-mediated immunity, wound healing, and other functions not directly related to IgE-mediated degranulation. Other stimuli, such as complement or certain cytokines, may also trigger degranulation.

The healthy human conjunctiva contains numerous mast cells localized in the substantia propria. In certain atopic and allergic disease states, such as vernal conjunctivitis, the number of mast cells increases in the substantia propria, and the epithelium—usually devoid of mast cells—becomes densely infiltrated. The uveal tract also contains numerous connective tissue–type mast cells, whereas the cornea has none.

Monocytes and macrophages

Monocytes, the circulating cells, and macrophages, the tissue-infiltrating equivalents, are important effectors in all forms of immunity and inflammation. Monocytes are relatively large cells (12–20 µm in suspension but up to 40 µm in tissues) that normally travel throughout the body. Most tissues have at least 2 identifiable macrophage populations: tissue-resident and blood-derived. Although exceptions exist, tissue-resident macrophages are monocytes that migrated into tissue during embryologic development and later acquired tissue-specific properties and cellular markers. Various resident macrophages have been given tissue-specific names: Kupffer cells in the liver, alveolar macrophages in the lung, and microglia in the brain and retina. Blood-derived macrophages are monocytes that have recently migrated from the blood into a fully developed tissue site.

Macrophages are extremely important effector cells in adaptive and innate immunity. They are often detectable in acute ocular infections, even if other cell types such as neutrophils are more numerous. Macrophages serve 3 primary functions:

1. as scavengers to clear cell debris and pathogens
2. as antigen-presenting cells (APCs) for T lymphocytes
3. as inflammatory effector cells

Resting monocytes can be primed through various signals into efficient APCs and, upon additional signals, activated into effector cells. Effective activation stimuli include exposure to bacterial products such as lipopolysaccharide, phagocytosis of antibody-coated or complement-coated pathogens, or exposure to mediators released during inflammation, such as IL-1 or interferon gamma.

Only after full activation do macrophages become most efficient at the synthesis and release of inflammatory mediators and the killing and degradation of phagocytosed pathogens. Macrophages may undergo a morphologic change into *epithelioid cells,* which may be altered further by fusing into multinucleated *giant cells,* characteristic of granulomatous inflammation such as that of sarcoidosis.

Dendritic cells and Langerhans cells

Dendritic cells (DCs) are terminally differentiated, bone marrow–derived, circulating mononuclear cells that are distinct from macrophages and monocytes. Up to 1% of blood mononuclear cells are DCs. In tissue sites, DCs are enlarged (15–30 µm), with cytoplasmic veils that form extensions 2 to 3 times the diameter of the cell, and resemble the dendritic structure of neurons. Through defined migration pathways, many organs recruit DCs, which form a system of APCs. In these sites, DCs share features of structure and function as accessory cells important to the processing and presentation of antigens to T lymphocytes; the distinctive function of DCs is to initiate responses in quiescent lymphocytes. Thus, DCs may act as the most potent leukocytes for generating primary T-lymphocyte–dependent immune responses.

Epidermal Langerhans cells (LCs) are the best-characterized subset of DCs. LCs account for up to 8% of the cells in most human epithelia, including the skin and mucosa of the conjunctiva, nasopharynx, vagina, and rectum. LCs are identified by their many dendrites, electron-dense cytoplasm, and Birbeck granules. At rest, they are not active APCs, but activity develops after in vitro culture with certain cytokines. On activation, LCs lose their granules and transform to resemble blood and lymphoid DCs. Evidence suggests that LCs can leave the skin and move along the afferent lymph vessels to the draining lymphoid organs. LCs are important components of the immune system and play roles in antigen presentation, control of lymphoid cell traffic, differentiation of T lymphocytes, and induction of delayed hypersensitivity. Elimination of LCs from skin before an antigen challenge inhibits induction of the contact hypersensitivity response. In the conjunctiva and limbus, LCs are the only cells that constitutively express major histocompatibility (MHC) class II molecules. LCs are present in the peripheral cornea, and any stimulation to the central cornea results in central migration of the peripheral LCs.

Lymphocytes

Lymphocytes are small (10–20 μm) cells with large, dense nuclei that are also derived from stem cell precursors within the bone marrow. Unlike other leukocytes, however, lymphocytes require subsequent maturation in peripheral lymphoid organs. Lymphocytes can be subdivided by the expression of specific cell-surface proteins (ie, *surface markers*). These markers are in turn related to the functional and molecular activity of individual subsets. Three broad categories of lymphocytes have been identified: T lymphocytes; B lymphocytes; and non-T, non-B lymphocytes. These subsets are discussed in greater detail in Chapter 2.

Abbas AK, Lichtman AH, Pillai S. *Basic Immunology: Functions and Disorders of the Immune System.* 4th ed. Philadelphia, PA: Elsevier Saunders; 2012.

Overview of the Innate Immune System

The innate immune response can be thought of as a "preprogrammed" reaction to foreign substances such as bacterial cell wall structures or foreign proteins. The innate immune response requires no prior exposure to the foreign substance and is similar for all encountered triggers. The result is the generation of biochemical mediators and cytokines that recruit innate effector cells, especially macrophages and neutrophils, to remove the offending stimulus through phagocytosis or enzymatic degradation.

The receptors of innate immunity are highly conserved within a species and respond to similarly conserved molecular motifs on triggering stimuli, such as specific amino acid sequences, certain lipoproteins, and certain phospholipids expressed by microbes. For example, in endophthalmitis, bacteria-derived toxins or host cell debris stimulates the recruitment of neutrophils and monocytes, leading to the production of inflammatory mediators and phagocytosis of the bacteria. Responses to *Staphylococcus* organisms, for example, are nearly identical to those mounted against any other bacteria.

Immunity Versus Inflammation

An immune response is the process for removing an offending stimulus. When this response becomes clinically evident, it is termed an *inflammatory response.* An inflammatory response is triggered by immunity (innate or adaptive) and consists of a sequence of molecular and cellular events resulting in 5 cardinal clinical manifestations: pain, hyperemia, edema, heat, and loss of function. These signs are the consequence of 2 physiologic changes within a tissue: cellular recruitment and altered vascular permeability. The following pathologic findings are typical in inflammation:

- infiltration of effector cells resulting in the release of biochemical and molecular mediators of inflammation, such as cytokines (eg, interleukins and chemokines) and lipid mediators (eg, prostaglandins and platelet-activating factors)
- production of oxygen metabolites (eg, superoxide and nitrogen radicals)
- release of granule products as well as catalytic enzymes (eg, collagenases and elastases)
- activation of plasma-derived enzyme systems (eg, complement components and fibrin)

These effector systems are described in greater detail later in this chapter.

Adaptive and innate immune responses are a constant presence, though usually at a subclinical level. For example, ocular surface allergen exposure, occurring daily in humans, or bacterial contamination during cataract surgery, occurring in most eyes, are usually cleared by innate or adaptive mechanisms *without* overt inflammation. The physiologic changes induced by innate and adaptive immunity may be indistinguishable. Compare the hypopyon of bacterial endophthalmitis, which results from innate immunity against bacterial toxins, with the hypopyon of lens-associated uveitis, presumably a result of an adaptive immune response against lens antigens. These hypopyons cannot be distinguished clinically or histologically.

Delves PJ, Martin SJ, Burton DR, Roitt IM. *Roitt's Essential Immunology.* 12th ed. Hoboken, NJ: Wiley-Blackwell; 2011.

Triggers of Innate Immunity

Innate immune responses generally use direct triggering mechanisms, of which 4 of the most important are reviewed here (Table 1-1).

Bacteria-Derived Molecules That Trigger Innate Immunity

Bacterial lipopolysaccharide

Bacterial lipopolysaccharide (LPS), also known as *endotoxin,* is an intrinsic component of the cell walls of most gram-negative bacteria. Among the most important triggering molecules of innate immunity, LPS consists of 3 components: lipid A, O polysaccharide, and core oligosaccharide. The exact structures of each component vary among species of bacteria, but all are recognized by the innate immune system. The primary receptors are the toll-like receptors (TLRs), principally TLR4 and TLR2, which are expressed on macrophages, neutrophils, and dendritic cells, as well as on B cells and T cells. Lipid A is the most potent component, capable of activating effector cells at concentrations of a few picograms per milliliter.

The effects of LPS are pleiotropic and include activation of monocytes and neutrophils, leading to upregulation of genes for various cytokines (IL-1, IL-6, tumor necrosis factor [TNF]); degranulation; alternative pathway complement activation; and direct

Table 1-1 Effector Reactivities of the Innate Immune Response in the Eye

Bacteria-derived molecules that trigger innate immunity
Lipopolysaccharide
Other cell wall components
Exotoxins and secreted toxins
Nonspecific soluble molecules that trigger or modulate innate immunity
Plasma-derived enzymes
Acute-phase reactants
Cytokines produced by parenchymal cells within a tissue site
Innate mechanisms for recruitment and activation of neutrophils
Cell adhesion and transmigration
Activation mechanisms
Phagocytosis of bacteria
Innate mechanisms for recruitment and activation of macrophages
Cell adhesion and transmigration
Activation mechanisms
Scavenging
Priming

impact on the vascular endothelium. LPS is the major cause of shock, fever, and other pathophysiologic responses to bacterial sepsis and thus is an important cause of morbidity and mortality during gram-negative bacterial infections. Interestingly, footpad injection of LPS in rodents results in an acute anterior uveitis; this animal model is called *endotoxin-induced uveitis* (EIU; see Chapter 4). See Clinical Examples 1-1 and 1-2.

Other bacterial cell wall components

The bacterial cell wall and membrane are complex, containing numerous polysaccharide, lipid, and protein structures that can initiate an innate immune response independent of adaptive immunity. Killed lysates of many types of gram-positive bacteria or mycobacteria have been demonstrated to directly activate macrophages, making them useful as adjuvants. Some of these components have been implicated in various models for arthritis and uveitis. In many cases, the molecular mechanisms are probably similar to those of LPS.

CLINICAL EXAMPLE 1-1

Lipopolysaccharide-induced uveitis Humans are intermittently exposed to low levels of LPS that are released from the gut, especially during episodes of diarrhea and dysentery, and exposure to LPS may play a role in dysentery-related uveitis, arthritis, and reactive arthritis. Systemic administration of a low dose of LPS in rabbits, rats, and mice produces a mild acute uveitis; this effect occurs at doses of LPS lower than those that cause apparent systemic shock. In rabbits, a breakdown of the blood–ocular barrier occurs because of loosening of the tight junctions between the nonpigmented ciliary epithelial cells, which allows leakage of plasma proteins through uveal vessels. Rats and mice exhibit an acute neutrophilic and monocytic infiltrate in the iris and ciliary body within 24 hours.

The precise mechanism of the LPS-induced ocular effects after systemic administration is unknown. One possibility is that LPS circulates and binds to the vascular endothelium or other sites within the anterior uvea. Alternatively, LPS might cause activation of uveal macrophages or circulating leukocytes, leading them to preferentially adhere to the anterior uveal vascular endothelium. It is clear that toll-like receptor 2 (TLR2) recognizes LPS, and binding of LPS by TLR2 on macrophages results in macrophage activation and secretion of a wide array of inflammatory cytokines. Degranulation of platelets is among the first histologic changes in LPS uveitis and is likely mediated by eicosanoids, platelet-activating factors, and vasoactive amines. The subsequent intraocular generation of several mediators, especially leukotriene B_4, thromboxane B_2, prostaglandin E_2, and IL-6, correlates with the development of the cellular infiltrate and vascular leakage.

Not surprisingly, direct injection of LPS into various ocular sites can initiate a severe localized inflammatory response. For example, intravitreal injection of LPS triggers a dose-dependent neutrophilic and monocytic infiltration of the uveal tract, retina, and vitreous. Injection of LPS into the central cornea causes development of a ring infiltrate as a result of the infiltration of neutrophils circumferentially from the limbus.

CLINICAL EXAMPLE 1-2

Role of bacterial toxin production in the severity of endophthalmitis As described in Clinical Example 1-1, intraocular injection of LPS is highly inflammatory and accounts for much of the enhanced pathogenicity of gram-negative infections of the eye. Using clinical isolates or bacteria genetically altered to diminish production of the various types of bacterial toxins, investigators have demonstrated that toxin elaboration in gram-positive or gram-negative endophthalmitis greatly influences inflammatory cell infiltration and retinal cytotoxicity. This effect suggests that sterilization through antibiotic therapy alone, in the absence of antitoxin therapy, may not prevent activation of innate immunity, ocular inflammation, and vision loss in eyes infected by toxin-producing strains.

Booth MC, Atkuri RV, Gilmore MS. Toxin production contributes to severity of *Staphylococcus aureus* endophthalmitis. In: Nussenblatt RB, Whitcup SM, Caspi RR, Gery I, eds. *Advances in Ocular Immunology: Proceedings of the 6th International Symposium on the Immunology and Immunopathology of the Eye.* New York, NY: Elsevier; 1994:269–272.

Jett BD, Parke DW 2nd, Booth MC, Gilmore MS. Host/parasite interactions in bacterial endophthalmitis. *Zentralbl Bakteriol.* 1997;285(3):341–367.

Exotoxins and other secretory products of bacteria

Certain bacteria secrete products known as *exotoxins* into their surrounding microenvironment. Many of these products are enzymes that, although not directly inflammatory, can cause tissue damage that subsequently results in inflammation and tissue destruction. Examples of these products include

- collagenases
- hemolysins such as streptolysin O, which can kill neutrophils by causing cytoplasmic and extracellular release of their granules
- phospholipases such as the *Clostridium perfringens* α-toxins, which kill cells and cause necrosis by disrupting cell membranes

For a specific example, intravitreal injection of a purified hemolysin BL toxin derived from *Bacillus cereus* can cause direct necrosis of retinal cells and retinal detachment. In animal studies, the toxin produced by as few as 100 *B cereus* is capable of causing complete loss of retinal function in 12 hours. In addition to being directly toxic, bacterial exotoxins can also be strong triggers of an innate immune response.

Callegan MC, Jett BD, Hancock LE, Gilmore MS. Role of hemolysin BL in the pathogenesis of extraintestinal *Bacillus cereus* infection assessed in an endophthalmitis model. *Infect Immun.* 1999;67(7):3357–3366.

Murphy K, Travers P, Walport M. *Janeway's Immunobiology.* 8th ed. London: Garland Science; 2012.

Other Triggers or Modulators of Innate Immunity

Another form of innate immunity is the mechanism by which trauma or toxins interact directly with nonimmune ocular parenchymal cells—especially iris or ciliary body epithelium, retinal pigment epithelium, retinal Müller cells, or corneal or conjunctival epithelium—which can result in synthesis of a wide range of mediators, cytokines, and eicosanoids. For example, phagocytosis of staphylococci by corneal epithelium, microtrauma to the ocular surface epithelium by contact lenses, chafing of iris or ciliary epithelium by an intraocular lens (IOL), or laser treatment of the retina can stimulate ocular cells to produce mediators that assist in the recruitment of innate effector cells such as neutrophils or macrophages. See Clinical Example 1-3.

Innate Mechanisms for the Recruitment and Activation of Neutrophils

Neutrophils are highly efficient effectors of innate immunity. They are categorized as either *resting* or *activated,* according to their secretory and cell membrane activity. Recruitment of resting, circulating neutrophils by the innate immune response occurs rapidly in a tightly controlled process consisting of 2 events:

1. neutrophil adhesion to the vascular endothelium through cell-adhesion molecules (CAMs) on leukocytes as well as on endothelial cells primarily in postcapillary venules
2. transmigration of the neutrophils through the endothelium and its extracellular matrix, mediated by chemotactic factors

CLINICAL EXAMPLE 1-3

Uveitis-glaucoma-hyphema syndrome One cause of postoperative inflammation after cataract surgery, uveitis-glaucoma-hyphema (UGH) syndrome, is related to the physical presence of certain IOL styles. Although UGH syndrome was more common when rigid anterior chamber lenses were used during the early 1980s, it has also been reported with posterior chamber lenses. The pathogenesis of UGH syndrome appears related to mechanisms for activation of innate immunity. A likely mechanism is cytokine and eicosanoid synthesis triggered by mechanical chafing or trauma to the iris or ciliary body. Plasma-derived enzymes, especially complement or fibrin, can enter the eye through vascular permeability altered by surgery or trauma and can then be activated by the surface of IOLs. Adherence of bacteria and leukocytes to the surface has also been implicated. Toxicity caused by contaminants on the lens surface during manufacturing is rare. Nevertheless, even noninflamed eyes with IOLs can demonstrate histologic evidence of low-grade, foreign-body reactions around the haptics.

Activation of vascular endothelial cells is triggered by various innate immune stimuli, such as LPS, physical injury, thrombin, histamine, or leukotriene release. *Neutrophil rolling*—a process by which neutrophils bind loosely but reversibly to nonactivated endothelial cells—involves molecules on both cell types belonging to at least 3 sets of CAM families:

1. *selectins,* especially L-, E-, and P-selectin
2. *integrins,* especially leukocyte function–associated antigen 1 (LFA-1) and macrophage-1 antigen (Mac-1)
3. *immunoglobulin superfamily molecules,* especially intercellular adhesion molecule 1 (ICAM-1) and ICAM-2

The primary events are mediated largely by members of the selectin family and occur within minutes of stimulation (Fig 1-1). Nonactivated neutrophils express L-selectin, which mediates a weak bond to endothelial cells by binding to specific selectin ligands. Upon exposure to the triggering molecules described in the previous section, endothelial cells become activated, expressing in turn at least 2 other selectins (E and P) by which they can bind to the neutrophils and help stabilize the interaction by a process called *adhesion.* Subsequently, other factors, such as platelet-activating factor (PAF), various cytokines, and bacterial products, can induce upregulation of the β-integrin family. As integrins are expressed, the selectins are shed, and neutrophils then bind firmly to endothelial cells through the immunoglobulin superfamily molecules.

Subsequent to adhesion, various chemotactic factors are required to induce *transmigration* of neutrophils across the endothelial barrier and extracellular matrix into the tissue site. Chemotactic factors are short-range signaling molecules that diffuse in a declining concentration gradient from the source of production within a tissue to the vessel. Neutrophils have receptors for these molecules and are induced to undergo membrane

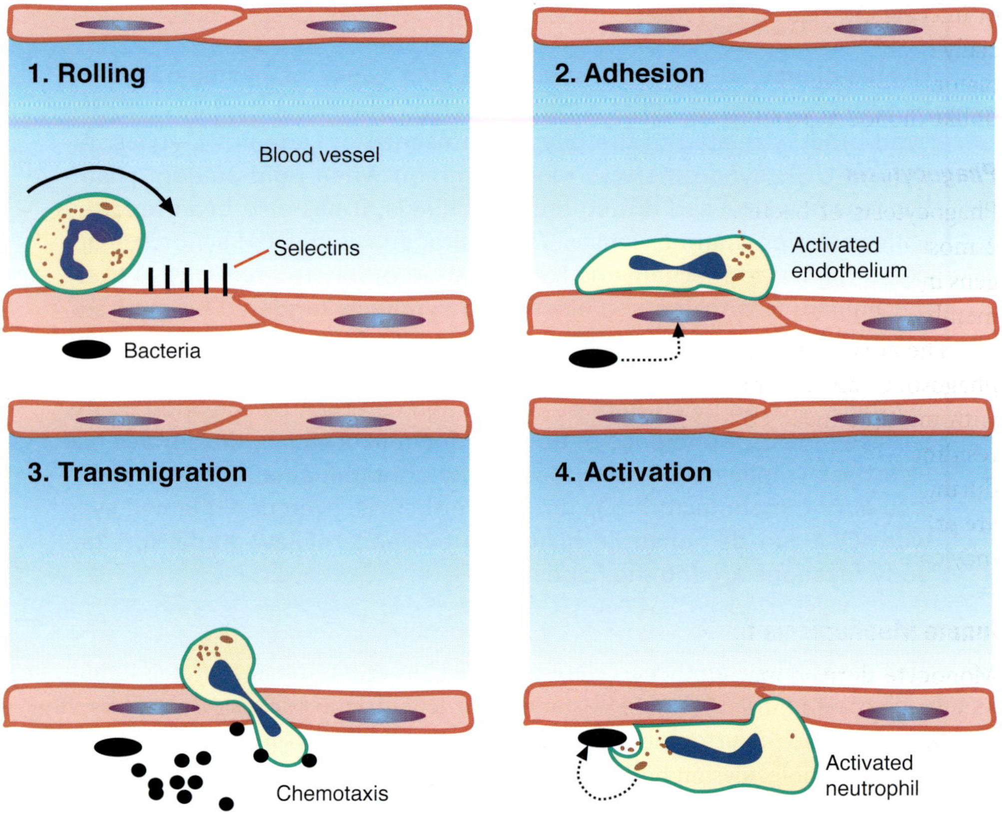

Figure 1-1 Four steps of neutrophil migration and activation. **1,** In response to innate immune stimuli, such as bacterial invasion of tissue, *rolling* neutrophils within the blood vessel bind loosely and reversibly to nonactivated endothelial cells by selectins. **2,** Exposure to innate activating factors and bacterial products *(dotted arrow)* activates endothelial cells, which in turn express E- and P-selectins, β-integrins, and immunoglobulin superfamily molecules to enhance and stabilize the interaction by a process called *adhesion.* **3,** Chemotactic factors triggered by the infection induce *transmigration* of neutrophils across the endothelial barrier into the extracellular matrix of the tissue. **4,** Finally, neutrophils are fully *activated* into functional effector cells upon stimulation by bacterial toxins and phagocytosis. *(Illustration by Barb Cousins, modified by Joyce Zavarro.)*

changes that cause migration in the direction of highest concentration. Numerous such factors have been identified:

- complement products, such as the anaphylatoxin C5a
- fibrin split products
- certain neuropeptides, such as substance P
- bacteria-derived formyl tripeptides, such as *N*-formyl-methionyl-leucyl-phenylalanine (fMLP)
- leukotrienes
- α-chemokines, such as IL-8

Activation of neutrophils into functional effector cells begins during adhesion and transmigration but is fully achieved upon interaction with specific signals within the injured or infected site. The most effective triggers of activation are bacteria and their toxins, especially LPS. Other innate or adaptive mechanisms (especially complement) and chemical mediators (such as leukotrienes and PAF) also contribute to neutrophil activation. Neutrophils, unlike monocytes or lymphocytes, do not leave a tissue to recirculate but remain and die.

Phagocytosis

Phagocytosis of bacteria and other pathogens is a process mediated by receptors, the 2 most important of which are *antibody Fc receptors* and *complement receptors.* Pathogens in complex with antibody or activated complement components bind to cell-surface-membrane–expressed Fc or complement (C) receptors.

The area of membrane to which the pathogen is bound invaginates and becomes a phagosome, and cytoplasmic granules fuse with the phagosomes. Phagocytes are endowed with multiple means of destroying microorganisms, notably, antimicrobial polypeptides residing within the cytoplasmic granules, reactive oxygen radicals generated from oxygen during the respiratory burst, and reactive nitrogen radicals. Although these mechanisms are primarily designed to destroy pathogens, released contents such as lysosomal enzymes may contribute to the amplification of inflammation and tissue damage.

Innate Mechanisms for the Recruitment and Activation of Macrophages

Monocyte-derived macrophages are the second important type of effector cell for the innate immune response that follows trauma or acute infection. The various molecules involved in monocyte adhesion and transmigration from blood into tissues are probably similar to those for neutrophils, although they have not been studied as thoroughly. The functional activation of macrophages, however, is more complex than that of neutrophils. Macrophages exist in different levels or stages of metabolic and functional activity, each representing different "programs" of gene activation and synthesis of macrophage-derived cytokines and mediators:

- resting (immature or quiescent)
- primed
- activated

A fourth category of macrophages, often called *stimulated, reparative,* or *inflammatory,* is used by some immunologists to refer to macrophages that are not quite fully activated. This multilevel model is oversimplified, but it does provide a framework for conceptualizing different levels of macrophage activation in terms of acute inflammation (Fig 1-2).

Resting and scavenging macrophages

Host cell debris is cleared from a tissue site by phagocytosis in the process called *scavenging.* Resting macrophages are the classic scavenging cell, capable of phagocytosis and uptake of the following:

- dead cell membranes
- chemically modified extracellular protein, through acetylated or oxidized lipoproteins
- sugar ligands, through mannose receptors
- naked nucleic acids as well as bacterial pathogens

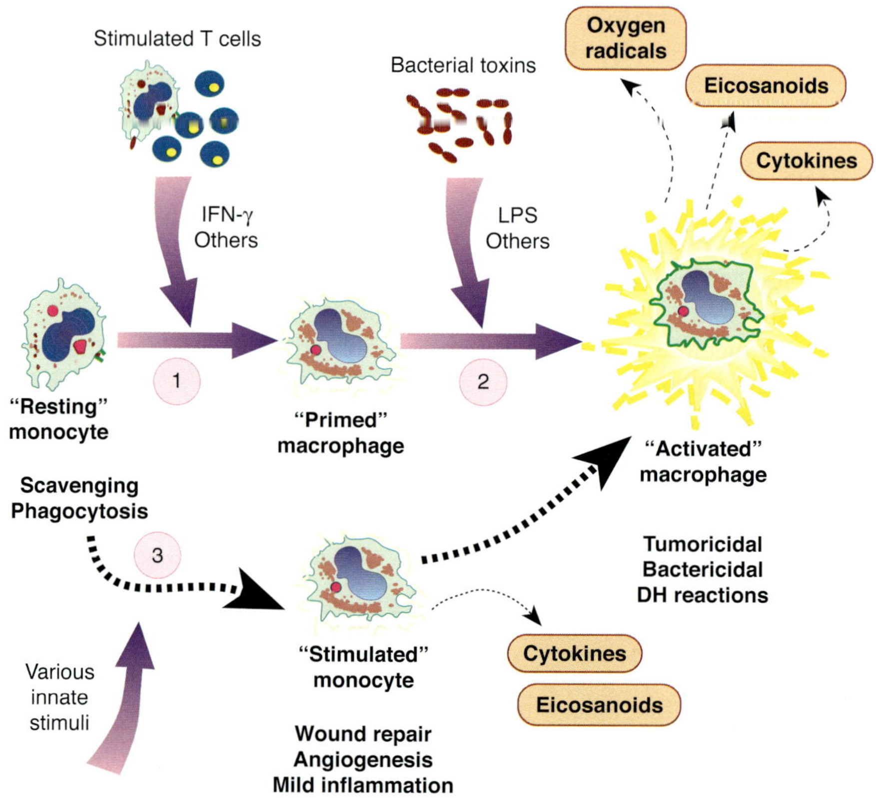

Figure 1-2 Schematic representation of macrophage activation pathway. Classically, *resting monocytes* are thought to be the principal noninflammatory scavenging phagocyte. **1,** Upon exposure to low levels of interferon gamma (IFN-γ) from T lymphocytes, monocytes become primed, upregulating major histocompatibility complex (MHC) class II molecules and performing other functions. *Primed macrophages* function in antigen presentation. **2,** *Fully activated macrophages,* after exposure to bacterial lipopolysaccharide and interferon, are tumoricidal and bactericidal and mediate severe inflammation. **3,** *Stimulated monocytes* result from resting monocyte activation by other innate stimuli, without exposure to IFN-γ. These cells are incompletely activated, producing low levels of cytokines and eicosanoids but not reactive oxygen intermediates. These cells participate in wound healing, angiogenesis, and low-level inflammatory reactions. DH = delayed hypersensitivity; LPS = lipopolysaccharide. *(Illustration by Barb Cousins, modified by Joyce Zavarro.)*

Resting monocytes express at least 3 types of scavenging receptors but synthesize very low levels of proinflammatory cytokines. Scavenging can occur in the absence of inflammation. See Clinical Example 1-4.

Primed macrophages

Resting macrophages become primed by exposure to certain cytokines. Upon priming, these cells become positive for MHC class II antigen and capable of functioning as APCs to T lymphocytes (see Chapter 2). Priming implies activation of specialized lysosomal enzymes such as cathepsins D and E for degrading proteins into peptide fragments; upregulation of certain specific genes such as MHC class II and costimulatory molecules such as B7.1; and increased cycling of proteins between endosomes and the surface membrane.

CLINICAL EXAMPLE 1-4

Phacolytic glaucoma Mild infiltration of scavenging macrophages centered around retained lens cortex or nucleus fragments occurs in nearly all eyes with lens injury, including those subjected to routine cataract surgery. This infiltrate is notable for the *absence* of both prominent neutrophil infiltration and significant nongranulomatous inflammation. An occasional giant cell may be present, but granulomatous changes are not extensive.

Phacolytic glaucoma is a variant of scavenging macrophage infiltration in which leakage of lens protein occurs through the intact capsule of a hypermature cataract. Lens protein–engorged scavenging macrophages present in the anterior chamber block the trabecular meshwork outflow channels, resulting in elevated intraocular pressure. Other signs of typical lens-associated uveitis are conspicuously absent. Experimental studies suggest that lens proteins may be chemotactic stimuli for monocytes.

Primed macrophages thus resemble dendritic cells. They can exit tissue sites by afferent lymphatic vessels to reenter the lymph node.

Activated and stimulated macrophages

Activated macrophages are classically defined as macrophages producing the full spectrum of inflammatory and cytotoxic cytokines; thus, they mediate and amplify acute inflammation, tumor killing, and major antibacterial activity. *Epithelioid cells* and *giant cells* represent the terminal differentiation of the activated macrophage. Activated macrophages synthesize numerous mediators to amplify inflammation:

- inflammatory or cytotoxic cytokines, such as IL-1, IL-6, and TNF-α
- reactive oxygen or nitrogen intermediates
- lipid mediators
- other products

Macrophages can be activated by many different innate stimuli, including

- cytokines derived from T lymphocytes and other cell types
- chemokines
- bacterial cell walls or toxins from gram-positive or acid-fast organisms
- complement activated through the alternative pathway
- foreign bodies composed of potentially toxic substances, such as talc or beryllium
- exposure to certain surfaces, such as some plastics

As noted, macrophages that are partially activated to produce some inflammatory cytokines are termed *stimulated* or *reparative* macrophages. Such partially activated macrophages contribute to fibrosis and wound healing through the synthesis of mitogens such as platelet-derived growth factors (PDGFs), metalloproteinases, and other matrix degradation factors as well as to angiogenesis through synthesis of angiogenic factors such as vascular endothelial growth factor (VEGF).

Mediator Systems That Amplify Immune Responses

Although innate or adaptive effector responses may directly induce inflammation, in most cases this process must be amplified to produce overt clinical manifestations. Molecules generated within the host that induce and amplify inflammation are termed *inflammatory mediators,* and mediator systems include several categories of these molecules (Table 1-2). Most act on target cells through receptor-mediated processes, although some act in enzymatic cascades that interact in a complex fashion.

Plasma-Derived Enzyme Systems

Complement

Complement is an important inflammatory mediator in the eye. Complement components account for approximately 5% of plasma protein and comprise more than 30 different proteins. Complement is activated by 1 of 3 pathways, and this activation generates products that contribute to the inflammatory process (Fig 1-3):

1. *Classic pathway activation* occurs upon fixation of complement C1 by antigen–antibody (immune) complexes formed by IgM, IgG1, and IgG3. This pathway results in a connection between innate and adaptive immunity.
2. *Alternative pathway activation* occurs continuously but is restricted by host complement regulatory components.
3. The *mannose-binding lectin pathway* is activated by certain carbohydrate moieties on the cell wall of microorganisms.

Complement serves the following 4 basic functions during inflammation:

1. coats antigenic or pathogenic surfaces with C3b to enhance phagocytosis (opsonization)
2. promotes lysis of cell membranes through pore formation by the membrane attack complex (MAC)
3. recruits neutrophils and induces inflammation through generation of the anaphylatoxins C3a and C5a
4. modulates antigen-specific immune responses by complement activation products such as iC3b and MACs

Table 1-2 Mediator Systems That Amplify Innate and Adaptive Immune Responses

Plasma-derived enzyme systems: complement, kinins, and fibrin
Vasoactive amines: serotonin and histamine
Lipid mediators: eicosanoids and platelet-activating factors
Cytokines
Reactive oxygen intermediates
Reactive nitrogen products
Neutrophil-derived granule products

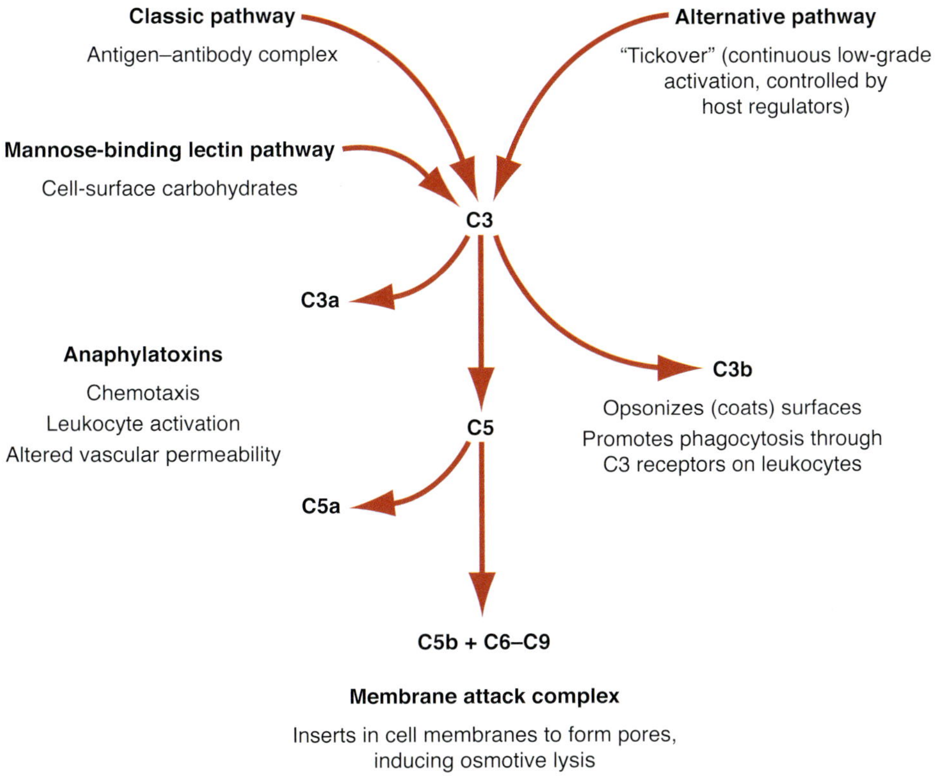

Figure 1-3 Overview of the essential intermediates of the complement pathway. C3a, C3b, C5a, and C5b are complement split products. C5b combines with intact C6, C7, C8, and C9 from the serum.

Anaphylatoxin effects include chemotaxis, changes in cell adhesiveness, and degranulation and release of mediators from mast cells and platelets. C5a stimulates oxidative metabolism and the production and release of toxic oxygen radicals from leukocytes, as well as the extracellular discharge of leukocyte granule contents.

Walport MJ. Complement. First of two parts. *N Engl J Med.* 2001;344(14):1058–1066.

Walport MJ. Complement. Second of two parts. *N Engl J Med.* 2001;344(15):1140–1144.

Fibrin and other plasma factors

Fibrin is the final deposition product of the coagulation pathway, and its deposition during inflammation promotes hemostasis, fibrosis, angiogenesis, and leukocyte adhesion. Fibrin is released from its circulating zymogen precursor, *fibrinogen,* upon cleavage by thrombin. In situ polymerization of smaller units gives rise to the characteristic fibrin plugs or clots. Fibrin dissolution is mediated by *plasmin,* which is activated from its zymogen precursor, *plasminogen,* by plasminogen activators such as tissue plasminogen activator. Thrombin, which is derived principally from platelet granules, is released after any vascular injury that causes platelet aggregation and release. Fibrin may be observed in severe anterior uveitis (the "plasmoid aqueous"), and it contributes to complications such as synechiae, cyclitic membranes, and tractional retinal detachment.

Histamine

Histamine is present in the granules of mast cells and basophils, and it is actively secreted after exposure to a wide range of stimuli. Histamine acts by binding to 1 of at least 3 known types of receptors that are differentially present on target cells. The best-studied pathway for degranulation is antigen crosslinking of IgE bound to mast-cell Fc IgE receptors, but many other inflammatory stimuli can stimulate secretion, including complement, direct membrane injury, and certain drugs. Classically, histamine release has been associated with allergy. The contribution of histamine to intraocular inflammation remains subject to debate.

Lipid Mediators

Two groups of lipid molecules synthesized by stimulated cells act as powerful mediators and regulators of inflammatory responses: the arachidonic acid (AA) metabolites, or *eicosanoids,* and the acetylated triglycerides, usually called *platelet-activating factors.* Both groups of molecules may be rapidly generated from the same lysophospholipid precursors by the enzymatic action of cellular phospholipases such as phospholipase A_2 (Fig 1-4).

Eicosanoids

All eicosanoids are derived from AA. AA is liberated from membrane phospholipids by phospholipase A_2, which is activated by various agonists. AA is oxidized by 2 major pathways to generate the various mediators:

1. the cyclooxygenase (COX) pathway, which produces prostaglandins, thromboxanes, and prostacyclins
2. the 5-lipoxygenase pathway, which produces 5-hydroperoxyeicosatetraenoic acid, lipoxins, and leukotrienes

The COX-derived products are evanescent compounds induced in virtually all cells by a variety of stimuli. In general, they act in the immediate environment of their release to directly mediate many inflammatory activities, including effects on vascular permeability, cell recruitment, platelet function, and smooth-muscle contraction.

Depending on conditions, COX-derived products can either upregulate or downregulate the production of cytokines, enzyme systems, and oxygen metabolites. The two forms of COX are COX-1 and COX-2. COX-1 is thought to be constitutively expressed by many cells, especially cells that use prostaglandin for basal metabolic functions, such as cells of the gastric mucosa and renal tubular epithelium. COX-2 is inducible by many inflammatory stimuli, including other inflammatory mediators (eg, PAF and some cytokines) and innate stimuli (eg, LPS).

Prostaglandins may be the cause of cystoid macular edema (CME) in association with anterior segment surgery or inflammation. Posterior diffusion of one or more of the eicosanoids through the vitreous is assumed to alter the permeability of the perifoveal

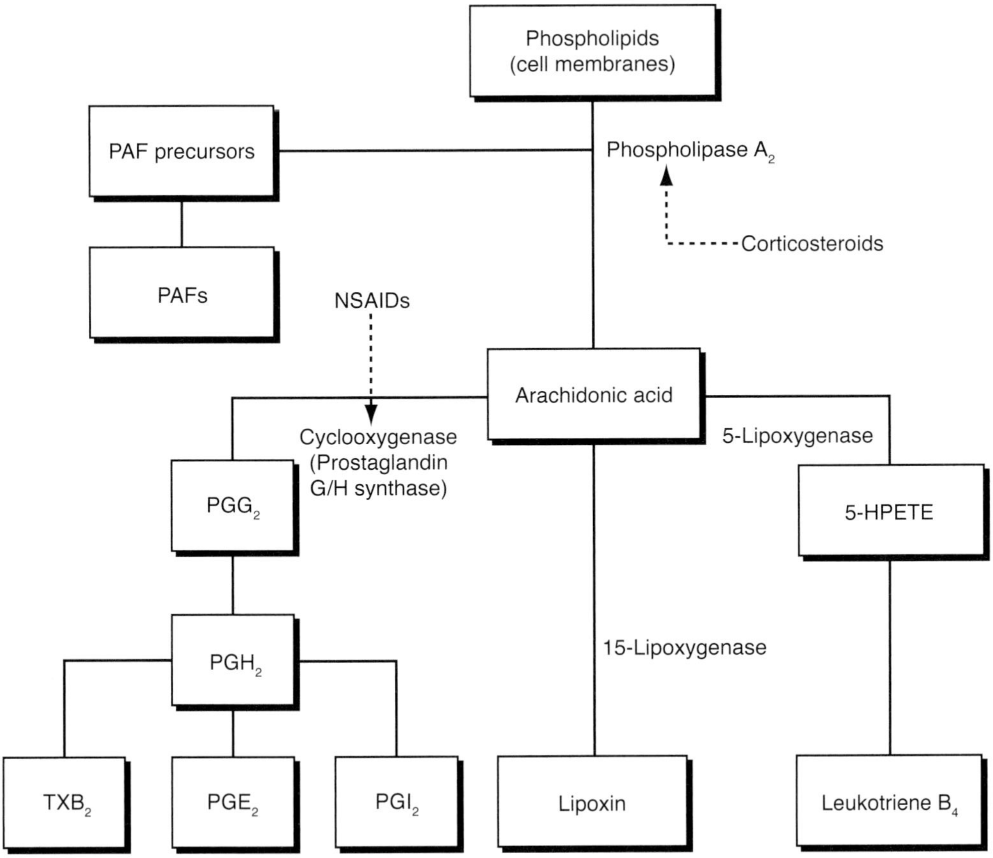

Figure 1-4 Overview of the essential intermediates of the eicosanoid and platelet-activating factor (PAF) pathways. 5-HPETE = 5-hydroperoxyeicosatetraenoic acid; NSAIDs = nonsteroidal anti-inflammatory drugs. *(Modified with permission from Pepose JS, Holland GN, Wilhelmus KR, eds.* Ocular Infection and Immunity. *St Louis, MO: Mosby; 1996.)*

capillary network, leading to CME. Clinical trials in humans have shown that topical treatment with COX inhibitors reduces the incidence of CME after cataract surgery.

Derivatives of 5-lipoxygenase, an enzyme found mainly in granulocytes and some mast cells, have been detected in the brain and retina. *Leukotrienes* probably contribute significantly to inflammatory infiltration; some leukotrienes have 1000 times the effect of histamine on vascular permeability. Another lipoxygenase product, lipoxin, is a potent stimulator of superoxide anion.

Platelet-activating factors

Platelet-activating factors are a family of phospholipid-derived mediators that appear to be important stimuli in the early stage of inflammation. PAFs also serve physiologic functions unrelated to inflammation, especially in reproductive biology, the physiology of secretory epithelium, and neurobiology. In these physiologic roles, a de novo biosynthetic pathway has been identified. However, the *remodeling pathway* is the one implicated in PAF inflammatory actions.

Phospholipase A_2 metabolizes phosphocholine precursors in cell membranes, releasing AA and PAF precursors, which are acetylated into multiple species of PAF. PAF release is stimulated by various innate immune triggers, such as bacterial toxins, trauma, and cytokines. PAFs activate not only platelets but also most leukocytes, which in turn produce and release additional PAFs. PAFs function by binding to one or more guanosine triphosphate protein–associated receptors on target cells.

In vitro, PAFs induce an impressive repertoire of responses, including phagocytosis, exocytosis, superoxide production, chemotaxis, aggregation, proliferation, adhesion, eicosanoid generation, degranulation, and calcium mobilization, as well as diverse morphologic changes. PAFs are a major regulator of cell adhesion and vascular permeability in many forms of acute inflammation, trauma, shock, and ischemia.

The precise role of PAFs in intraocular inflammation remains unknown, but synergistic interactions probably exist among PAFs, nitric oxide, eicosanoids, and cytokines. Therapeutically, PAF antagonists are in development and undergoing testing in clinical trials, though caution regarding their use in uveitis must be followed, as intravitreal injection of PAFs in animals induces an acute retinitis and photoreceptor toxicity.

Cytokines

Cytokines are soluble polypeptide mediators synthesized and released by cells for the purposes of intercellular signaling and communication. Table 1-3 lists examples of cytokines associated with ocular inflammation. Various types of intercellular signaling occur, including *paracrine* (signaling of neighboring cells at the same site), *autocrine* (stimulation of a receptor on its own surface, and *endocrine* (action on a distant site through release into the blood).

Traditionally, investigators have subdivided cytokines into families with related activities, sources, and targets, using terms such as *growth factors, interleukins, lymphokines, interferons, monokines,* and *chemokines.* Thus, *growth factor* traditionally refers to cytokines mediating cell proliferation and differentiation. The terms *interleukin* and *lymphokine* identify cytokines thought to mediate intercellular communication among lymphocytes or other leukocytes. Interferons are cytokines that limit or interfere with the ability of a virus to infect a cell; monokines are immunoregulatory cytokines secreted by monocytes and macrophages; and chemokines are chemotactic cytokines. Although some cytokines are specific for particular cell types, most have such multiplicity and redundancy of source, function, and target that this focus on specific terminology is not particularly useful for the clinician. For example, activated macrophages in an inflammatory site synthesize growth factors, interleukins, interferons, and chemokines.

Both innate and adaptive responses result in the production of cytokines. T lymphocytes are the classic cytokine-producing cell of adaptive immunity, but macrophages, mast cells, and even neutrophils also synthesize a wide range of cytokines upon stimulation. Cytokine interactions can be additive, combinatorial, synergistic, or antagonistic. Elimination of the action of a single molecule may have an unpredictable outcome; for example, monoclonal antibodies directed against tumor necrosis factor α (TNF-α) result in

Table 1-3 Cytokines of Relevance to Ocular Immunology

Family	Example	Major Cell Source	Major Target Cells	Major General Actions	Specific Ocular Actions
Interleukins	IL-1α	Macrophages Many others	Most leukocytes Various ocular cells	Many actions on T and B lymphocytes Systematic toxicity (fever, shock)	Altered vascular permeability Neutrophil and macrophage infiltration Langerhans migration to central cornea
	IL-2	Th0 or Th1 CD4 T lymphocytes	T lymphocytes B lymphocytes NK cells	Activates CD4 and CD8 T lymphocytes Induces Th1	Detectable levels in some forms of uveitis
	IL-4	Th2 CD4 T lymphocytes Basophils, mast cells	T lymphocytes B lymphocytes	Induces Th2, blocks Th1 Induces B lymphocytes to make IgE	? Role in atopic and vernal conjunctivitis
	IL-5	Th2 CD4 T lymphocytes		Recruits eosinophils	? Role in atopic and vernal conjunctivitis
	IL-6	Macrophages T lymphocytes Mast cells Mast ocular epithelium	Most leukocytes Various ocular cells	Many actions on B lymphocytes Systematic toxicity (fever, shock)	Altered vascular permeability Neutrophil infiltration High levels in many forms of uveitis and nonuveitic diseases
Alpha chemokines	IL-8	Many cell types	Endothelial cells Neutrophils Many others	Recruits and activates neutrophils Upregulates CAM on endothelium	Altered vascular permeability Neutrophil infiltration
Beta chemokines	Macrophage chemotactic protein-1	Macrophages Endothelium RPE	Endothelial cells Macrophages T lymphocytes	Recruits and activates macrophages, some T lymphocytes	Recruits macrophages and T lymphocytes to eye
Tumor necrosis factors	TNF-α or -β	Macrophages (TNF-α) T lymphocytes (TNF-β)		Tumor apoptosis Macrophage and neutrophil activation Cell adhesion and chemotaxis Fibrin deposition and vascular injury Systemic toxicity (fever, shock)	Altered vascular permeability Mononuclear cell infiltration

(Continued)

Table 1-3 *(continued)*

Family	Example	Major Cell Source	Major Target Cells	Major General Actions	Specific Ocular Actions
Interferons	Interferon gamma (IFN-γ)	Th1 T lymphocytes NK cells		Activates macrophages	Neutrophil and macrophage infiltration
	IFN-α	Most leukocytes	Most parenchymal cells	Prevents viral infection of many cells Inhibits hemangioma, conjunctival intraepithelial neoplasia, and other tumors	Innate protection of ocular surface from viral infection, treatment of ocular surface neoplasms
Growth factors	Transforming growth factor β (TGF-β)	Many cells Leukocytes, T lymphocytes RPE and NPE of ciliary body Pericytes Fibroblasts	Macrophages T lymphocytes RPE Glia Fibroblasts	Suppresses T-lymphocyte and macrophage inflammatory functions Fibrosis of wounds	Regulator of immune privilege and ACAID
	Platelet-derived growth factors	Platelets Macrophages RPE	Fibroblasts Glia Many others	Fibroblast proliferation	Role in inflammatory membranes, subretinal fibrosis
Neuropeptides	Substance P	Ocular nerves Mast cells	Leukocytes Others	Pain Altered vascular permeability	Altered vascular permeability Leukocyte infiltration, photophobia
	Vasoactive intestinal peptide	Ocular nerves	Leukocytes Others	Suppresses macrophage and T-lymphocyte inflammatory function	Role in ACAID and immune privilege

ACAID = anterior chamber–associated immune deviation; NK = natural killer; NPE = nonpigmented epithelium; RPE = retinal pigment epithelium; Th = T helper.

substantial suppression of immune responses but also increase susceptibility to multiple sclerosis. Finally, not only do innate and adaptive immune responses use cytokines as mediators and amplifiers of inflammation, but cytokines also modulate the initiation of immune responses; the function of most leukocytes is altered by preexposure to various cytokines. Thus, for many cytokines, their regulatory role may be as important as their actions as mediators of inflammation.

Reactive Oxygen Intermediates

Under certain conditions, oxygen can undergo chemical modification into highly reactive substances with the potential to damage cellular molecules and inhibit functional properties in pathogens or host cells. BCSC Section 2, *Fundamentals and Principles of Ophthalmology,* discusses the processes involved in greater detail in Part IV, Biochemistry and Metabolism. See especially Chapter 14, Free Radicals and Antioxidants.

Three of the most important oxygen intermediates are the superoxide anion, hydrogen peroxide, and the hydroxyl radical:

$O_2 + e^- \rightarrow O_2^-$	superoxide anion
$O_2^- + O_2^- + 2H^+ \rightarrow O_2 + H_2O_2$	superoxide dismutase catalyzes anions to form hydrogen peroxide
$H_2O_2 + e^- \rightarrow OH^- + OH\bullet$	hydroxyl anion and hydroxyl radical

Oxygen metabolites triggered by immune responses and generated by leukocytes, especially neutrophils and macrophages, are the most important source of free radicals during inflammation. A wide variety of stimuli can trigger leukocyte oxygen metabolism, including

- innate triggers such as LPS or fMLP
- adaptive effectors such as complement-fixing antibodies or certain cytokines produced by activated T lymphocytes
- other chemical mediator systems, such as C5a, PAF, and leukotrienes

Reactive oxygen intermediates can also be generated as part of noninflammatory cellular biochemical processes, especially by electron transport in the mitochondria, detoxification of certain chemicals, or interactions with environmental light or radiation. These reactive intermediates are highly toxic to both living pathogens and to pathogenic mediators such as exotoxins and lipids.

Reactive Nitrogen Products

Nitric oxide (NO) is a highly reactive chemical species that, like reactive oxygen intermediates, is involved in various important biochemical functions in microorganisms and host cells. The formation of NO depends on the enzyme nitric oxide synthetase (NOS), which is located in the cytosol and dependent on NADPH (the reduced form of nicotinamide-adenine dinucleotide phosphate). NO is formed from the terminal guanidino-nitrogen atoms of L-arginine. Several types of NOS are known, including various forms of constitutive NOS and an inducible NOS. Many cells produce basal levels of NO via the calcium-dependent, constitutive form of the enzyme (constitutive NOS, or cNOS). Activation induces enhanced production of NO in certain cells, especially macrophages via the induced synthesis of a second, calcium-independent form of NOS (inducible NOS, or iNOS). Many innate and adaptive stimuli modulate induction of iNOS, especially cytokines and bacterial toxins.

Neutrophil-Derived Granule Products

Neutrophils are also a source of specialized products that can amplify immune responses. Many antimicrobial polypeptides are present in neutrophilic granules; the principal ones are bactericidal/permeability-increasing protein, defensins, lysozyme, lactoferrin, and the serine proteases.

In addition to antimicrobial polypeptides, neutrophils contain numerous other molecules that may contribute to inflammation. These compounds include hydrolytic enzymes, elastase, metalloproteinases, gelatinase, myeloperoxidase, vitamin B_{12}–binding protein, cytochrome b_{558}, and others. Granule contents are considered to remain inert and membrane-bound when the granules are intact but to become active and soluble when granules fuse to the phagocytic vesicles or plasma membrane.

An example of a neutrophil-derived granule product is collagenase; various forms of collagenase contribute to corneal injury and liquefaction during bacterial keratitis and scleritis, especially in infections with *Pseudomonas* species. Collagenases also contribute to peripheral corneal melting syndromes secondary to rheumatoid arthritis–associated peripheral keratitis.

CHAPTER 2

Immunization and Adaptive Immunity: The Immune Response Arc and Immune Effectors

The term *antigen* refers to substances recognized by the immune system. The term *epitope* refers to each specific portion of an antigen to which the immune system can respond. Antigenic epitopes exist on both native "self" tissues as well as foreign "nonself" tissues. A complex 3-dimensional protein has multiple antigenic epitopes that may be recognized as well as many other sites that remain "invisible" to the immune system.

The adaptive immune response, unlike the innate immune response discussed in Chapter 1, is a "learned" response to these highly variable but specific antigenic epitopes rather than a response to conserved patterns. The entire purpose of the adaptive immune system is to continuously sample antigenic epitopes, determine if they are self or nonself, and then either avoid mounting or mount, respectively, an immune response so that foreign antigens are eliminated from the system. Several immunologic concepts, especially those of the immune response arc, the primary adaptive immune response, and the secondary adaptive immune response, are involved in this process. See Clinical Example 2-1.

CLINICAL EXAMPLE 2-1

Primary and secondary response to tuberculosis The afferent phase of the primary response begins after the inhalation of live organisms, which proliferate slowly within the lung. Alveolar macrophages ingest the bacteria and transport the organisms to the hilar lymph nodes, where the processing phase begins. Over the next few days, as T and B lymphocytes are primed, the hilar nodes become enlarged because of the increased number of dividing T and B lymphocytes as well as the generalized increased trafficking of other lymphocytes through the nodes. The

(Continued on next page)

(continued)

effector phase begins when the primed T lymphocytes recirculate and enter the infected lung. The T lymphocytes interact with the macrophage-ingested bacteria, and cytokines are released that activate neighboring macrophages to fuse into giant cells, forming caseating granulomas. Meanwhile, some of the effector T lymphocytes home to other lymph nodes throughout the body, where they become inactive memory T lymphocytes, trafficking and recirculating throughout the secondary lymphoid tissue.

A secondary response in the skin is the basis of the tuberculin skin test used to diagnose tuberculosis (TB). The afferent phase of the secondary response begins when a purified protein derivative (PPD) reagent (antigens purified from mycobacteria) is injected into the dermis. These antigens are taken up by dermal macrophages. The secondary processing phase begins when these PPD-stimulated macrophages migrate into the draining lymph node, where they encounter memory T lymphocytes from the previous lung infection, leading to reactivation of memory T lymphocytes. The secondary effector phase commences when these reactivated memory T lymphocytes recirculate and home back into the dermis, where they encounter additional antigen and macrophages at the injection site, causing the T lymphocytes to become fully activated and release cytokines. Within 24–72 hours, these cytokines induce infiltration of additional lymphocytes and monocytes as well as fibrin clotting. This process produces the typical indurated dermal lesion of the TB skin test, called the *tuberculin form* of delayed hypersensitivity (DH). *Mycobacterium tuberculosis* is difficult for macrophages to digest and process, sometimes resulting in a less robust immune response, explaining the situation of a negative PPD result in the face of active infection. A disadvantage of skin testing is the need to examine the injection site 48–72 hours later. The interferon-gamma release assays eliminate this disadvantage. In this testing method, peripheral blood is collected and exposed to tuberculin antigens. If a patient has been exposed to TB, circulating T lymphocytes that are TB antigen specific should be present. As described above, when exposed to TB antigen, these cells release interferon gamma, which can be measured either as the concentration of interferon gamma or as the number of cells releasing interferon gamma.

Overview of the Immune Response Arc

Analogous to the neural reflex arc, the immune response arc—the interaction between antigen and the adaptive immune system—can be subdivided into 3 phases: afferent, processing, and effector (Fig 2-1).

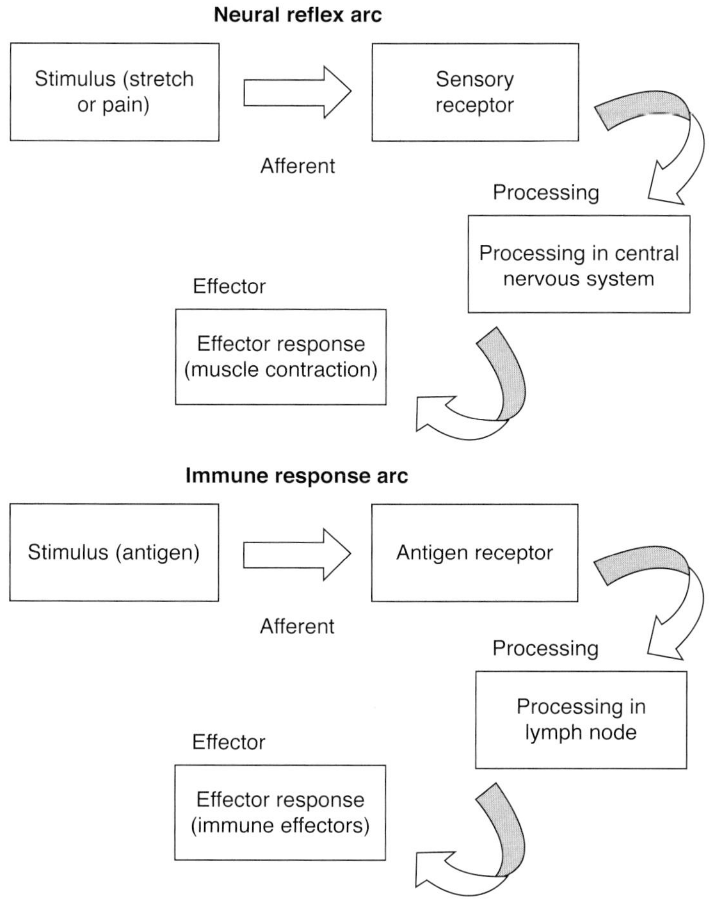

Figure 2-1 Comparison between the neural reflex arc and the immune response arc.

Phases of the Immune Response Arc

Afferent Phase

The afferent phase of the immune response arc comprises the initial recognition, transport, and presentation of antigenic substances to the adaptive immune system. Recognition starts with antigen-presenting cells (APCs), which are specialized cells that bind and phagocytize antigen at a site. Phagocytosis occurs following receipt by the APC of stimulatory signals, such as exposure to complement, as discussed in Chapter 1. Following ingestion of antigen, APCs migrate via afferent lymphatics to lymph nodes. Afferent lymphatic channels, usually simply termed *lymphatics,* are veinlike structures that drain extracellular fluid (ie, lymph) from a site into a regional lymph node. Lymphatics serve 2 major purposes: to convey immune cells and to carry whole antigen from the site of inoculation to a lymph node. In the APCs, enzymatic digestion of proteins within endocytic vesicles produces short amino acid chains of 7–11 amino acids: the antigenic epitopic fragments. Each antigenic fragment is combined with a groove-shaped HLA peptide residing on the APC surface, and this surface complex forms a unique epitope. The combination of peptide and HLA protein is recognized by the T-lymphocyte receptors CD4 and CD8. HLA molecules vary in their capacity to bind various antigenic peptide fragments within their groove, and thus the HLA type determines the repertoire of peptide antigens capable of being presented to T lymphocytes. Specific HLA alleles are important risk factors for certain forms of uveitis. See Chapter 4 for a more thorough discussion of HLA molecules and disease susceptibility.

Major histocompatibility complex (MHC) class I molecules (ie, HLA-A, -B, and -C) serve as the antigen-presenting platform for $CD8^+$ T lymphocytes (Fig 2-2). $CD8^+$ T lymphocytes include natural killer T cells and regulatory T cells. Class I molecules are present on

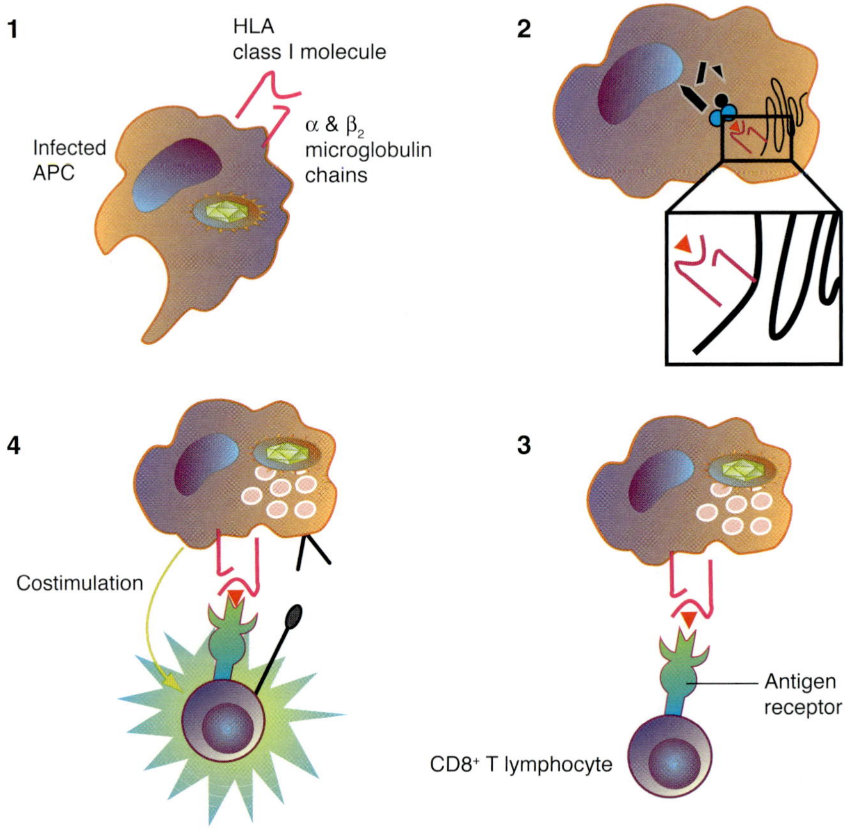

Figure 2-2 Class I–dependent antigen-presenting cells (APCs). **1,** APC is infected by a virus, which causes the cell to synthesize virus-associated peptides that are present in the cytosol. **2,** The viral antigen must be transported (through specialized transporter systems) into the endosomal compartment, where the antigen encounters class I human leukocyte antigen (HLA) molecules. The fragment is placed into the pocket formed by the α chain of the class I HLA molecule. Unlike class II molecules, the second chain, called β_2-microglobulin, is constant among all class I molecules. **3,** The CD8 T-lymphocyte receptor recognizes the fragment–class I complex. **4,** With the help of costimulatory molecules such as CD28-B7 and cytokines, the $CD8^+$ T lymphocyte becomes primed, or partially activated. A similar mechanism is used to recognize tumor antigens that are produced by cells after malignant transformation. *(Illustration by Barb Cousins, modified by Joyce Zavarro.)*

almost all nucleated cells and generally function in the processing of peptide antigens that have been synthesized by the host cell itself. If these presented antigens are recognized as self (ie, normal host protein), no immune reaction occurs. However, if there is an alteration of the normal host peptide (termed "altered self"), such as would occur with tumor or viral peptides after host cell invasion, an immune response is initiated. This process serves to provide surveillance for cancer or viral infection within the host. One could thus envision how a viral infection, a neoplasm, or simply a genetic mutation that alters protein structure could induce autoimmunity by stimulating an immune response that encompasses host tissue.

MHC class II molecules (ie, HLA-DR, -DP, and -DQ) serve as the antigen-presenting platform for CD4⁺, or *helper,* T lymphocytes (Fig 2-3). The antigen receptor on the helper T lymphocyte can recognize peptide antigens only if the antigens are presented with class II molecules simultaneously. However, only certain cell types express MHC class II molecules. Macrophages and dendritic cells are the most important of these types, though B lymphocytes can also function as class II–dependent APCs, especially within a lymph

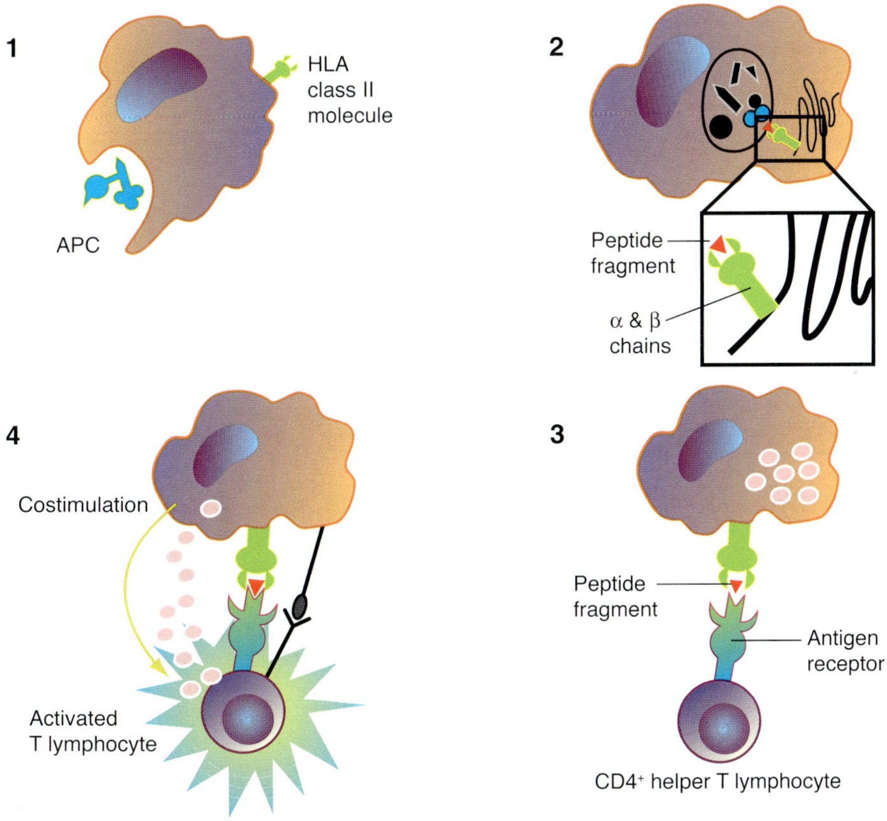

Figure 2-3 Class II–dependent antigen-presenting cells. **1,** APCs endocytose exogenous antigens into the endosomal compartment. **2,** There, the antigen is digested into peptide fragments and placed into the groove formed by the α and β chains of the HLA class II molecule. **3,** The $CD4^+$ T-lymphocyte receptor recognizes the fragment–class II complex. **4,** With the help of costimulatory molecules such as CD28-B7 and cytokines, the $CD4^+$ T lymphocyte becomes primed, or partially activated. *(Illustration by Barb Cousins, modified by Joyce Zavarro.)*

node. Class II–dependent APCs are considered the most efficient "professional" APCs for processing extracellular protein antigens, that is, antigens that have been phagocytosed from the external environment (eg, bacterial or fungal antigens).

Processing Phase

The conversion of an antigenic stimulus into an immunologic response occurs through *priming* of naive B and T lymphocytes (B lymphocytes and T lymphocytes that have not yet encountered their specific antigen) within lymph nodes and the spleen. This conversion is also called *activation,* or *sensitization,* of lymphocytes. Processing involves regulation of the interaction between antigen and naive lymphocytes, followed by lymphocyte activation (Fig 2-4).

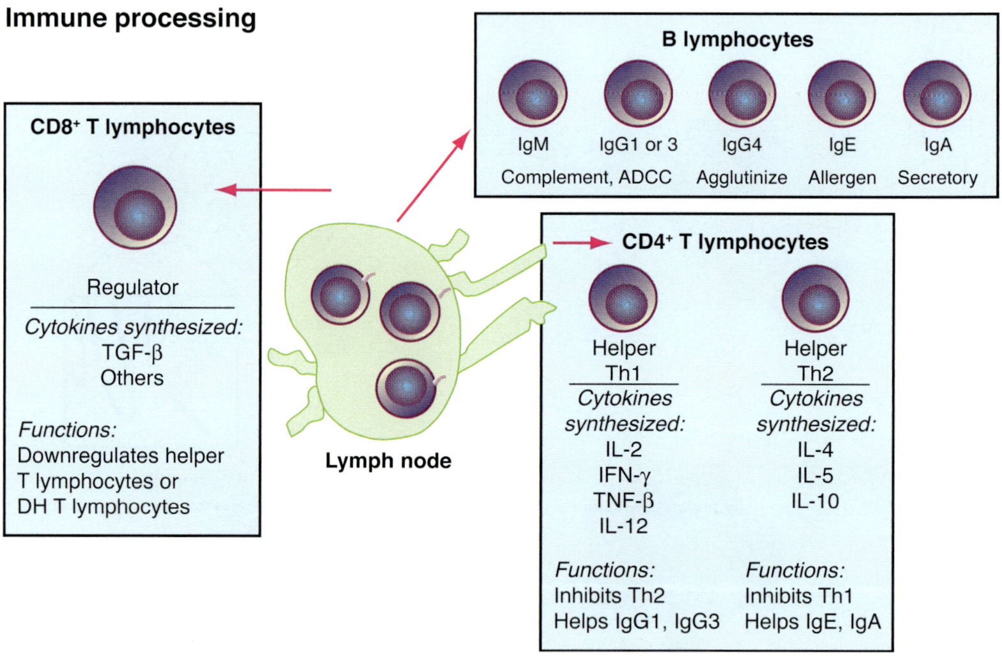

Figure 2-4 Schematic illustration of immune processing of antigen within the lymph node. On exposure to antigen and APCs within the lymph node, the 3 major lymphocyte subsets—B lymphocytes, $CD4^+$ T lymphocytes, and $CD8^+$ T lymphocytes—are activated to release specific cytokines and perform specific functional activities. B lymphocytes are stimulated to produce one of the various antibody isotypes, whose functions include complement activation, antibody-dependent cellular cytotoxicity (ADCC), agglutinization, allergen recognition, and release into secretions. $CD4^+$ T lymphocytes become activated into T helper-1 (Th1) or T helper-2 (Th2) subsets. Th1 lymphocytes function to help B lymphocytes secrete immunoglobulin G1 (IgG1) and IgG3; inhibit Th2; and release cytokines such as interleukin-2 (IL-2), interferon gamma (IFN-γ), tumor necrosis factor β (TNF-β), and IL-12. Th2 lymphocytes function to help B lymphocytes secrete IgE and IgA; inhibit Th1 lymphocytes; and synthesize cytokines such as IL-4, IL-5, and IL-10. $CD8^+$ T lymphocytes become activated into regulatory T lymphocytes that function by inhibiting other $CD4^+$ T lymphocytes, often by secreting cytokines such as transforming growth factor β (TGF-β). DH = delayed hypersensitivity. *(Illustration by Barb Cousins, modified by Joyce Zavarro.)*

Preconditions necessary for processing

$CD4^+$ helper T lymphocytes are the principal cell type for immune processing. These lymphocytes have a receptor that detects antigen only when a trimolecular complex consisting of an HLA molecule, a processed antigen fragment, and a T-lymphocyte antigen receptor is formed. The $CD4^+$ molecule stabilizes binding and enhances signaling between the HLA complex on the APC and the T-lymphocyte receptor. When helper T lymphocytes recognize their specific antigen, they become primed and partially activated, acquiring new functional properties, including cell division, cytokine synthesis, and cell membrane expression of *accessory molecules* such as cell-adhesion molecules and costimulatory molecules. The synthesis and release of immune cytokines, especially interleukin-2 (IL-2), by T lymphocytes is crucial for the progression of initial activation and the functional differentiation of T lymphocytes through autocrine stimulation.

Helper T-lymphocyte differentiation

At the stage of initial priming, $CD4^+$ T lymphocytes are classified as T helper-0, or Th0, cells. Th0 cells can differentiate into functional subsets based on the pattern of cytokines to which they are exposed. One subset, T helper-1 (Th1), secretes interferon gamma (IFN-γ), tumor necrosis factor β (TNF-β), but *not* IL-4, IL-5, or IL-10. Another subset, T helper-2 (Th2), secretes IL-4, IL-5, and IL-10 but not Th1 cytokines. Th17 cells produce IL-17, IL-21, and IL-22. Th17 cells have been implicated in a number of autoimmune conditions, including some forms of uveitis. T regulatory (Treg) cells are identified by their simultaneous expression of CD4, CD25, and Foxp3 (a transcriptional regulator protein) and not by their cytokine-secretion profile. Treg cells appear to be generated in the thymus during development and are essential to self-tolerance, the process by which autoreactive T cells are minimized and their function downregulated, although Treg cells can be induced as well.

The cytokine profiles produced by these various ThX cell types determine subsequent immune processing, B-lymphocyte antibody synthesis, and cell-mediated effector responses (discussed in the following section). For example, IFN-γ, produced by Th1 lymphocytes, blocks the differentiation and activation of Th2 lymphocytes, whereas IL-4, produced by Th2 lymphocytes, blocks the differentiation of Th1 lymphocytes. The process determining whether a Th1 or a Th2 response develops consequent to exposure to a particular antigen is not entirely understood, but presumed variables include cytokines preexisting in the microenvironment, the nature and amount of antigen encountered, and the type of APC involved. For example, IL-12, which is produced by macrophage APCs, might preferentially induce Th1 responses.

Amadi-Obi A, Yu CR, Liu X, et al. Th17 cells contribute to uveitis and scleritis and are expanded by IL-2 and inhibited by IL-27/STAT1. *Nat Med.* 2007;13(6):711–718.

Caspi R. Autoimmunity in the immune privileged eye: pathogenic and regulatory T cells. *Immunol Res.* 2008;42(1–3):41–50.

B-lymphocyte activation

A major function of helper T lymphocytes is B-lymphocyte activation. B lymphocytes are responsible for producing antibodies (glycoproteins that bind to a specific antigen, the epitope). These antibodies contain an epitope-specific binding site, termed *paratope*, on the Fab (*f*ragment, *a*ntigen-*b*inding) portion of the molecule. B lymphocytes begin as naive lymphocytes, with immunoglobulin M (IgM) and IgD on their cell surfaces serving as B-lymphocyte antigen receptors. Through these surface antibodies, B lymphocytes detect epitopes on intact antigens without the requirement of antigen processing by APCs. After appropriate stimulation of the B-lymphocyte antigen receptor, helper T lymphocyte–B lymphocyte interaction occurs, leading to further B-lymphocyte activation and differentiation. B lymphocytes acquire new functional properties, such as cell division, cell surface expression of accessory molecules, and synthesis of large quantities of antibody. Most important, activated B lymphocytes acquire the ability to change antibody class from IgM to another class (eg, to IgG, IgA, or IgE). This class shift requires a molecular change in the immunoglobulin heavy chain, a process regulated by specific cytokines released by the helper T lymphocyte. For example, treatment of an antigen-primed B lymphocyte with IFN-γ induces a switch from IgM to IgG1 production. Treatment with IL-4 induces a switch from IgM to IgE production. The terminal form of B lymphocyte differentiation is the plasma cell.

Role of regulatory T lymphocytes

Regulatory T lymphocytes are potentially important therapeutically, as they may provide a means for induction of tolerance to specific antigens. Originally, regulatory T lymphocytes were thought to express the CD8 marker and to become activated during the initial phases of processing. More recently, $CD4^+$ $CD25^+$ $Foxp3^+$ T lymphocytes have also been observed to have regulatory functions. In many cases, both $CD8^+$ and $CD4^+$ regulatory T lymphocytes appear to operate by the release of immunomodulatory cytokines such as transforming growth factor β that can inhibit or alter the effector function of other T lymphocytes.

Effector Phase

The purpose of the adaptive immune response (ie, the elimination or neutralization of foreign antigen) is accomplished during the effector phase. Antigen-specific effectors exist in 2 major subsets:

1. T lymphocytes
2. B lymphocytes plus their antibodies

Effector lymphocytes require 2 exposures to antigen for maximum effectiveness. The initial (*priming,* or *activation*) exposure occurs in the lymph node. The second *(restimulation)* exposure occurs in the peripheral tissue, from which the antigen originated.

Effector T lymphocytes consist primarily of 2 types, as determined by their different responses on experimental assays and different cell surface molecules (Fig 2-5). *Delayed hypersensitivity* (DH) T lymphocytes usually express CD4 (and so recognize antigen with MHC class II) and release IFN-γ and TNF-β. They function by encountering antigen presented by APCs in a tissue site, becoming fully activated, and releasing cytokines and mediators that recruit nonspecific, antigen-independent effector cells such as neutrophils, basophils, or monocytes (discussed in Chapter 1). As with helper T lymphocytes, Th1 and Th2 types of DH effector cells have been identified. *Cytotoxic* T lymphocytes express

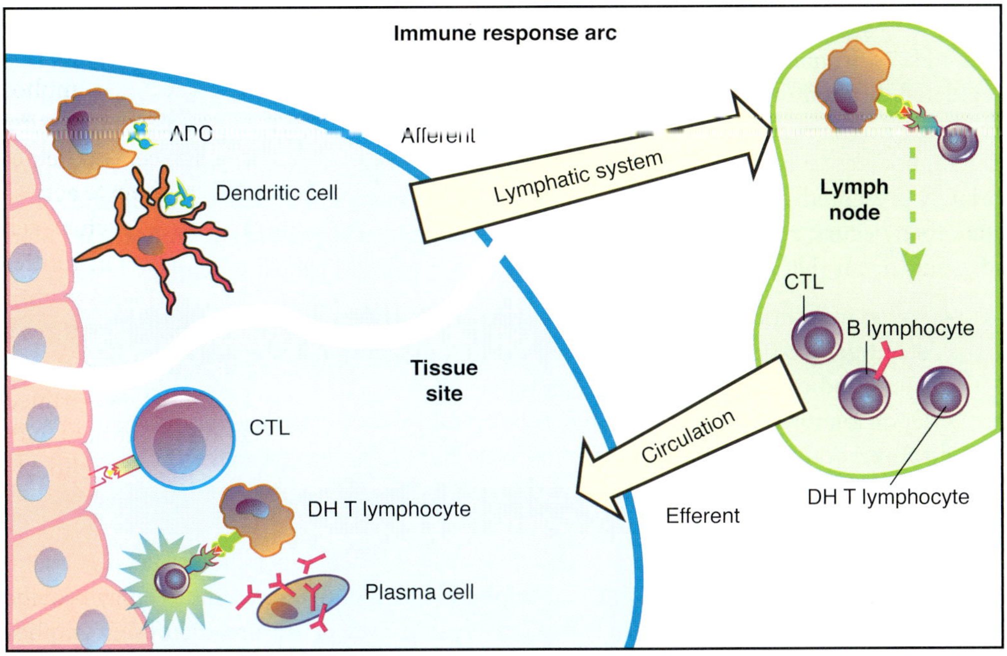

Figure 2-5 Schematic representation of effector mechanisms during adaptive immunity. The tissue site *(left)* is not only where the immune response is initiated but is also ultimately where the immune response arc is completed—when effectors encounter antigen within tissue after their release into the circulation from the lymph node *(right)*. The 3 most important effector mechanisms of adaptive immunity are cytotoxic T lymphocytes (CTLs), delayed hypersensitivity (DH) T lymphocytes, and antibody-producing B lymphocytes, especially plasma cells. *(Illustration by Barb Cousins, modified by Joyce Zavarro.)*

CD8 and serve to kill tumor cells and virally infected host cells. They accomplish this function through release of cytotoxic cytokines or specialized pore-forming molecules. A third subset of effector lymphocytes, grouped as non-T, non-B lymphocytes, includes natural killer cells, lymphokine-activated cells, and killer cells.

Antibodies, or *immunoglobulins,* are produced by B lymphocytes after appropriate antigenic stimulation with T-lymphocyte help. B lymphocytes initially secrete IgM antibodies, followed later by secretion of other isotypes after antibody-class switching. Antibodies are released into the efferent lymph fluid (downstream from lymph nodes), draining into the venous circulation. Once bound to their specific epitope, antibodies mediate a variety of immune effector activities, including opsonization for phagocytosis and complement activation via the classical pathway.

Immune Response Arc and Primary or Secondary Immune Response

Immunologic memory is the most distinctive feature of adaptive immunity, with protective immunization the prototypical example of this powerful phenomenon.

Differences in Primary and Secondary Responses

The idea of an *anamnestic response* posits that the second encounter with an antigen is regulated differently from the first. During the processing phase of the primary response, relatively rare antigen-specific B lymphocytes (perhaps 1 in 100,000 B lymphocytes) and T lymphocytes (perhaps 1 in 10,000 T lymphocytes) must come in contact with appropriately presented antigen. Stimulation of these cells from a completely resting and naive state then occurs, a process that requires days. Following the primary response, a number of events occur that set the stage for a subsequent rapid and robust secondary response:

- Following stimulation, lymphocytes divide, dramatically increasing the population of antigen-responsive T and B lymphocytes. In addition, these cells migrate to other sites of potential encounter with antigen.
- Upon removal of antigen, T and B lymphocytes activated during the primary response gradually return to a resting state but are no longer naive. They retain the capacity to become reactivated within 12–24 hours of antigen exposure and thus are now termed *memory cells.*
- IgM produced during the primary response is often too large (molecular mass, 900 kDa) to leak passively into a peripheral site. Following antibody-class switching, IgG or other isotypes can leak passively into a site or are already present because they were produced at the site; thus, they can immediately combine with antigen, causing the secondary response triggered by antibody to be very rapid *(immediate hypersensitivity).*
- In some cases, such as in mycobacterial infection, low doses of antigen may remain in the node or site, producing a chronic, low-level, continuous antigenic stimulation of T and B lymphocytes.

Homing

Memory also requires that lymphocytes demonstrate a complex migratory pattern called *homing.* Thus, lymphocytes pass from the circulation into various tissues, from which they subsequently depart, and then pass by way of lymphatics to reenter the circulation. Homing involves the dynamic interaction between lymphocytes and endothelial cells using multiple cell-adhesion molecules. Usually, the major types of lymphocytes that migrate into tissue sites are memory lymphocytes that express higher levels of certain cell-adhesion molecules, such as the integrins, than do naive cells. In contrast, naive lymphocytes tend to migrate to lymphoid tissues, where they have the chance of meeting their cognate antigen. Inflammation, however, changes the rules and serves to break down homing patterns. At inflammatory sites, the volume of lymphocyte migration is far greater and selection much less precise, although migration of memory cells or activated lymphocytes still exceeds that of naive cells.

Effector Reactivities of Adaptive Immunity

Traditionally, 4 mechanisms of adaptive immune-triggered inflammatory responses were recognized: anaphylaxis, cytotoxic antibodies, immune complex reactions, and cell-mediated reactions. These mechanisms were elaborated by Coombs and Gell in 1962, with a fifth category, *stimulatory hypersensitivity,* added later (Table 2-1). This system was developed before T lymphocytes had been discovered, at a time when understanding was limited to antibody-triggered mechanisms. It is thus primarily of historical importance, but familiarity with it is important for interpretation of much older literature.

Delves PJ, Martin SJ, Burton DR, Roitt IM. *Roitt's Essential Immunology.* 12th ed. Hoboken, NJ: Wiley-Blackwell; 2011.

Kindt TJ, Goldsby RA, Osborne BA. *Kuby Immunology.* 6th ed. New York, NY: WH Freeman; 2006.

Antibody-Mediated Immune Effector Responses

Structural and functional properties of antibody molecules

Structural features of immunoglobulins Five major classes of immunoglobulin (M, G, A, E, and D) exist, with 9 subclasses or isotypes (IgG1, IgG2, IgG3, IgG4, IgM, IgA1, IgA2, IgE, and IgD). The basic immunoglobulin structure is composed of 4 covalently bonded glycoprotein chains that form a monomer of approximately 150,000–180,000 daltons (Fig 2-6). Each antibody monomer contains 2 identical light chains, either kappa (κ) or lambda (λ),

Table 2-1 Types of Hypersensitivity (Coombs and Gell)

Type I	Anaphylaxis (immediate hypersensitivity)
Type II	Cytotoxic antibodies
Type III	Immune complex reactions
Type IV	Cell-mediated reactions
Type V	Stimulatory hypersensitivity

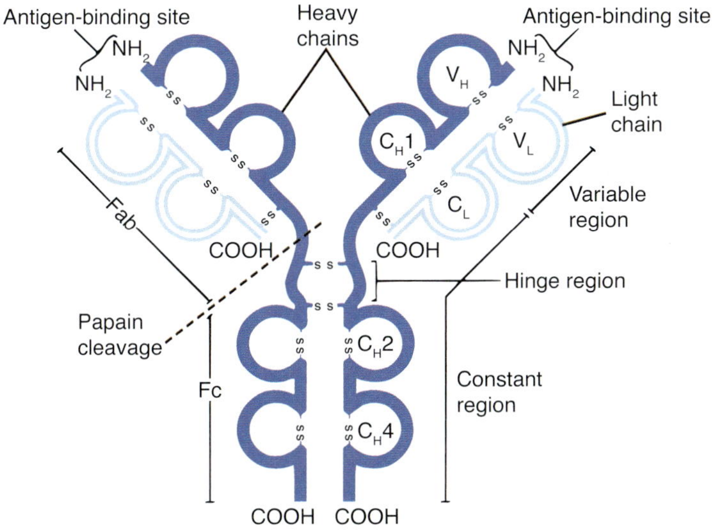

Figure 2-6 Schematic representation of an immunoglobulin (Ig) molecule. The *solid lines* indicate the identical 2 heavy chains; the *open lines* indicate the identical light chains; *-s s-* indicates intrachain and interchain covalent disulfide bonds. Fab = the *f*ragment, *a*ntigen-*b*inding region; Fc = *f*ragment *c*rystallizable region (attachment site for effector cells). *(Reprinted with permission from* Dorland's Illustrated Medical Dictionary. *32nd ed. Philadelphia, PA: Elsevier Saunders; 2012:921.)*

and 2 identical heavy chains from 1 of the 9 distinct subclasses of immunoglobulins; the type of heavy chain defines the specific isotype. IgM can form pentamers or hexamers in vivo, and IgA can form dimers in secretions, so the molecular size of these 2 classes in vivo is much larger than that of the others.

Antibodies contain regions called *domains* that carry out the specific functions of the antibody molecule. The Fab region (2 of which are present on each molecule) contains the antigen-binding domain, called the *hypervariable region.* The opposite end of the molecule, on the heavy chain portion, contains the attachment site for effector cells (the *Fc portion,* for *f*ragment *c*rystallizable); it also contains the site of other effector functions, such as complement fixation (for IgG3) or binding to a secretory component for transportation through epithelia and secretion into tears (for IgA). Table 2-2 summarizes the important structural differences among immunoglobulin isotypes.

Functional properties of immunoglobulins Immunoglobulin isotypes differ in how they mediate effector functions of antibody activity. Human IgM and IgG3 are good complement activators, whereas IgG4 is not. Only IgA1 and IgA2 can bind the secretory component and be actively passed into mucosal secretions. The importance of these differences is that 2 antibodies with identical capacity to bind to an antigen—but of different isotype—will produce different effector and inflammatory outcomes.

Terminology

Clonality Each individual B cell creates, via genetic recombination, a unique Fab fragment that recognizes a single, unique antigenic configuration. Proliferation of that individual B cell via cell division produces daughter cells that contain the exact same antigenic configuration. Continual clonal expansion results in a population of identical cells all recognizing the same epitope, termed a *monoclonal* population. As previously discussed, however, a foreign substance will have many antigenic epitopes present. Thus, a multitude of B cells will recognize various epitopes on the same substance, each undergoing simultaneous clonal expansion. The sum reactivity of all these antibodies is termed a *polyclonal response* and is the typical immune response. Modern molecular biologic techniques, however, allow the amplification of a single B-cell clone and production of large amounts of monoclonal antibodies. "Biologic" drugs such as infliximab, adalimumab, and rituximab are recombinant monoclonal antibodies.

Idiotypes Because they are proteins, antibodies themselves can be antigenic. Their antigenic sites are called *idiotopes,* as distinguished from *epitopes,* the antigenic sites on foreign molecules. Antibodies to idiotopes are called *idiotypes.* Anti-idiotypic antibodies may function as feedback mechanisms for immune regulation and have clinical significance for modern biologic therapies. Infliximab, for example, is a monoclonal chimeric (mouse and human) antibody to TNF-α used to treat some forms of uveitis. Efficacy of this drug may be limited by the development of anti-idiotype antibodies that neutralize the antigen binding site for TNF-α.

Infiltration of B lymphocytes into tissues and local production of antibody

B-lymphocyte infiltration B lymphocytes can infiltrate the site of an immunologic reaction in response to persistent antigenic stimulus. If the process becomes chronic, plasma cell

Table 2-2 Structural and Functional Properties of Immunoglobulin Isotypes

	Structural Properties			Functional Properties		
Immunoglobulin (Ig) Isotype (Heavy Chain)	% of Total Serum Igs	Relative Size	Other Structural Features	Activates Complement	Fc Receptor Binding Preferences	Other Functions
IgD δ	<1%	Monomer	Mostly on surface of B lymphocytes	No	NA	B-lymphocyte antigen receptor
IgM μ	5%	Pentamer or hexamer	Mostly on B lymphocytes or intravascular	Strong (classic pathway)	NA	B-lymphocyte antigen receptor, agglutinization, neutralization, intravascular cytolysis
IgG1 γ	50%	Monomer	Intravascular, in tissues, crosses placenta	Moderate (classic pathway)	Monocytes	Cytolysis
IgG2 γ	18%	Monomer	Same as IgG1	Weak (classic pathway)	Neutrophil monocytes, killer lym-phocytes	ADCC
IgG3 γ	6%	Monomer	Same as IgG1	Strong (classic pathway)	Neutrophil monocytes, killer lym-phocytes	ADCC, agglutinization, cytolysis
IgG4 γ	3%	Monomer	Same as IgG1	No	NA	Neutralization
IgE ϵ	<<1%	Monomer	Mostly in skin or mucosa, bound to mast cells	No	Mast cells	Mast-cell degranulation
IgA1 α	15%	Mostly monomer in serum, dimer in secretions	In mucosal secretions, binds secretory component in subepithelial tissues for transepithelial transport and protection from proteolysis	Moderate (alternative pathway)	NA	Mucosal immunity, neutralization
IgA2 α	3%	Same as IgA1	Same as IgA1	Same as IgA1	NA	NA

ADCC = antibody-dependent cellular cytotoxicity; NA = not applicable.

formation occurs, with local production of antibody specific for the inciting antigen(s). If the antigen is known, as for certain presumed infections, assessment of local antibody production can be used as a diagnostic test.

Differentiation between local production of antibody and passive leakage from the blood involves determination of the *Goldmann-Witmer* (GW) *coefficient,* calculated by comparing the ratio of specific antibody present in intraocular fluid to that in serum versus the ratio of total Ig level in intraocular fluid to the level in serum. Although a GW coefficient greater than 1.0 should theoretically indicate ocular antibody production, in practice, quotients greater than 3.0 are used to improve specificity and positive predictive value. See Clinical Example 2-2.

Local antibody production within a tissue and chronic inflammation Persistence of antigen within a site, coupled with infiltration of specific B lymphocytes and local antibody formation, can produce a chronic inflammatory reaction with a complicated histologic pattern, often demonstrating lymphocytic infiltration, plasma cell infiltration, and granulomatous features. This process is sometimes called the *chronic Arthus reaction.* This mechanism may contribute to the pathophysiology of certain chronic autoimmune disorders, such as rheumatoid arthritis, which feature formation of pathogenic antibodies.

Foster CS, Streilein JW, Coma MC. Immune-mediated tissue injury. In: Albert DM, Jakobiec FA, Azar DT, Gragoudas ES, eds. *Principles and Practice of Ophthalmology.* 3rd ed. Philadelphia, PA: WB Saunders; 2008:chap 9.

Lymphocyte-Mediated Effector Responses

Delayed hypersensitivity T lymphocytes

Delayed hypersensitivity (Coombs and Gell type IV) represents the prototypical adaptive immune mechanism for lymphocyte-triggered inflammation. It is especially powerful

CLINICAL EXAMPLE 2-2

Identification of rubella virus reactivity in Fuchs heterochromic uveitis Fuchs heterochromic uveitis (FHU) is a typically unilateral chronic anterior uveitis that frequently features elevated intraocular pressure, early cataract, and iris atrophy leading to heterochromia. By sampling aqueous at the time of cataract surgery, Quentin and Rieber demonstrated markedly elevated intraocular IgG titers to rubella virus in 52 eyes of patients with FHU compared with levels found in 50 control participants. The average Goldmann-Witmer coefficient (local antibody titer) was 20.6 in patients with FHU compared with less than 1.4 in controls. The authors found that a cutoff of 1.5 identified all patients with FHU and no controls (although studies of other diseases suggest a cutoff of 3.0 may have better specificity).

Quentin CD, Reiber H. Fuchs heterochromic cyclitis: rubella virus antibodies and genome in aqueous humor. *Am J Ophthalmol.* 2004;138(1):46–54.

in secondary immune responses. Previously primed DH CD4+ T lymphocytes leave the lymph node, home into local tissues where antigen persists, and become activated by restimulation with the specific priming antigen and MHC class II–expressing APCs. Fully activated DH T lymphocytes secrete mediators and cytokines, leading to the recruitment and activation of macrophages and/or other nonspecific leukocytes (Fig 2-7). The term *delayed* for this type of hypersensitivity refers to the fact that the reaction becomes maximal 12–48 hours after antigen exposure.

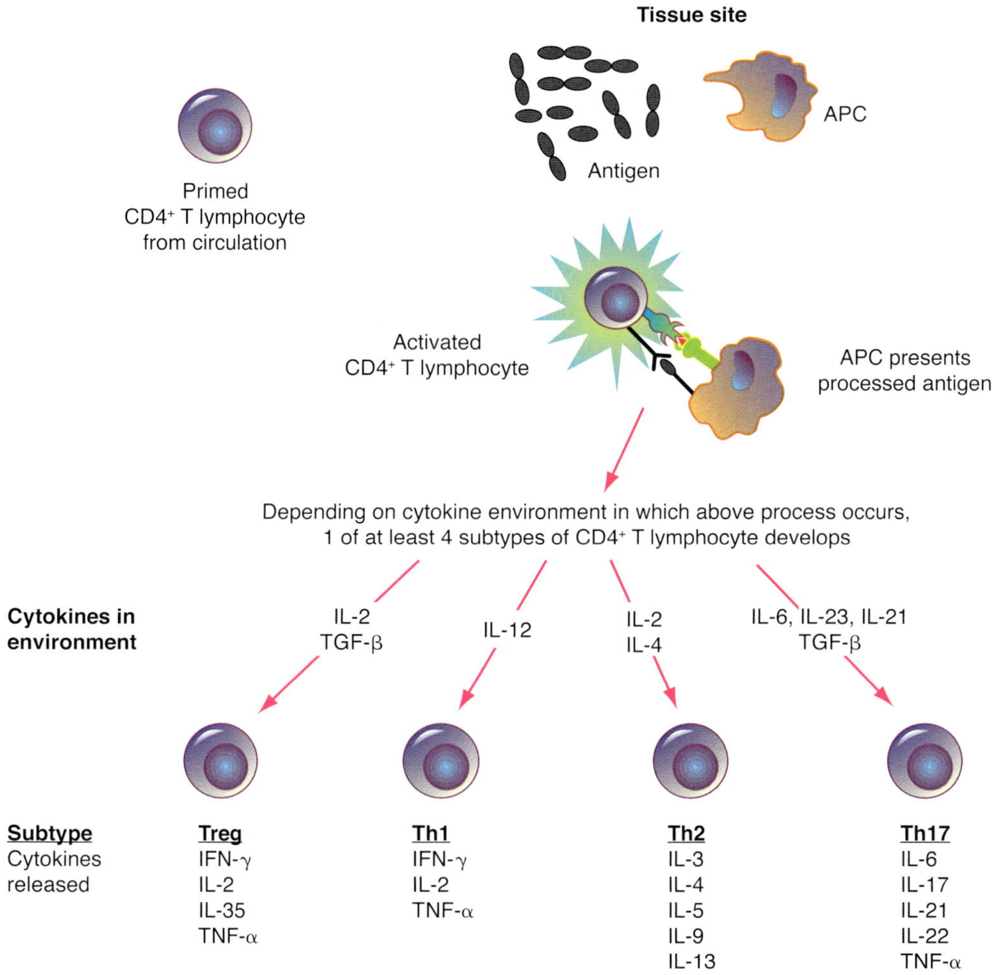

Figure 2-7 Schematic representation of CD4+ T lymphocyte development. After initial priming in the lymph node, CD4+ T lymphocytes enter the tissue site, where they again encounter APCs containing processed antigen. Upon restimulation, and depending on the cytokines present in the local environment at the time of restimulation, they become activated into 1 of at least 4 subtypes. T regulatory lymphocytes (Tregs) suppress other T-cell responses. Th1 lymphocytes are the classic delayed-hypersensitivity effector cells and mediate IFN-γ–driven responses. Th2 lymphocytes are thought to be less intensively inflammatory and have been associated with parasite-induced granulomas and atopic diseases. Th-17 lymphocytes mediate and sustain inflammation. *(Illustration developed by Russell W. Read, MD, PhD.)*

Analysis of experimental animal models and the histologic changes of human inflammation suggest that different subtypes of DH might exist. One of the most important determinants of the pattern of DH reaction is the subtype of DH $CD4^+$ effector T cells that mediate the reaction. Just as helper T lymphocytes can be differentiated into 2 groups—Th1 and Th2 subsets—according to the spectrum of cytokines secreted, DH T lymphocytes can also be grouped by the same criteria. Experimentally, the Th1 subset of cytokines, especially IFN-γ (also known as *macrophage-activating factor*) and TNF-β, activates macrophages to secrete inflammatory mediators and kill pathogens, thus amplifying inflammation. Th1-mediated DH mechanisms, therefore, are thought to produce the following effects:

- the classic DH reaction (eg, the PPD skin reaction)
- immunity to intracellular infections (eg, to mycobacteria or *Pneumocystis* organisms)
- immunity to fungi
- most forms of severe T-lymphocyte–mediated autoimmune diseases
- chronic transplant rejection

Table 2-3 summarizes ocular inflammatory diseases thought to require a major contribution of Th1 DH effector mechanisms.

The Th2 subset of DH cells secretes IL-4, IL-5, and other cytokines. IL-4 can induce B lymphocytes to synthesize IgE, and IL-5 can recruit and activate eosinophils within a site. IL-4 can also induce macrophage granulomas in response to parasite-derived antigens. Thus, Th2-mediated DH mechanisms are thought to play a major role in the following:

- response to parasite infections
- late-phase responses of allergic reactions
- asthma
- atopic dermatitis or other manifestations of atopic diseases

Table 2-3 Ocular Inflammatory Diseases Likely Involving Th1-Mediated DH Effector Mechanisms

Site	Disease	Presumed Antigen
Conjunctiva	Contact hypersensitivity to contact lens solutions	Thimerosal or other chemicals
	Giant papillary conjunctivitis	Unknown
	Phlyctenulosis	Bacterial antigens
Cornea and sclera	Chronic allograft rejection	Histocompatibility antigens
	Marginal infiltrates of blepharitis	Bacterial antigens
	Disciform keratitis after viral infection	Viral antigens
Anterior uvea	Acute anterior uveitis	Uveal autoantigens, bacterial antigens
	Sarcoidosis-associated uveitis	Unknown
	Intermediate uveitis	Unknown
Retina and choroid	Sympathetic ophthalmia	Retinal or uveal autoantigens
	Vogt-Koyanagi-Harada syndrome	Retinal or uveal autoantigens
	Birdshot uveitis	Retinal or uveal autoantigens
Orbit	Acute thyroid orbitopathy	Unknown
	Giant cell arteritis	Unknown

The persistence of certain infectious agents, especially bacteria within intracellular compartments of APCs and certain extracellular parasites, can cause destructive induration with granuloma formation and giant cells, termed the *granulomatous* form of DH. However, immune complex deposition and innate immune mechanisms in response to heavy metal or foreign-body reactions can also cause granulomatous inflammation, in which the inflammatory cascade (resulting in DH) is triggered in the absence of specific T lymphocytes. Unfortunately, for most clinical entities in which T-lymphocyte responses are suspected, especially autoimmune disorders such as multiple sclerosis or rheumatoid arthritis, the precise immunologic mechanisms remain highly speculative. See Clinical Examples 2-3.

CLINICAL EXAMPLES 2-3

***Toxocara* granuloma (Th2 DH)** *Toxocara canis* is a nematode parasite that infects up to 2% of all children worldwide and may occasionally produce inflammatory vitreoretinal manifestations. Although the ocular immunology of this disorder is not clearly delineated, animal models and a study of the immunopathogenesis of human nematode infections at other sites suggest the following scenario. The primary immune response begins in the gut after ingestion of viable eggs, which mature into larvae within the intestine. The primary processing phase produces a strong Th2 response, leading to a primary effector response that includes production of IgM, IgG, and IgE antibodies, as well as Th2-mediated DH T lymphocytes. Accidental avoidance of immune effector mechanisms may result in hematogenous dissemination of a few larvae to the choroid or retina, followed by invasion into the retina and/or vitreous. There, a Th2-mediated T-lymphocyte effector response recognizes larva antigens and releases Th2-derived cytokines to induce eosinophil and macrophage infiltration, causing the characteristic eosinophilic granuloma seen in the eye. In addition, antilarval B lymphocytes can infiltrate the eye and are induced to secrete various immunoglobulins, especially IgE. Finally, eosinophils, in part by attachment through Fc receptors, can recognize IgE or IgG bound to parasites and release cytotoxic granules containing the antiparasitic cationic protein directly in the vicinity of the larvae, using a mechanism similar to antibody-dependent cellular cytotoxicity.

Grencis RK. Th2-mediated host protective immunity to intestinal nematode infections. *Philos Trans R Soc Lond B Biol Sci.* 1997;352(1359): 1377–1384.

Sympathetic ophthalmia (Th1 DH) Sympathetic ophthalmia is a bilateral panuveitis that follows penetrating trauma to 1 eye (see Chapter 6 for a more detailed discussion). This disorder represents one of the few human diseases in which autoimmunity can be directly linked to an initiating event. In most cases, penetrating injury activates the afferent phase. It is unclear whether the injury causes a de novo primary immunization to

(Continued on next page)

(continued)

self-antigens—perhaps because of externalization of sequestered uveal antigens through the wound and exposure to the afferent immune response arc of the conjunctiva or extraocular sites—or if the injury instead somehow changes the immunologic microenvironment of the retina, retinal pigment epithelium (RPE), and uvea so that a secondary afferent response is initiated that serves to alter preexisting tolerance to retinal and uveal self-antigens.

The inflammatory effector response is generally thought to be dominated by a Th1-mediated DH mechanism generated in response to uveal or retinal antigens. $CD4^+$ T lymphocytes predominate early in the disease course, although $CD8^+$, or suppressor, T lymphocytes can be numerous in chronic cases. Activated macrophages are also numerous in granulomas, and Th1 cytokines have been identified in the vitreous or produced by T lymphocytes recovered from the eyes of affected patients. Although the target antigen for sympathetic ophthalmia is unknown, cutaneous immunization in experimental animals with certain retinal antigens (arrestin, rhodopsin, interphotoreceptor retinoid-binding protein), RPE-associated antigens, and melanocyte-associated tyrosinase can induce autoimmune uveitis with physiology or features suggestive of sympathetic ophthalmia. Th1-mediated DH is thought to mediate many forms of ocular inflammation. Table 2-3 lists other examples.

Boyd SR, Young S, Lightman S. Immunopathology of the noninfectious posterior and intermediate uveitides. *Surv Ophthalmol.* 2001;46(3):209–233.

Cytotoxic lymphocytes

Cytotoxic T lymphocytes Cytotoxic T lymphocytes (CTLs) are a subset of antigen-specific T lymphocytes, usually bearing the CD8 marker, that are especially good at killing tumor cells and virus-infected cells. CTLs can also mediate graft rejection and some types of autoimmunity. In most cases, the ideal antigen for CTLs is an intracellular protein that either occurs naturally or is produced as a result of viral infection. CTLs appear to require help from $CD4^+$ helper T-lymphocyte signals to fully differentiate. Primed *precursor* CTLs leave the lymph node and migrate to the target tissue, where they are restimulated by the interaction of the CTL antigen receptor and foreign antigens within the antigen pocket of MHC class I molecules (HLA-A, -B, or -C) on the target cell. Additional $CD4^+$ T lymphocytes help at the site, and expression of other accessory costimulatory molecules on the target is often required to obtain maximal killing.

CTLs kill cells in 1 of 2 ways: "assassination" or "suicide" induction (Fig 2-8). *Assassination* refers to CTL-mediated lysis of targets; a specialized pore-forming protein called *perforin* is released that inserts into cell membranes and causes osmotic lysis of the cell. *Suicide induction* refers to the capability of CTLs to stimulate programmed cell death of target cells, called *apoptosis,* using the CD95 ligand (FasL) to activate the CD95 receptor

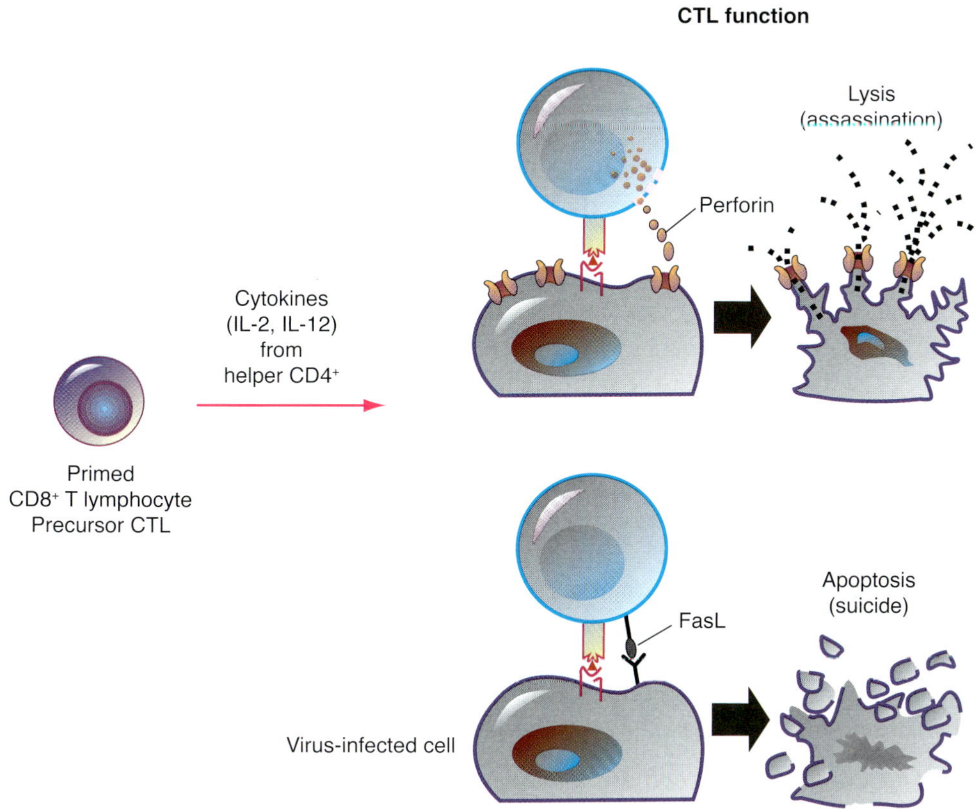

Figure 2-8 Schematic representation of the 2 major mechanisms of $CD8^+$ T-lymphocyte cytotoxicity. $CD8^+$ T lymphocytes, having undergone initial priming in the lymph node, enter the tissue site, where they again encounter antigen in the form of infected target cells. Upon restimulation, usually requiring $CD4^+$ helper T-lymphocyte factors, they become activated into fully cytolytic T lymphocytes. CTLs can kill by lysing the infected cell using a pore-forming protein called perforin or by inducing programmed cell death, called *apoptosis,* using either FasL or cytokine-mediated mechanisms. *(Illustration by Barb Cousins, modified by Joyce Zavarro.)*

(Fas) on target cells. Alternatively, CTLs can release cytotoxic cytokines such as TNF to induce apoptosis. CTLs produce low-grade lymphocytic infiltrate within tumors or infected tissues and usually kill without causing significant inflammation.

Natural killer cells Natural killer (NK) cells are a subset of non-T, non-B lymphocytes. They kill tumor cells and virus-infected cells, but unlike CTLs, NK cells do not have a specific antigen receptor. Instead, they are triggered by a less well-characterized NK cell receptor. Once triggered, however, NK cells kill target cells using the same molecular mechanisms as CTLs. Because NK cells are not antigen-specific, they theoretically have the advantage of no time delay awaiting induction of the adaptive, antigen-specific CTL immune response. However, NK cells do require some of the same effector activation signals at the tissue site, especially cytokine stimulation. Thus, NK cells are probably most effective in combination with adaptive effector responses.

Combined Antibody and Cellular Effector Mechanisms

Antibody-dependent cellular cytotoxicity

An antibody can combine with a cell-associated antigen such as a tumor or viral antigen, but if the antibody is not a subclass that activates complement, it may not induce cytotoxicity. However, because the Fc tail of the antibody is exposed, various leukocytes recognize the Fc domain and are directed to the cell through the antibody. Binding to the antibody then activates various leukocyte cytotoxic mechanisms, including degranulation and cytokine production.

Because human leukocytes express various types of Fc receptors—IgG subclasses have 3 different Fcg receptors, IgE has 2 different Fce receptors, and so on—leukocyte subsets differ in their capacity to recognize and bind different antibody isotypes. Classically, *antibody-dependent cellular cytotoxicity* (ADCC) was observed to be mediated by a subset of large granular (non-T, non-B) lymphocytes, called *killer cells,* that induce cell death in a manner similar to CTLs. The killer cell itself is nonspecific but gains antigen specificity through interaction with specific antibody. Macrophages, NK cells, certain T lymphocytes, and neutrophils can also participate in ADCC using other Fc receptor types. An IgE-dependent form of ADCC may also exist for eosinophils.

ADCC is presumed to be important in tumor surveillance, antimicrobial host protection, graft rejection, and certain autoimmune diseases such as cutaneous systemic lupus erythematosus. However, this effector mechanism probably does not play an important role in uveitis, although it might contribute to antiparasitic immunity.

Acute IgE-mediated mast-cell degranulation

Mast cells bind IgE antibodies to their surface through a high-affinity Fc receptor specific for IgE molecules, positioning the antigen-recognition site of the bound IgE externally (Fig 2-9). The combining of 2 adjacent IgE antibody molecules with a specific allergen (see Clinical Examples 2-4) causes degranulation of the mast cell and release of mediators

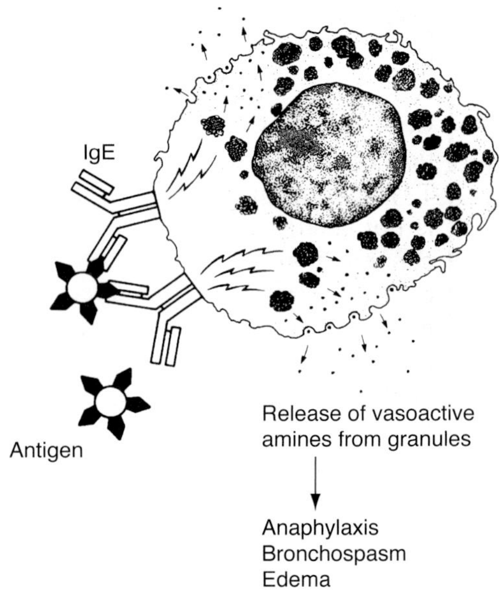

Figure 2-9 Schematic representation of IgE-mediated mast cell degranulation.

CLINICAL EXAMPLES 2-4

Allergic conjunctivitis Allergic conjunctivitis is an atopic (out of place or inappropriate) immune response to a family of antigens called *allergens,* ordinarily harmless and tolerated by most humans, that induce predominantly an acute IgE–mast-cell effector response in individuals genetically destined to be "allergic" to such substances. The primary response presumably occurred during a prior exposure to the allergen, often within the nasopharynx, during which afferent and processing phases were initiated. During this primary response, allergen-specific B lymphocytes were distributed to specialized areas in various mucosa-associated lymphoid tissue (MALT) sites. At these sites, the B lymphocytes, with T-lymphocyte help, switch from IgM-antiallergen production to IgE-antiallergen production. IgE released at the site then combines with the Fc receptors of mast cells, thereby "arming" the mast cells with a specific allergen receptor (ie, the antigen-recognizing Fab portion of the IgE). Thus, 1 mast cell may have bound IgE specific for numerous different allergens.

When reexposure to allergen occurs, it must permeate beyond the superficial conjunctival epithelium to the subepithelial region, where the antigen binds allergen-specific IgE on the surface of mast cells. Degranulation occurs within 60 minutes, leading to the release of mediators, most particularly histamine, causing chemosis and itching. A late response, within 4–24 hours, is characterized by the recruitment of lymphocytes, eosinophils, and neutrophils. The role of Th2 DH or helper T lymphocytes in the effector response has not been confirmed for allergic conjunctivitis, but presumably both types of lymphocytes are involved, especially in B-lymphocyte differentiation, because the IgE is thought to be produced locally within the conjunctiva.

Atopic keratoconjunctivitis Atopic keratoconjunctivitis (AKC) is a complex, vision-threatening ocular allergy involving chronic inflammation of the palpebral and bulbar conjunctiva with both immediate and delayed cell-mediated inflammation (see BCSC Section 8, *External Disease and Cornea*). Analysis of biopsy specimens reveals the inflammatory infiltration to consist of mast cells and eosinophils as well as activated $CD4^+$ T lymphocytes and B lymphocytes. Although the immunopathogenesis is not clearly defined, a mechanism similar to that of atopic dermatitis can be inferred, combining poorly understood genetic mechanisms, chronic mast-cell degranulation, and features of Th2-type DH. The immunopathogenesis of vernal conjunctivitis and giant papillary conjunctivitis is probably also similar. The eosinophil, with its highly toxic cytokines, eosinophil major basic protein and eosinophil cationic protein, is the effector cell most responsible for corneal damage and vision loss in patients with AKC.

within minutes, producing an acute inflammatory reaction called *immediate hypersensitivity* (Coombs and Gell type I, or *anaphylaxis*), characterized by local plasma leakage and itching. When severe, this response can produce a systemic reaction, with manifestations ranging from generalized skin lesions such as erythema, urticaria, or angioedema to severely altered vascular permeability with plasma leakage into tissues and airway obstruction or hypotensive shock.

CHAPTER 3

Ocular Immune Responses

Regional Immunity and Immunologic Microenvironments

The concept that many organs and tissue sites possess modifications to the classic immune response arc is called *regional immunity.* Regional immunity can affect all 3 phases of the response arc—afferent, processing, and effector. Regional differences in immune response occur because of differences in the immunologic microenvironments of various tissue sites. These regional differences can occur down to the level of specific locations within and around the eye (Table 3-1), such as the

- conjunctiva
- anterior chamber, anterior uvea (iris and ciliary body), and vitreous
- cornea and sclera
- retina, retinal pigment epithelium (RPE), and choriocapillaris
- choroid

Immune Responses of the Conjunctiva

Features of the Immunologic Microenvironment

The conjunctiva shares many of the features typical of mucosal sites. It is composed of 2 layers: an epithelial layer and a connective tissue layer called the *substantia propria.* The conjunctiva is well vascularized and has good lymphatic drainage to preauricular and submandibular nodes. The tissue contains numerous Langerhans cells, other dendritic cells, and macrophages that serve as potential antigen-presenting cells (APCs). Conjunctival follicles that enlarge after certain types of ocular surface infection or inflammation represent collections of T lymphocytes, B lymphocytes, and APCs. By analogy with similar sites, such as Peyer patches of the intestine, these follicles are likely sites for localized immune processing of antigens that permeate through the thin overlying epithelium.

The conjunctiva, especially the substantia propria, is richly populated with potential effector cells, predominately mast cells. All antibody isotypes are represented, with IgA the most abundant type in the tear film. Local antibody production presumably occurs as well as passive leakage. Soluble molecules of the innate immune system, especially complement, are also present. The conjunctiva appears to support most adaptive and innate immune effector responses, especially antibody-mediated and lymphocyte-mediated responses, although IgE-mediated mast-cell degranulation is one of the most common and

Table 3-1 Comparison of Immune Microenvironments in Various Normal Ocular Sites

	Conjunctiva	Cornea, Sclera	Anterior Chamber, Anterior Uvea, Vitreous	Subretinal space, RPE, Choroid
Anatomical features	Lymphatics, follicles	Lymphatics at limbus, none centrally Macromolecules diffuse through stroma	No lymphatics, antigen clearance through trabecular meshwork Partial blood–uvea barrier	No lymphatics Blood–retina barrier Uveal circulation permeable
Resident APCs	Dendritic and Langerhans cells, macrophages	Langerhans cells at limbus No APCs in central cornea No APCs in sclera Epithelium/endothelium can be induced to express class II MHC	Many dendritic cells and macrophages in iris and ciliary body Hyalocytes are macrophage-derived	Microglia in the retina Dendritic cells and macrophages in choriocapillaris RPE can be induced to express class II MHC
Specialized immune compartments for localized immune processing	?? Follicles	None	None	None
Resident effector cells	Mast cells, T lymphocytes, B lymphocytes, plasma cells, rare neutrophils	Centrally—none Sclera—none	Rare to no T lymphocytes or B lymphocytes, rare mast cells	Retina—normally no lymphocytes Choroid—mast cells, some lymphocytes
Resident effector molecules	All antibody isotypes, especially IgE, IgG subclasses, IgA in tears Complement and kininogen precursors present	Peripherally—Igs but minimal IgM Centrally—minimal antibody, some complement present Sclera—low antibody concentration, minimal IgM	Kallikrein but not kininogen precursors Some complement present, but less than in blood Minimal Igs in iris, some IgG in ciliary body and aqueous humor	Retina—minimal to no Igs Choroid—IgG and IgA
Immunoregulatory systems	Mucosa-associated lymphoid tissue	Immune privilege—Fas ligand, avascularity, lack of central APCs	Immune privilege—anterior chamber–associated immune deviation, immunosuppressive factors in aqueous, Fas ligand	Immune privilege—?? mechanisms Complement regulator expression

APC = antigen-presenting cell; Ig = immunoglobulin; MHC = major histocompatibility complex; RPE = retinal pigment epithelium.

important. See also BCSC Section 8, *External Disease and Cornea,* for further information on conjunctival immune responses.

Immunoregulatory Systems

The conjunctiva contains *mucosa-associated lymphoid tissue* (MALT), an interconnected network of mucosal sites in the body (the epithelial lining of the respiratory tract, gut, and genitourinary tract and the ocular surface and its adnexae) that share certain immunologic features:

- rich investment of APCs
- specialized structures for localized antigen processing (eg, Peyer patches and tonsils)
- unique effector cells (eg, intraepithelial T lymphocytes and abundant mast cells)

The most distinctive feature of MALT is the homing of effector T and B lymphocytes to all MALT sites following immunization at 1 site. This migration occurs because of the shared expression of specific cell-adhesion molecules on postcapillary venules of the mucosal vasculature. MALT immune response arcs favor T helper-2 (Th2)–dominated responses that result in the production of predominantly immunoglobulin A (IgA) and IgE antibodies. Processing of soluble antigens through MALT, especially in the gut sites, often produces oral tolerance, presumably by activating Th2-like regulatory T lymphocytes that suppress T helper-1 (Th1)–delayed hypersensitivity (DH) effector cells.

Clinical Example 3-1 gives an example of an immune response to conjunctivitis.

CLINICAL EXAMPLE 3-1

Immune response to viral conjunctivitis Conjunctivitis caused by adenovirus infection is a common ocular infection (see BCSC Section 8, *External Disease and Cornea*). Although precise details of the immune response after conjunctival adenovirus infection are still being discovered, they can be inferred from knowledge of viral infection at other mucosal sites and from animal studies. After infection with adenovirus, the epithelial cells begin to die within 36 hours. Innate immune mechanisms that can assist in limiting infection become activated soon after infection. For example, infected cells produce cytokines such as interferons that limit spread of the infectious virus and recruit nonspecific effector cells such as macrophages and neutrophils.

However, the adaptive immune response to adenovirus infection is considered more important in viral clearance. The primary adaptive response begins when macrophages and dendritic cells become infected or take up cell debris and viral antigens. Both antigen-presenting cells (APCs) and extracellular antigenic material are conveyed to the preauricular and submandibular nodes along lymphatic channels, where helper T-lymphocyte and antibody responses are activated, producing characteristic lymphadenopathy. Local immune processing may also occur

(Continued on next page)

(continued)

within the follicle if virus invades the epithelial capsule. During the early effector phase of the primary B-lymphocyte response, immunoglobulin M (IgM) antibodies are released into the blood that are *not* very effective in controlling surface infection, although they combat widespread viremia. However, IgM-bearing B lymphocytes eventually infiltrate the conjunctival stroma and may release antibodies locally in the conjunctiva. Later, during the primary effector response, class switching to IgG or IgA may occur to mediate local effector responses, such as neutralization or complement-mediated lysis of infected cells.

The most active effector response later in acute viral infection comes from CD8-positive natural killer cells and cytotoxic T lymphocytes (CTLs), which kill infected epithelium. However, adenovirus can block the expression of major histocompatibility complex (MHC) class I on infected cells and thereby escape being killed by CTLs. Adaptive immunity can also activate macrophages by antiviral delayed hypersensitivity (DH) mechanisms later during infection. DH response to viral antigens is thought to contribute to the development of the corneal subepithelial infiltrates that occur in some patients late in adenovirus infection.

The secondary response of the conjunctiva, assuming a prior primary exposure to the same virus at some other mucosal site, differs in that antibody-mediated effector mechanisms dominate. Because of mucosa-associated lymphoid tissue (MALT), antivirus IgA is present not only in blood but also in tear film as a result of differentiated IgA-secreting B lymphocytes in the lacrimal gland, the substantia propria, and follicles. Thus, recurrent infection is often prevented by preexisting neutralizing antibodies that had disseminated into tears or follicles following the primary infection. However, if the inoculum of recurrent virus overwhelms this antibody barrier, or if the virus has mutated its surface glycoproteins recognized by antibodies, then epithelial infection does occur. Additional immune processing can occur in the follicle and draining nodes. Specific memory effector CTLs are effective in clearing infection within a few days.

Hendricks RL. Immunopathogenesis of viral ocular infections. *Chem Immunol.* 1999;73:120–136.

Nathanson N. *Viral Pathogenesis and Immunity.* 2nd ed. London: Academic Press; 2007.

Immune Responses of the Anterior Chamber, Anterior Uvea, and Vitreous

Features of the Immunologic Microenvironment

Numerous specialized anatomical features of the anterior region of the eye affect ocular immune responses. The anterior chamber is a fluid-filled cavity; circulating aqueous humor provides a unique medium for intercellular communication among cytokines, immune cells, and resident tissue cells of the iris, ciliary body, and corneal endothelium. Although aqueous humor is relatively protein-depleted compared with serum (containing about 0.1%–1.0% of the total serum protein concentration), even normal aqueous humor contains a complex mixture of biological factors, such as immunomodulatory cytokines, neuropeptides, and complement inhibitors that influence immunologic events within the eye.

A partial blood–ocular barrier is present. Fenestrated capillaries in the ciliary body allow a size-dependent concentration gradient of plasma macromolecules to permeate the interstitial tissue; smaller plasma-derived molecules are present in higher concentration than are larger molecules. The tight junctions between the pigmented and nonpigmented ciliary epithelium provide a more exclusive barrier, preventing interstitial macromolecules from permeating directly through the ciliary body into the aqueous humor. Nevertheless, a small number of plasma macromolecules bypass the nonpigmented epithelium barrier and may permeate by diffusion anteriorly through the uvea to enter the anterior chamber through the anterior iris surface.

Few resident T lymphocytes and some mast cells are present in the normal anterior uvea; B lymphocytes, eosinophils, and neutrophils are normally not present. Very low concentrations of IgG and complement components occur in normal aqueous humor. The iris and ciliary body contain significant numbers of macrophages and dendritic cells that serve as APCs and possible effector cells. Immune processing is unlikely to occur locally. Rather, because the inner eye does not contain well-defined lymphatic channels, clearance of soluble substances depends on aqueous humor outflow channels; clearance of particulates depends on endocytosis by trabecular meshwork endothelial cells or macrophages. Nevertheless, antigen inoculation into the anterior chamber results in efficient communication with the systemic immune response. Intact soluble antigens gain entrance to the venous circulation, through which they are transported to the spleen.

The vitreous has not been studied as extensively as the anterior chamber but likely has most of the same properties, with several notable exceptions. The vitreous gel can electrostatically bind charged protein substances and may thus serve as an antigen depot as well as a substrate for leukocyte cell adhesion. Because the vitreous contains type II collagen, it may serve as a depot of potential autoantigen as well.

Immunoregulatory Systems

Relatively mild degrees of inflammation that would be harmless in the skin, for example, can cause severe vision loss if they occur in the eye. A variety of immunoregulatory mechanisms have thus evolved to modulate intraocular immune responses. This concept, termed *immune privilege,* arose from the observation that tumor implants or allografts survive better within an immunologically privileged region, whereas a similar implant or graft is rapidly rejected by immune mechanisms within the skin or other nonprivileged sites. Other immune-privileged sites include the subretinal space, brain, and testes.

Ocular immune privilege has been observed with a wide variety of antigens, including alloantigens (eg, transplantation antigens), tumor antigens, haptens, soluble proteins, autoantigens, bacteria, and viruses. The best-studied model of immune privilege in the eye is called *anterior chamber–associated immune deviation* (ACAID). Whereas subcutaneous immunization with antigen elicits a strong, delayed-type sensitivity, immunization into the anterior chamber with the identical antigen results in a robust antibody response but a virtual absence of delayed-type hypersensitivity. In fact, preexisting delayed-type hypersensitivity can be suppressed by the ACAID response.

Once ACAID is induced by injection of antigen into the anterior chamber, specialized macrophages residing in the iris recognize and phagocytose the antigen. The APC function of these uveal macrophages has been altered by exposure to immunoregulatory cytokines present within aqueous humor and uveal tissue, especially transforming growth factor β_2 (TGF-β_2). These TGF-β_2–exposed, antigen-stimulated, ocular macrophages exit via the trabecular meshwork and Schlemm canal to enter the venous circulation, by which they migrate to the spleen. Within the spleen, the antigen signal is processed, resulting in activation of not only helper T lymphocytes and B lymphocytes but also regulatory T lymphocytes. These $CD8^+$ regulatory cells serve to alter $CD4^+$ helper T-lymphocyte responses in the spleen and downregulate $CD4^+$ T-lymphocyte DH responses to the specific immunizing antigen at all body sites. Thus, the resulting effector response is characterized by a selective suppression of antigen-specific DH and a selectively diminished production of complement-fixing isotypes of antibodies. Splenectomy eliminates ACAID, demonstrating the importance of this site for generation of immune deviation.

ACAID represents an attenuated effector arc. The eye is further protected from severe inflammation by another modulating system termed *effector blockade,* by which Th1 lymphocytes, cytotoxic T lymphocytes, natural killer cells, and complement activation appear to function less effectively in the anterior uvea than elsewhere. For instance, the anterior uvea is *relatively* resistant to induction of a secondary purified protein derivative DH response after primary immunization with mycobacteria in the skin. There are several mechanisms of effector blockade, but one of the most important and best studied involves the *Fas ligand* (FasL, or CD95 ligand). The FasL is constitutively expressed on the iris and corneal endothelium and is a potent trigger of programmed cell death, or *apoptosis,* of lymphocytes expressing the Fas receptor. Thus, even if an immune response develops to an ocular antigen, the inflammation can be downregulated by this mechanism of effector blockade.

It should be noted that ACAID and other effector blockades can be overcome by sufficient immune stimulation. Following an episode of inflammation, ACAID may be only partly restored, thus potentially reducing the eye's immune protection.

Foster CS, Suelves AM. Basic immunology. In: Foster CS, Vitale AT, eds. *Diagnosis and Treatment of Uveitis.* Philadelphia, PA: WB Saunders; 2013:44–100.

Niederkorn JY. The induction of anterior chamber–associated immune deviation. *Chem Immunol Allergy.* 2007;92:27–35.

Sugita S, Ng TF, Lucas PJ, Gress RE, Streilein JW. $B7^+$ iris pigment epithelium induce $CD8^+$ T regulatory cells; both suppress CTLA-4^+ T cells. *J Immunol.* 2006;176(1):118–127.

Immune Responses of the Cornea

Features of the Immunologic Microenvironment

The cornea is unique in that the peripheral and central portions of the tissue represent distinctly different immunologic microenvironments (Fig 3-1). In normal eyes, only the

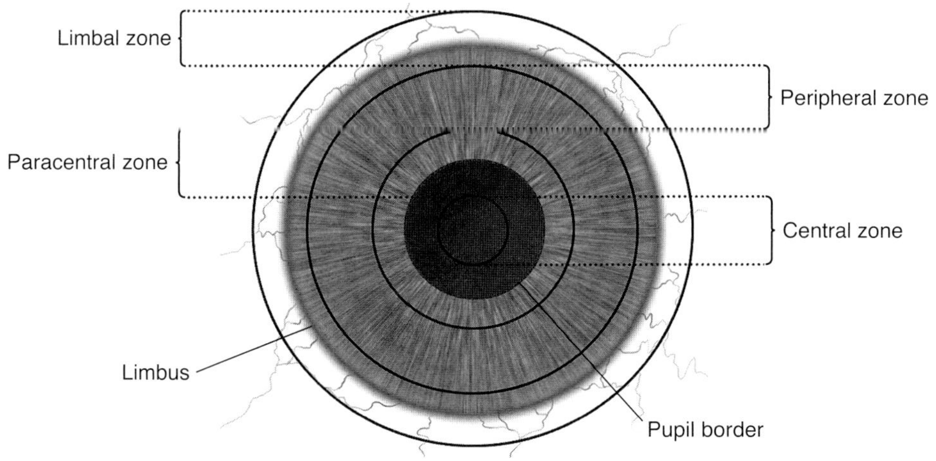

Figure 3-1 Topographic zones of the cornea. *(Illustration by Christine Gralapp.)*

limbus is vascularized and richly invested with Langerhans cells. The paracentral and central cornea are normally devoid of APCs and are avascular. Various stimuli, such as mild trauma, certain cytokines (eg, interleukin-1), or infection, can recruit APCs to the central cornea. Plasma-derived proteins such as complement, IgM, and IgG are present in moderate concentrations in the periphery, but only low levels of IgM are present centrally.

Corneal cells also appear to synthesize various antimicrobial and immunoregulatory proteins. Effector cells are absent or scarce in the normal cornea, but neutrophils, monocytes, and lymphocytes can readily migrate through the stroma if appropriate chemotactic stimuli are activated. Lymphocytes, monocytes, and neutrophils can also adhere to the endothelial surface during inflammation, giving rise to keratic precipitates or the classic Khodadoust line of endothelial rejection (Fig 3-2). Localized immune processing probably does not occur in the cornea. See also BCSC Section 8, *External Disease and Cornea.*

Immunoregulatory Systems

The cornea demonstrates a form of immune privilege different from that observed in the anterior uvea. Immune privilege of the cornea is multifactorial. Normal limbal physiology is a major component, especially the maintenance of avascularity and lack of APCs in the mid- and central cornea. The absence of APCs and lymphatic channels partially inhibits afferent recognition in the central cornea, and the absence of postcapillary venules centrally can limit the efficiency of effector recruitment, although both effector cells and molecules can ultimately infiltrate even avascular cornea. Another factor is the presence of intact immunoregulatory systems of the anterior chamber (eg, ACAID), to which the corneal endothelium is exposed. Finally, effector blockade likely provides relative immune privilege to the cornea. Allografts tolerated between different strains of wild-type mice are rejected in mice that genetically lack either Fas or FasL.

See Clinical Example 3-2.

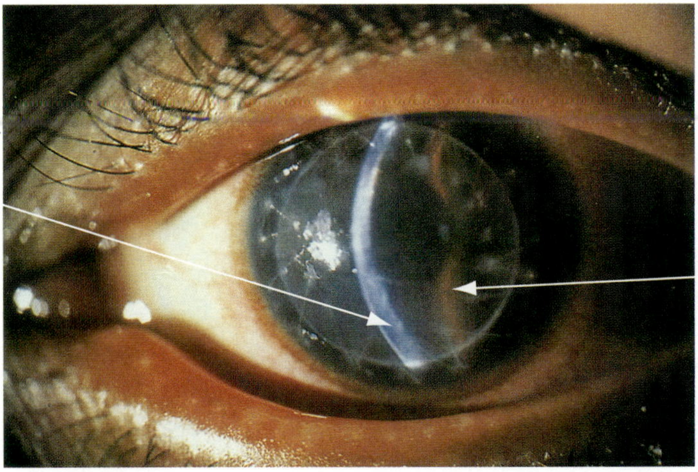

Figure 3-2 Endothelial graft rejection with stromal and epithelial edema on the trailing aspect of the migrating Khodadoust line.

CLINICAL EXAMPLE 3-2

Corneal allograft rejection Penetrating keratoplasty, or the transplantation of corneal allografts, has an extremely high success rate (>90%) even in the absence of systemic immunomodulation. This rate is substantially superior to acceptance rates after transplantation of other donor tissues. The mechanisms of corneal graft survival have been attributed to immune privilege. In experimental models, factors contributing to rejection include the following:

- presence of central corneal vascularization
- induction of MHC molecule expression, which is normally low, by the stroma
- contamination of the donor graft with donor-derived APCs prior to transplantation
- MHC disparity between the host and the donor
- preimmunization of the recipient to donor transplantation antigens

Loss of the immunoregulatory systems of the anterior chamber can influence corneal allograft immunity, and the expression of FasL on corneal endothelium has been observed to be essential for allograft protection in animal models. Rapid replacement of donor epithelium by host epithelium removes this layer as an antigenic stimulus. Once activated, however, antibody-dependent DH and CTL-related mechanisms can target transplantation antigens in all corneal layers.

Klebe S, Coster DJ, Williams KA. Rejection and acceptance of corneal allografts. *Curr Opin Organ Transplant.* 2009;14(1):4–9.

Immune Responses of the Retina, RPE, Choriocapillaris, and Choroid

Features of the Immunologic Microenvironment

The immunologic microenvironments of the retina, RPE, choriocapillaris, and choroid have not been well described. The retinal circulation establishes an inner blood–ocular barrier at the level of tight junctions between adjacent endothelial cells, while tight junctions between the cells of the RPE provide an outer barrier between the choroid and the retina. The vessels of the choriocapillaris are highly permeable to macromolecules and allow transudation of most plasma macromolecules into the extravascular spaces of the choroid and choriocapillaris. Well-developed lymphatic channels are absent, although both the retina and the choroid have abundant potential APCs. In the retina, resident microglia (bone marrow–derived cells related to dendritic cells) are interspersed within all layers and can undergo physical changes and migration in response to various stimuli. The choriocapillaris and choroid contain an abundance of certain potential APCs, especially macrophages and dendritic cells.

The RPE can be induced to express major histocompatibility complex (MHC) class II molecules, suggesting that the RPE may interact with T lymphocytes in some circumstances. The presence of T lymphocytes or B lymphocytes within the normal posterior segment has not been carefully studied, but effector cells appear to be absent from the normal retina. A moderate density of mast cells is present in the choroid, especially around the arterioles, but lymphocytes are present only in very low number. Eosinophils and neutrophils appear to be absent. Under various clinical or experimental conditions, however, high densities of T lymphocytes, B lymphocytes, macrophages, and neutrophils can infiltrate the choroid, choriocapillaris, and retina. The RPE and various cell types within the retina and the choroid (eg, pericytes) can synthesize many different cytokines (eg, TGF-β) that may alter the subsequent immune response. Local immune processing does not seem to occur. See also BCSC Section 12, *Retina and Vitreous.*

Detrick B, Hooks JJ. Immune regulation in the retina. *Immunol Res.* 2010;47(1–3):153–161.

Immunoregulatory Systems

A form of immune privilege, likely similar to ACAID, is present after subretinal injection of antigen. This observation may be important because of growing interest in retinal transplantation, stem cell therapies, and gene therapy. (See Clinical Examples 3-3.) The capacity of the choriocapillaris and choroid to function as unique environments for the afferent or effector phases has not yet been evaluated. The RPE expresses the complement regulatory protein CD46 on its basolateral surface, likely providing protection from complement activation occurring in the subjacent choroid.

Vogt SD, Barnum SR, Curcio CA, Read RW. Distribution of complement anaphylatoxin receptors and membrane-bound regulators in normal human retina. *Exp Eye Res.* 2006; 83(4):834–840.

CLINICAL EXAMPLES 3-3

Retinal transplantation Transplantation of retina, retinal pigment epithelium (RPE), or embryonic stem cell–derived retinal tissue is being investigated as a method for restoring retinal function in various disorders. In experimental animal models, subretinal transplantation of fetal retinal tissue or various kinds of RPE allografts often show longer survival than the same grafts implanted elsewhere, even without systemic immunomodulation. The afferent phase recognition of alloantigens is likely performed by retinal microglia or blood-derived macrophages recruited from the choriocapillaris whose function has been altered by the subretinal microenvironment. This environment is probably altered further in retinal diseases, such as retinitis pigmentosa or macular degeneration, as a result of changes in the blood–retina barrier arising from retinal cell and RPE injury. However, injured RPE can still synthesize immunomodulatory and inflammatory cytokines. Although the site of immune processing is unknown, the spleen or other secondary compartment outside of the eye is likely involved.

In mice with fetal retinal grafts, immune rejection occurs by an unusual, slowly progressive cytotoxic mechanism not involving typical antibody-mediated cytolysis or DH T lymphocytes. In humans and nonhuman primates, rejection of RPE allografts has occurred in both subacute and chronic forms.

Retinal gene therapy Retinal gene therapy is the intentional transfection of neural retina cells or RPE with a replication-defective virus that has been genetically altered to carry a replacement gene of choice. This gene becomes expressed in any cell infected by the virus. Immune clearance of the virus has been shown to cause loss of expression of the transferred gene in other body sites. Two applications of gene therapy in primates (including humans) have been successfully completed. In one, an adeno-associated viral vector targeting the RPE was used to replace the defective *RPE65* gene responsible for Leber congenital amaurosis. Immunomodulatory therapy was given along with the gene therapy. In the second application, dichromatic New World monkeys underwent cone photoreceptor gene therapy with an adeno-associated virus encoding the missing cone gene, which resulted in the new cone pigment being expressed in photoreceptors. Because photoreceptors are within the privileged site of the retina, no additional immunomodulation is given.

Mancuso K, Hauswirth WW, Li Q, et al. Gene therapy for red-green colour blindness in adult primates. *Nature.* 2009;461(7265):784–787.

CHAPTER 4

Special Topics in Ocular Immunology

Animal Models of Human Uveitis

Many models of uveitis exist, using a variety of species, antigens, adjuvants, and protocols to produce disease that ranges from transient to persistent and mild to severe. None is an exact corollary to human disease, but all have contributed substantially to the understanding of ocular immunology.

Experimental Autoimmune Uveoretinitis

Experimental autoimmune uveoretinitis (EAU) is the most widely used and well-studied animal model of human uveitis. In the original model, a retinal extract administered intradermally with Freund complete adjuvant in rats and rabbits results in a panuveitis approximately 1–2 weeks later. Features include inflammation in the anterior segment, vitreous, and choroid. Refinements of the model have occurred over time; purified arrestin (also called *S-antigen*) has been used in rats, and the model was expanded to mice, using immunization with interphotoreceptor retinoid-binding protein (IRBP)–derived peptides. The mouse model manifests initially as a vasculitis and papillitis, followed by intraretinal infiltration. Only in the most severe cases does true uveitis occur, evidenced by choroidal infiltration.

Endotoxin-Induced Uveitis

Endotoxin-induced (also termed *experimental immune*) uveitis (EIU) is a transient uveitis model induced by footpad, intraperitoneal, or intravitreal injection of lipopolysaccharide in mice and rats (see Chapter 1). Sixteen to 48 hours after administration, a transient anterior uveitis develops. This model has been especially useful for studies of the dynamics of leukocyte function in the anterior chamber. It is not clear how or even if this model correlates with human disease.

Equine Recurrent Uveitis

This spontaneous uveitis occurs in horses. It is typically a bilateral uveitis featuring anterior and posterior segment inflammation. The disease affects up to 10% of horses. Immunologic studies have indicated the presence of autoantibodies and autoreactive T cells in this disease.

AIRE-Deficient Mice

AIRE (for *autoimmune regulator*) is a transcription factor used by the thymus in the process of establishing thymic tolerance. Early in life, the thymus expresses many cell-type–specific proteins; T-cell clones reactive to these proteins are deleted. This mechanism is important in the development of self-tolerance. Mice deficient in AIRE do not express these proteins during development; thus, autoreactive T cells escape deletion, and the mice spontaneously develop a posterior uveitis. Recent work has suggested that the major antigen targeted in this autoimmune uveitis is IRBP—the same protein used to generate mouse models of EAU.

IRBP-Specific T-Cell Receptor Transgenic Mice

As described earlier, immunization of mice with a peptide sequence from IRBP induces autoimmune uveitis in mice. Mice bred to be transgenic for an IRBP-specific T-cell receptor develop a spontaneous uveitis that begins around 4 weeks of age and progresses to an incidence of 100% by age 12 weeks. These mice provide an additional model to study disease that negates the need for peripheral immunization and produces a chronic course, in contrast to the more acute disease of EAU.

Caspi RR, Silver PB, Luger D, et al. Mouse models of experimental autoimmune uveitis. *Ophthalmic Res.* 2008;40(3–4):169–174.

DeVoss J, Hou Y, Johannes K, et al. Spontaneous autoimmunity prevented by thymic expression of a single self-antigen. *J Exp Med.* 2006;203(12):2727–2735.

Forrester JV, Klaska IP, Yu T, Kuffova L. Uveitis in mouse and man. *Int Rev Immunol.* 2013;32(1):76–96.

Horai R, Silver PB, Chen J, et al. Breakdown of immune privilege and spontaneous autoimmunity in mice expressing a transgenic T cell receptor specific for a retinal autoantigen. *J Autoimmun.* 2013;44:21–33.

HLA Associations and Disease

Normal Function of HLA Molecules

All animals with white blood cells express a family of cell-surface glycoproteins called *major histocompatibility complex* (MHC) proteins. In humans, the MHC proteins are called *human leukocyte antigen* (HLA) molecules. As discussed in Chapter 2, 6 different families of HLA molecules have been identified:

- 3 MHC class I: HLA-A, -B, -C
- 3 MHC class II: HLA-DR, -DP, -DQ

A seventh category, HLA-D, does not exist as a specific molecule but instead represents a functional classification as determined by an in vitro assay.

The important role MHC molecules play in immunologic function is discussed in Chapter 2. HLA genes are also considered human immune response genes because the HLA type determines the capacity of the antigen-presenting cell (APC) to bind peptide fragments and thus determines T-lymphocyte immune responsiveness.

Allelic Variation

Within the human population, a large variety of alleles exist for each of the 6 HLA types: more than 25 alleles for HLA-A, 50 for HLA-B, 10 for HLA-C, 100 for HLA-DR, and so on. Because there are 6 HLA types and each person has a pair of each HLA type (codominantly expressed), or 1 *haplotype*, an APC expresses 6 pairs of MHC molecules. Thus, with the exception of identical twins, only rarely will all 12 potential haplotypes match between 2 individuals.

Allelic diversity provides protection through *population-wide immunity.* Each HLA haplotype covers a theoretical set of antigens against which a particular individual can respond. The presence of many different HLA alleles within a population should thus ensure that the collective adaptive immune system will be able to respond to a wide range of potential pathogens. The converse also holds true: some individuals may be at increased risk for immunologic diseases because of either an aberrantly strong immune response to a benign pathogen or an autoimmune disease arising from inappropriate recognition of host peptides in the context of a particular HLA as foreign. See Clinical Example 4-1.

CLINICAL EXAMPLE 4-1

HLA-B27–associated acute anterior uveitis Approximately 50% of patients with acute anterior uveitis (AAU) express the HLA-B27 haplotype, and many of these patients also experience other immunologic disorders, such as reactive arthritis, ankylosing spondylitis, inflammatory bowel disease, and psoriatic arthritis (see Chapter 6). Although the immunopathogenesis remains unknown, various animal models permit some informed speculation. Many cases of uveitis or reactive arthritis follow gram-negative bacillary dysentery or chlamydial infection. The possible role of bacterial lipopolysaccharide and innate mechanisms was discussed in Chapter 1. Experiments in rats and mice genetically altered to express human HLA-B27 molecules seem to suggest that bacterial infection of the gut predisposes rats to arthritis and a reactive arthritis–like syndrome, although uveitis is uncommon.

One suggestion is that chronic intracellular chlamydial infection of a joint, and presumably the eye, stimulates an adaptive immune response using the endogenous (class I) antigen-processing pathway of the B27 molecule, in which a $CD8^+$ T-lymphocyte effector mechanism is activated to kill the microbe but indirectly injures the eye. Another speculation is that B27 amino acid sequences might present *Klebsiella* species peptide antigens to $CD8^+$ T lymphocytes, although the method by which a presumed exogenous bacterial antigen would be presented through the class I pathway is unknown. Another hypothesis posits that molecular mimicry may exist between bacterial antigens and some amino acid sequences of HLA-B27. Analysis of human AAU fluids and various animal models of AAU and arthritis suggests that anterior uveitis might be

(Continued on next page)

(continued)

a CD4+ Th1-mediated delayed hypersensitivity response, possibly in response to bacteria-derived antigens (such as bacterial cell wall antigens or heat shock proteins trapped in the uvea) or to endogenous autoantigens of the anterior uvea (possibly melanin-associated antigens, type I collagen, or myelin-associated proteins). How a CD4-predominant mechanism would relate to a class I immunogenetic association is unclear.

Clinical detection and classification of different alleles

Determination of HLA type has evolved from prior antisera reactions to molecular techniques that determine the nucleic acid sequence of MHC alleles. HLA molecules are composed of 2 chains: α and β chains for class II, and the α chain and the β_2-microglobulin chain for class I. Genotyping specifies the chain, major genetic type, and specific minor molecular variant subtype. For example, genotype DRB1*0408 refers to the HLA-DR4 molecule β chain with the "–08" minor variant subtype. Haplotypes currently recognized as a single group will continue to be subdivided into new categories or new subtypes as research progresses. For example, at least 2 different A29 subtypes and 8 different HLA-B27 subtypes have been recognized.

Disease Associations

In 1973, the first association between an HLA haplotype and a disease—ankylosing spondylitis—was identified. Since then, more than 100 other disease associations have been established, including several for ocular inflammatory diseases (Table 4-1). An HLA–disease association is established when there is a statistically increased frequency of an HLA haplotype in persons with that disease compared with the frequency in a disease-free population. The ratio of the probability of the disease occurring in individuals with the HLA haplotype to that in individuals without the haplotype is termed *relative risk.* A relative risk of 1 denotes no difference in risk, <1 indicates a reduced risk, and >1 an increased risk. Several points are important when considering HLA–disease associations:

- The HLA association identifies individuals at risk, but it is not a diagnostic marker. The associated haplotype is not necessarily present in all people with the disease, nor does its presence in a person ensure the correct diagnosis.
- The association depends on the validity of the haplotyping. Older literature often reflects associations based on HLA classifications (some provisional) that might have changed.
- The association is only as strong as the clinical diagnosis. Diseases that are difficult to diagnose based on clinical features may obscure real associations.
- The concept of *linkage disequilibrium* proposes that if 2 genes are physically close together on a chromosome, they are likely to be inherited together rather than undergo genetic randomization in a population. Thus, HLA genes may be coinherited with a separate gene that confers the actual risk, and sometimes 2 HLA haplotypes can occur together more frequently than predicted by their independent frequencies in the population.

Table 4-1 HLA Associations and Ocular Inflammatory Disease

Disease	HLA Association	Relative Risk (RR), Other Associations
Uveitic diseases with strong HLA associations		
Tubulointerstitial nephritis and uveitis (TINU) syndrome	HLA-DRB1*0102	RR = 167
Birdshot uveitis	HLA-A29, -A29.2	RR up to 224 for North Americans and Europeans
Reactive arthritis	HLA-B27	RR = 60
Acute anterior uveitis	HLA-B27	RR = 8
Uveitic diseases with weaker HLA associations		
Juvenile idiopathic arthritis	HLA-A2, -DR5, -DR8, -DR11, -DP2.1	Acute systemic disease
Behçet disease	HLA-B51	RR = 4–6; Japanese and Middle Eastern descent
Intermediate uveitis	HLA-B8, -B51, -DR2, -DR15	RR = 6, possibly the DRB1*1501 genotype
Sympathetic ophthalmia	HLA-DR4	Unknown
Vogt-Koyanagi-Harada syndrome	HLA-DR4	RR = 2, Japanese and North Americans
Sarcoidosis	HLA-B8 HLA-B13	Acute systemic disease Chronic systemic disease but not for eye
Multiple sclerosis	HLA-B7, -DR2	Unknown
Retinal vasculitis	HLA-B44	Britons

For example, approximately 8% of the Caucasian population in the United States is HLA-A29 positive, but fewer than 1 in 10,000 US residents have birdshot uveitis (although nearly all patients with birdshot uveitis are HLA-A29 positive). Thus, the vast majority of individuals who are HLA-A29 positive will never have birdshot uveitis.

Several mechanisms have been proposed for HLA–disease associations. The most direct theory postulates that HLA molecules act as peptide-binding molecules for etiologic antigens or infectious agents. Thus, individuals bearing a specific HLA molecule might be predisposed to processing certain antigens, such as an infectious agent that cross-reacts with a self-antigen, and other individuals, lacking that haplotype, would not be so predisposed. Specific variations or mutations in the peptide-binding region would greatly influence this mechanism; these variations can be detected only by molecular typing. Preliminary data in support of this theory have been provided for patients with type 1 diabetes mellitus.

A second theory proposes molecular mimicry between bacterial antigens and an epitope on the HLA molecule (ie, an antigenic site on the molecule itself). An appropriate antibacterial effector response might inappropriately initiate a cross-reactive effector response with an epitope of the HLA molecule.

A third theory suggests that the T-lymphocyte antigen receptor (gene) is really the true susceptibility factor. Because a specific T-lymphocyte receptor uses a specific HLA haplotype, a strong correlation would exist between an HLA and the T-lymphocyte antigen receptor repertoire.

Levinson RD. Immunogenetics of ocular inflammatory disease. *Tissue Antigens.* 2007;69(2): 105–112.

PART II

Intraocular Inflammation and Uveitis

CHAPTER 5

Clinical Approach to Uveitis

This chapter includes related videos, which can be accessed by scanning the QR codes provided in the text or going to www.aao.org/bcscvideo_section09.

The uvea consists of the middle, pigmented, vascular layer of the eye and includes the iris, ciliary body, and choroid. *Uveitis* is broadly defined as inflammation (ie, *-itis*) of the uvea (from the Latin *uva,* meaning "grape"). Inflammation of the uvea may be accompanied by involvement of other ocular structures such as the retina, sclera, cornea, vitreous, and optic nerve.

Because uveitis is frequently associated with systemic disease, a careful, thorough history and review of systems is an essential first step in elucidating a cause. A comprehensive physical examination of the eye and pertinent organ systems must be done to characterize the type of inflammation present. The anatomical location of inflammation combined with information obtained from the history and physical examination help dictate which investigational studies to conduct. Laboratory studies can help determine the etiology of the intraocular inflammation but are never a substitute for a thorough history and physical examination. Determining a specific etiology of uveitis may guide the selection of therapy.

Classification of Uveitis

Several schemes for the classification of uveitis currently exist. Various methods are based on the anatomy (the portion of the uvea involved), clinical course (acute, chronic, or recurrent), etiology (infectious or noninfectious), and histology (granulomatous or nongranulomatous) of the uveitis. The rapid expansion of published clinical information on various uveitic entities from a myriad of global sources using different classification and grading systems—combined with the undeniable need for multicenter, randomized clinical trials to better understand the course, prognosis, and treatment of these entities—led the Standardization of Uveitis Nomenclature (SUN) Working Group in 2005 to develop an anatomical classification system, descriptors, standardized grading systems, and terminology. This system was adopted by leading uveitis specialists worldwide.

This text uses an etiologic division of uveitic entities into noninfectious (autoimmune) and infectious conditions and then further subcategorizes and describes them using the basic anatomical classification of uveitis into 4 groups (Table 5-1):

- anterior uveitis
- intermediate uveitis
- posterior uveitis
- panuveitis

The SUN Working Group recognized that clinical scenarios exist in which both anterior chamber and vitreous inflammation are present but the vitritis is more than expected in an isolated anterior uveitis. These cases should be referred to as "anterior and intermediate uveitis" and not as "panuveitis."

The SUN Working Group further refined this anatomical classification of uveitis by defining descriptors based on clinical onset, duration, and course (Table 5-2); in addition, the group recommended specific terminology for grading and monitoring uveitic activity (Table 5-3).

Jabs DA, Nussenblatt RB, Rosenbaum JT; Standardization of Uveitis Nomenclature (SUN) Working Group. Standardization of uveitis nomenclature for reporting clinical data. Results of the First International Workshop. *Am J Ophthalmol.* 2005;140(3):509–516.

Anterior Uveitis

The anterior chamber is the primary site where inflammation is observed in anterior uveitis—the result of inflammation of the iris and ciliary body. Anterior uveitis can have a range of presentations, from a quiet, white eye with a low-grade inflammatory reaction that is apparent only on close examination to a painful, red eye with moderate or severe

Table 5-1 The SUN Working Group Anatomical Classification of Uveitis

Type	Primary Site of Inflammation	Includes
Anterior uveitis	Anterior chamber	Iritis Iridocyclitis Anterior cyclitis
Intermediate uveitis	Vitreous	Pars planitis Posterior cyclitis Hyalitis
Posterior uveitis	Retina or choroid	Focal, multifocal, or diffuse choroiditis Chorioretinitis Retinochoroiditis Retinitis Neuroretinitis
Panuveitis	Anterior chamber, vitreous, and retina or choroid	

Reprinted with permission from Jabs DA, Nussenblatt RB, Rosenbaum JT; Standardization of Uveitis Nomenclature (SUN) Working Group. Standardization of nomenclature for reporting clinical data. Results of the First International Workshop. *Am J Ophthalmol.* 2005;140(3):510.

Table 5-2 The SUN Working Group Descriptors in Uveitis

Category	Descriptor	Comment
Onset	Sudden Insidious	
Duration	Limited Persistent	≤3 months' duration >3 months' duration
Course	Acute Recurrent Chronic	Episode characterized by sudden onset and limited duration Repeated episodes separated by periods of inactivity without treatment ≥3 months' duration Persistent uveitis with relapse in <3 months after discontinuing treatment

Reprinted with permission from Jabs DA, Nussenblatt RB, Rosenbaum JT; Standardization of Uveitis Nomenclature (SUN) Working Group. Standardization of nomenclature for reporting clinical data. Results of the First International Workshop. *Am J Ophthalmol.* 2005;140(3):511.

Table 5-3 The SUN Working Group Activity of Uveitis Terminology

Term	Definition
Inactive	Grade 0 cells (anterior chamber)
Worsening activity	2-step increase in level of inflammation (eg, anterior chamber cells, vitreous haze) or increase from grade 3+ to 4+
Improved activity	2-step decrease in level of inflammation (eg, anterior chamber cells, vitreous haze) or decrease to grade 0
Remission	Inactive disease for ≥3 months after discontinuing all treatments for eye disease

Reprinted with permission from Jabs DA, Nussenblatt RB, Rosenbaum JT; Standardization of Uveitis Nomenclature (SUN) Working Group. Standardization of nomenclature for reporting clinical data. Results of the First International Workshop. *Am J Ophthalmol.* 2005;140(3):513.

inflammation. If the inflammation is confined to the anterior chamber it may also be called *iritis;* whereas if there are cells in the retrolental (anterior vitreous) space, it may also be called *iridocyclitis.* Inflammatory processes that originate in the cornea with secondary involvement of the anterior chamber are called *keratouveitis,* and if the inflammatory reaction involves the sclera and uveal tract, it is called *sclerouveitis.* When more than one ocular structure is involved, the convention is that the primary site of inflammation is named first. Chapter 6 discusses anterior uveitis in greater detail. See Table 5-4.

Intermediate Uveitis

In intermediate uveitis, the major site where inflammation is apparent is the vitreous cavity. Inflammation in this middle portion (posterior ciliary body, pars plana) of the eye manifests primarily as floaters affecting vision; the eye frequently appears quiet externally. Vision loss is primarily a result of chronic cystoid macular edema (CME) or, less commonly, cataract formation. See Chapter 6 of this volume for discussion, as well as Table 5-4.

Table 5-4 Flowchart for Evaluation of Uveitis Patients

Type of Inflammation	Associated Factors	Suspected Disease	Laboratory Tests, Imaging
		Panuveitis	
See entities described below: sarcoidosis, toxoplasmosis, toxocariasis, endophthalmitis, VKH syndrome, sympathetic ophthalmia, syphilis, cysticercosis			
		Anterior Uveitis	
Acute/sudden onset, severe with or without fibrin membrane or hypopyon	Arthritis, back pain, GI/GU symptoms	Seronegative spondyloarthropathies (ankylosing spondylitis, reactive arthritis, inflammatory bowel disease, psoriatic arthritis)	HLA-B27; sacroiliac films; rheumatology, gastroenterology referrals
	Aphthous ulcers	Behçet disease	HLA-B5, -B51 (not essential, rarely obtained)
	Febrile illness, flank or abdominal pain	Tubulointerstitial nephritis and uveitis (TINU) syndrome	Renal function tests, urine beta$_2$-microglobulin, nephrology referral
	Postsurgical, posttraumatic	Infectious endophthalmitis	Vitreous culture, vitrectomy
	None	Idiopathic	HLA-B27
Moderate severity (red, painful)	Shortness of breath	Sarcoidosis	Serum ACE, lysozyme; chest x-ray; chest CT or gallium scan; biopsy
	Posttraumatic	Traumatic iritis	
	Increased IOP	Glaucomatocyclitic crisis, herpetic iritis	PCR of ocular fluid (optional)
	Poor response to steroids	Syphilis	RPR or VDRL; Syphilis IgG or FTA-ABS or MHA-TP (check 1 per category)
	Post–cataract extraction	Low-grade endophthalmitis, IOL-related iritis	Consider vitrectomy, culture
	None	Idiopathic	
Chronic; minimal redness, pain	Child, especially with arthritis	JIA-related anterior uveitis	ANA, ESR, rheumatoid factor
	Heterochromia, diffuse KP, unilateral	Fuchs heterochromic uveitis	None
	Postsurgical	Low-grade endophthalmitis (eg, *Propionibacterium acnes*); IOL-related	Consider vitrectomy, capsulectomy with culture
	None	Idiopathic	
		Intermediate Uveitis	
Mild to moderate	Shortness of breath	Sarcoidosis	Serum ACE, lysozyme; chest x-ray; chest CT or gallium scan; biopsy
	Tick exposure, erythema chronicum migrans rash	Lyme disease (can also be anterior, posterior/panuveitis)	ELISA, Western blot for confirmation

Type of Inflammation	Associated Factors	Suspected Disease	Laboratory Tests, Imaging
		Intermediate Uveitis (continued)	
	Neurologic symptoms	Multiple sclerosis	MRI of brain
	Over age 50 years	Intraocular lymphoma	Vitrectomy, cytology
	None	Pars planitis	
		Posterior Uveitis	
Chorioretinitis *with* vitritis			
Focal	Adjacent scar; raw meat ingestion	Toxoplasmosis	Serology for toxoplasmosis or PCR
	Child; history of geophagia	Toxocariasis	ELISA, complete blood count with differential
	HIV infection	CMV retinitis	
Multifocal	Shortness of breath	Sarcoidosis	Serum ACE, lysozyme; chest x-ray; chest CT or gallium scan; biopsy
		Tuberculosis	PPD, chest x-ray
	Peripheral retinal necrosis	Acute retinal necrosis (ARN)	VZV, HSV titers (ELISA), PCR of ocular fluids, possibly vitrectomy/retinal biopsy
		Progressive outer retinal necrosis if immunocompromised	Same as for ARN
	AIDS	Syphilis, toxoplasmosis	RPR or VDRL; Syphilis IgG or FTA-ABS or MHA-TP (check 1 per category); ELISA
	IV drug use	*Candida, Aspergillus* infection	Blood, vitreous cultures
	Visible intraocular parasite; from Africa or Central/South America	Cysticercosis	ELISA, MRI
		Onchocerciasis	Skin snip
	Over age 50 years	Intraocular lymphoma	Vitrectomy, cytology
	None	Birdshot uveitis	HLA-A29, fluorescein angiography (FA)
		Multifocal choroiditis with panuveitis	Rule out TB, sarcoidosis, syphilis

(Continued)

Table 5-4 *(continued)*

Type of Inflammation	Associated Factors	Suspected Disease	Laboratory Tests, Imaging
		Posterior Uveitis (continued)	
Diffuse	Dermatologic/CNS symptoms; serous RD	Vogt-Koyanagi-Harada (VKH) syndrome	FA, B-scan ultrasonography, lumbar puncture to document CSF pleocytosis
	Postsurgical/traumatic, bilateral	Sympathetic ophthalmia	FA
	Postsurgical/traumatic, unilateral	Infectious endophthalmitis	Consider vitrectomy, culture
	Child; history of geophagia	Toxocariasis	ELISA, complete blood count with differential
Chorioretinitis *without* vitritis			
Focal	None; history of carcinoma	Neoplastic	Metastatic workup
Multifocal	Ohio/Mississippi Valley	Ocular histoplasmosis	FA if macula involved
	Lesions confined to posterior pole	White dot syndromes (eg, APMPPE, MEWDS, PIC)	FA
	Geographic (maplike) pattern of scars	Serpiginous choroiditis	FA, PPD or interferon-gamma release assay, chest x-ray
Diffuse	From Africa, Central/South America	Onchocerciasis	Skin snip
Vasculitis			
	Aphthous ulcers, hypopyon	Behçet disease	HLA-B5, -B51 (not essential, rarely obtained)
	Malar rash, female, arthralgias	Systemic lupus erythematosus	ANA, anti-ds DNA, C3, C4
	Chronic sinusitis with hemorrhagic rhinorrhea, dyspnea, renal insufficiency, purpura	Granulomatosis with polyangiitis	c-ANCA (anti–proteinase 3)

ACE = angiotensin-converting enzyme; ANA = antinuclear antibody; anti-dsDNA = anti-double-stranded DNA antibody; APMPPE = acute posterior multifocal placoid pigment epitheliopathy; C3, C4 = complement 3, complement 4; c-ANCA = c-anti-neutrophil cytoplasmic antibody; CMV = cytomegalovirus; CNS = central nervous system; CSF = cerebrospinal fluid; CT = computed tomography; ELISA = enzyme-linked immunosorbent assay; ESR = erythrocyte sedimentation rate; FTA-ABS = fluorescent treponemal antibody absorption; GI = gastrointestinal; GU = genitourinary; HIV = human immunodeficiency virus; HSV = herpes simplex virus; IOL = intraocular lens; IOP = intraocular pressure; IV = intravenous; JIA = juvenile idiopathic arthritis; KP = keratic precipitates; MEWDS = multiple evanescent white dot syndrome; MHA-TP = microhemagglutination assay–*Treponema pallidum;* MRI = magnetic resonance imaging; PCR = polymerase chain reaction; PIC = punctate inner choroidopathy; PPD = purified protein derivative; RD = retinal disease; RPR = rapid plasma reagin; TB = tuberculosis; VZV = varicella zoster virus.

Posterior Uveitis

Posterior uveitis is defined as intraocular inflammation primarily involving the retina and/or choroid. Inflammatory cells may be observed diffusely throughout the vitreous cavity, overlying foci of active inflammation, or on the posterior vitreous face. Ocular examination reveals focal, multifocal, or diffuse areas of retinitis or choroiditis, with varying degrees of vitreous cellular activity; different entities may have a similar clinical appearance. Certain posterior uveitic syndromes present either as a focal or multifocal retinitis, whereas others localize predominantly to the choroid in a similar distribution, involving the retina secondarily, with or without vitreous cells and/or involvement of the retinal vasculature (Table 5-5; see Table 5-4). Macular edema, peripheral retinal vasculitis, and retinal or choroidal neovascularization are structural complications of certain uveitic entities and are *not* considered sufficient for the anatomical classification of posterior uveitis. Chapters 6 and 7 discuss noninfectious and infectious posterior uveitis, respectively, in greater detail.

Panuveitis

In panuveitis, inflammation is diffuse without a predominant site. Inflammation is observed in the anterior chamber, vitreous, and retina and/or choroid. Many systemic infectious and noninfectious diseases associated with uveitis may produce diffuse intraocular inflammation with concomitant anterior uveitis and posterior uveitis. Chapters 6 and 7 discuss noninfectious and infectious panuveitis, respectively, in greater depth, and Chapter 8 covers endophthalmitis. See also Table 5-4.

Retinal Vasculitis

Retinal vasculitis is defined by the presence of retinal vascular changes in association with ocular inflammation. The term is used in distinction to *vasculopathy*, in which there are vessel changes but no visible evidence of inflammation. Blood vessel changes include perivascular sheathing and vascular leakage or occlusion shown on fluorescein angiography studies. Peripheral retinal vasculitis may be observed in intermediate uveitis but is not

Table 5-5 Uveitis With Retinal Vasculitis

Primarily Arteritis	Primarily Phlebitis	Arteritis and Phlebitis
Systemic lupus erythematosus	Sarcoidosis	Toxoplasmosis
Polyarteritis nodosa	Multiple sclerosis	Relapsing polychondritis
Syphilis	Behçet disease	Granulomatosis with polyangiitis
HSV (ARN/BARN)	Birdshot uveitis	Crohn disease
VZV (PORN)	HIV paraviral syndrome	Frosted branch angiitis
IRVAN	Eales disease	
Churg-Strauss syndrome		

ARN = acute retinal necrosis; BARN = bilateral acute retinal necrosis; HIV = human immunodeficiency virus; HSV = herpes simplex virus; IRVAN = idiopathic retinal vasculitis, aneurysms, and neuroretinitis; PORN = progressive outer retinal necrosis; VZV = varicella-zoster virus.

Adapted with permission from Foster CS, Vitale AT. *Diagnosis and Treatment of Uveitis.* 2nd ed. Jaypee Brothers Medical Publishers, New Delhi, India; 2012:123–128.

sufficient for the anatomical classification of posterior/panuveitis, whereas diffuse retinal vasculitis is sufficient. See also Table 5-5.

Categorization by Clinical Course

Uveitis may be subcategorized as acute, chronic, or recurrent: *acute uveitis* is used to describe episodes of sudden onset and limited duration that usually resolve within 3 months or less, whereas *chronic uveitis* is persistent, with relapse occurring in less than 3 months after discontinuing treatment. *Recurrent uveitis* is characterized by repeated episodes separated by periods of inactivity without treatment that last 3 months or longer.

Whether the inflammation is severe or low grade can influence categorization and prognosis. The inflammatory process may occur in 1 or both eyes, or it may alternate between them. The distribution of ocular involvement—focal, multifocal, or diffuse—is also helpful to note when classifying uveitis.

Uveitis can be further characterized as either granulomatous or nongranulomatous. The physician should be aware, however, that the *clinical* appearance of uveitis as granulomatous or nongranulomatous may not necessarily correlate with the *histologic* description and may instead be related to the stage in which the disease is first evaluated, the amount of antigen at presentation, or the patient's state of immunocompromise (eg, a patient being treated with corticosteroids). *Nongranulomatous* inflammation typically has a lymphocytic and plasma cell infiltrate, whereas *granulomatous* reactions also include epithelioid and giant cells. Discrete granulomas are characteristic of sarcoidosis; diffuse granulomatous inflammation appears in Vogt-Koyanagi-Harada (VKH) syndrome and sympathetic ophthalmia. Zonal granulomatous disease can be observed in lens-induced uveitis.

Symptoms of Uveitis

Symptoms produced by uveitis depend on which part of the uveal tract is inflamed, the rapidity of onset (sudden or insidious), the duration of the disease (limited or persistent), and the course of the disease (acute, chronic, or recurrent).

Acute-onset anterior uveitis causes pain, photophobia, redness, and blurred vision. Pain usually results from the acute onset of inflammation in the region of the iris, or from secondary glaucoma. The pain associated with ciliary spasm in anterior uveitis may be a referred pain that radiates over the larger area served by cranial nerve V (the trigeminal nerve). Epiphora, redness, and photophobia are usually present when inflammation involves the iris, cornea, or iris–ciliary body.

In contrast, chronic anterior uveitis in patients with juvenile idiopathic arthritis (JIA) may not be associated with any symptoms at all. However, with chronic anterior uveitis, blurred vision may develop as a result of calcific band keratopathy, cataract, or CME.

Intermediate uveitis produces symptoms of floaters and blurred vision. Floaters result from the shadows cast by vitreous cells and "snowballs" on the retina. Blurred vision may be caused by CME or vitreous opacities in the visual axis.

Presenting symptoms in patients with posterior uveitis include painless decreased visual acuity, floaters, photopsia, metamorphopsia, scotomata, nyctalopia, or a combination

Table 5-6 Symptoms of Uveitis

Redness
Pain
Photophobia
Epiphora
Visual disturbances
Diffuse blur, caused by
Myopic or hyperopic shift
Inflammatory cells
Cataract
Scotomata (central or peripheral)
Floaters

of these symptoms. The blurred vision may be caused by the primary effects of uveitis, such as retinitis and/or choroiditis directly affecting macular function, or by complications of inflammation such as CME, epiretinal membrane, retinal ischemia, and choroidal neovascularization. Blurred vision may also result from refractive error such as a myopic or hyperopic shift associated with macular edema, hypotony, or a change in lens position. Other possible causes of blurred vision include opacities in the visual axis from inflammatory cells, fibrin, or protein in the anterior chamber; keratic precipitates (KPs); secondary cataract; vitreous debris; macular edema; and retinal atrophy. See Table 5-6.

Signs of Uveitis

The chemical mediators involved in inflammation (see Chapter 1) result in vascular dilation (ciliary flush), increased vascular permeability (aqueous flare), and chemotaxis of inflammatory cells into the eye (aqueous and vitreous cellular reaction). Table 5-7 lists the signs associated with uveitis.

Anterior Segment

Signs of uveitis in the anterior portion of the eye include

- keratic precipitates (Figs 5-1, 5-2)
- inflammatory cells
- flare (Fig 5-3)
- fibrin
- hypopyon
- pigment dispersion
- pupillary miosis
- iris nodules (Fig 5-4)
- synechiae, both anterior and posterior (Fig 5-5)
- band keratopathy (observed in long-standing uveitis)

Table 5-7 Signs of Uveitis

Eyelid and skin	**Intraocular pressure**
Vitiligo	Hypotony
Nodules	Secondary glaucoma
Conjunctiva	**Vitreous**
Perilimbal or diffuse injection	Inflammatory cells (single/clumped)
Nodules	Traction bands
Corneal endothelium	**Pars plana**
Keratic (cellular) precipitates (diffuse or gravitational)	Snowbanking
Fibrin	**Retina**
Pigment (nonspecific)	Inflammatory cells
Anterior/posterior chamber	Inflammatory cuffing of blood vessels
Inflammatory cells	Edema
Flare (proteinaceous influx)	Cystoid macular edema
Pigment (nonspecific)	Retinal pigment epithelium: hypertrophy/clumping/loss
Iris	Epiretinal membranes
Nodules	**Choroid**
Posterior synechiae	Inflammatory infiltrate
Atrophy	Atrophy
Heterochromia	Neovascularization
Angle	**Optic Nerve**
Peripheral anterior synechiae	Edema (nonspecific)
Nodules	Neovascularization
Vascularization	

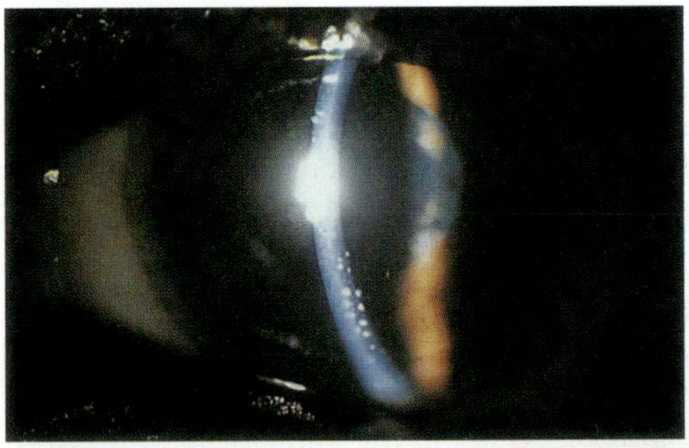

Figure 5-1 Keratic precipitates (medium and small) with broken posterior synechiae. *(Courtesy of H. Jane Blackman, MD.)*

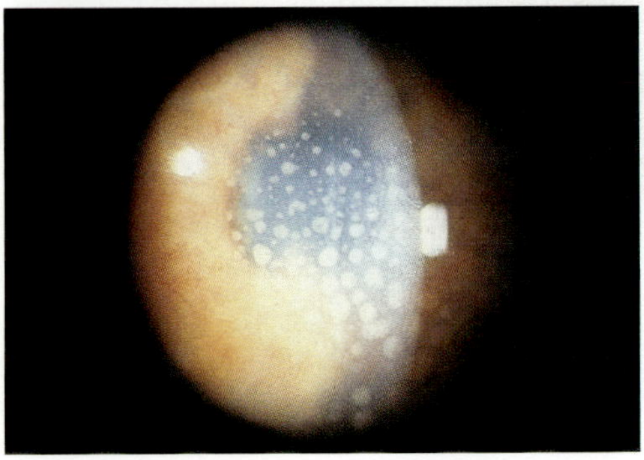

Figure 5-2 Large "mutton-fat" keratic precipitates in a patient with sarcoidosis. Large keratic precipitates such as these generally indicate a granulomatous disease process. *(Courtesy of David Forster, MD.)*

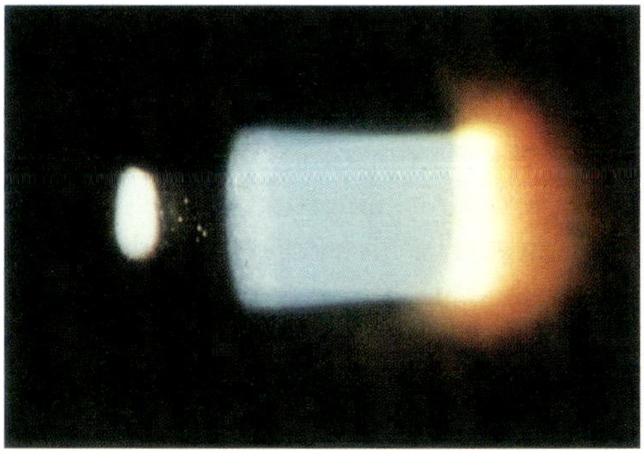

Figure 5-3 Aqueous flare (grade 4+) in a patient with acute anterior uveitis.

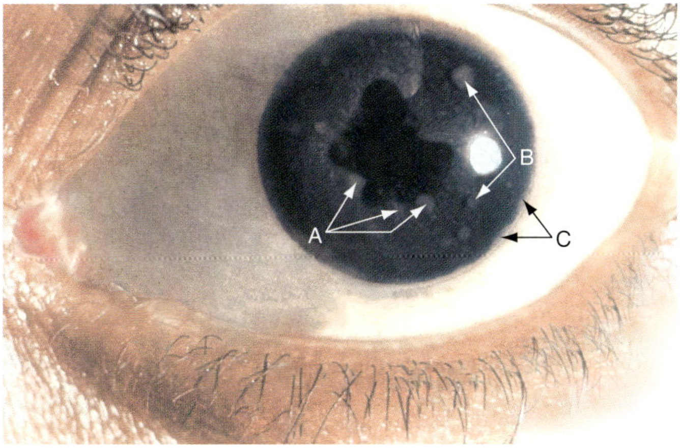

Figure 5-4 Posterior synechiae and iris nodules in a patient with sarcoidosis. Note the 3 types of iris nodules: **A,** Koeppe nodules (pupillary border); **B,** Busacca nodules (midiris); and **C,** Berlin nodules (iris angle). *(Courtesy of David Forster, MD.)*

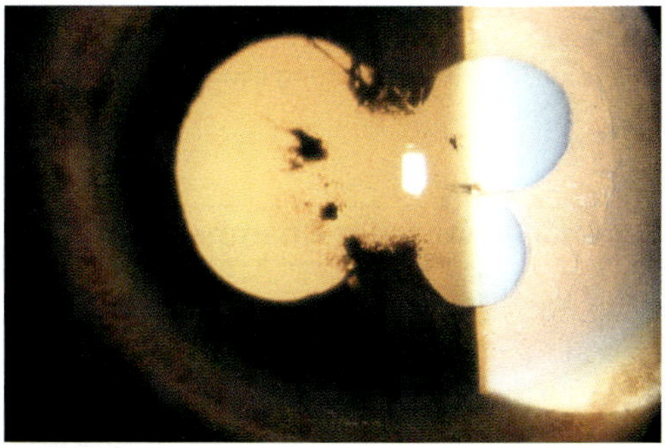

Figure 5-5 Multiple posterior synechiae preventing complete dilation of the pupil. *(Courtesy of David Forster, MD.)*

Keratic precipitates are collections of inflammatory cells on the corneal endothelium. When newly formed, they tend to be white and smoothly rounded, later transitioning to crenated (shrunken), pigmented, or glassy. Large, yellowish KPs are called *mutton-fat KPs* and are usually associated with granulomatous types of inflammation.

Perilimbal vascular engorgement (ciliary flush) or diffuse injection of the conjunctiva, episclera, or both is typical with acute anterior uveitis. With increased capillary permeability, the anterior chamber reaction can be described as

- serous (aqueous flare caused by protein influx)
- purulent (polymorphonuclear leukocytes and necrotic debris causing hypopyon)
- fibrinous (plasmoid, or intense fibrinous exudate)
- sanguinoid (inflammatory cells with erythrocytes, as manifested by hypopyon mixed with hyphema)

The SUN group recommends grading the intensity of anterior chamber cells and flare according to the number of inflammatory cells observed on slit-lamp examination in a field defined as a 1- × 1-mm high-power beam at full intensity at a 45°–60° angle in a dark room (Table 5-8). Flare may be graded similarly, and the SUN group adopted the method described previously by Hogan and colleagues (Table 5-9).

Iris involvement may manifest as either anterior or posterior synechiae, iris nodules (Koeppe nodules at the pupillary border, Busacca nodules within the iris stroma, and

Table 5-8 The SUN Working Group Grading Scheme for Anterior Chamber Cells

Grade	Cells in Field (High-Intensity 1- × 1-mm Slit Beam)
0	<1
0.5+	1–5
1+	6–15
2+	16–25
3+	26–50
4+	>50

Reprinted with permission from Jabs DA, Nussenblatt RB, Rosenbaum JT; Standardization of Uveitis Nomenclature (SUN) Working Group. Standardization of nomenclature for reporting clinical data. Results of the First International Workshop. *Am J Ophthalmol.* 2005;140(3):512.

Table 5-9 The SUN Working Group Grading Scheme for Anterior Chamber Flare

Grade	Description
0	None
1+	Faint
2+	Moderate (iris and lens details clear)
3+	Marked (iris and lens details hazy)
4+	Intense (fibrin or plasmoid aqueous)

Reprinted with permission from Jabs DA, Nussenblatt RB, Rosenbaum JT; Standardization of Uveitis Nomenclature (SUN) Working Group. Standardization of nomenclature for reporting clinical data. Results of the First International Workshop. *Am J Ophthalmol.* 2005;140(3):512.

Berlin nodules in the angle; see Fig 5-4), iris granulomas, heterochromia (eg, Fuchs heterochromic uveitis), or stromal atrophy (eg, herpetic uveitis).

With uveitic involvement of the ciliary body and trabecular meshwork, intraocular pressure (IOP) is often low, secondary to decreased aqueous production or increased uveoscleral outflow, but IOP may increase precipitously if the meshwork becomes clogged by inflammatory cells or debris or if the trabecular meshwork itself is the site of inflammation (trabeculitis). Pupillary block with iris bombé and secondary angle closure may also lead to an acute rise in IOP.

Hogan MJ, Kimura SJ, Thygeson P. Signs and symptoms of uveitis. I. Anterior uveitis. *Am J Ophthalmol.* 1959;47(5, part 2):155–170.

Intermediate Segment

Signs in the intermediate anatomical area of the eye include vitreal inflammatory cells, which are graded in density from 0 to 4+:

Grade	Number of cells
0	0
0.5+	1–5
1+	6–10
2+	11–20
3+	21–50
4+	>50

The SUN group did not achieve consensus regarding a grading system for vitreous cells. The vitreous grading scale shown here was used in the Multicenter Uveitis Steroid Treatment Trial. Vitreous cells are typically graded by observing the retrolental space in a dilated eye using the slit-lamp biomicroscope and a 1- × 0.5-mm beam. The consensus is that cells in the vitreous strands are old, and cells in the syneretic areas may be new.

The National Institutes of Health (NIH) grading system for vitreous haze, which was adopted by the SUN group, may be a better indicator of disease activity than cell counts alone. With this method, standardized photographs are used for comparison with clinical images to ultimately arrive at the level of vitreous haze. Additional uveitic changes may be observed in the vitreous, namely,

- *snowball opacities,* which are common in sarcoidosis or intermediate uveitis
- exudates over the pars plana *(snowbank).* Active snowbanks have a fluffy or shaggy appearance. As pars planitis becomes inactive, the pars plana appears gliotic or fibrotic and smooth; thus, these changes are not referred to as snowbanks.
- vitreal strands

Chronic uveitis may be associated with cyclitic membrane formation, secondary ciliary body detachment, and hypotony.

Posterior Segment

Signs in the posterior segment of the eye include

- retinal or choroidal inflammatory infiltrates
- inflammatory sheathing of arteries or veins
- exudative, tractional*, or rhegmatogenous* retinal detachment
- retinal pigment epithelial hypertrophy or atrophy*
- atrophy or swelling of the retina, choroid, or optic nerve head*
- preretinal or subretinal fibrosis*
- retinal or choroidal neovascularization*

An *asterisk* is used to indicate structural complications. Retinal and choroidal signs may be unifocal, multifocal, or diffuse.

Nussenblatt RB, Palestine AG, Chan CC, Roberge F. Standardization of vitreal inflammatory activity in intermediate and posterior uveitis. *Ophthalmology.* 1985;92(4):467–471.

Review of the Patient's Health and Other Associated Factors

Many aspects of the patient's medical history other than ocular symptoms and signs can help in the classification or identification of uveitis (Table 5-10). A comprehensive history and review of systems is of paramount importance in helping to elucidate the cause of

Table 5-10 Medical History Factors in Diagnosis of Uveitis

Modifying Factors	Associated Factors Suggesting Systemic Conditions
Time course of disease	Immune system status
Acute	Systemic medications
Recurrent	Trauma history
Chronic	Travel history
Onset	Social history
Sudden	Eating habits
Insidious	Pets
Duration	Sexual practices
Limited (≤3 months)	Occupation
Persistent (>3 months)	Drug use
Severity	Tobacco exposure
Severe	
Inactive	
Distribution of uveitis	
Unilateral	
Bilateral	
Alternating	
Focal	
Multifocal	
Diffuse	
Patient's sex	
Patient's age	
Patient's race	

uveitis. In this regard, a diagnostic survey for uveitis as shown in the appendix can be very helpful. The age, sex, sexual practices, and racial background of the patient are important elements in some uveitic syndromes.

Although ocular inflammation may be an isolated process involving only the eye, it can also be associated with a systemic condition. However, ocular inflammation frequently does not correlate with inflammatory activity elsewhere in the body, so it is important for the clinician to carefully review systems. In some cases, the uveitis may actually precede the development of inflammation at other body sites. Immunocompromise, use of intravenous drugs, hyperalimentation, and certain occupations are just a few risk factors that can direct the investigation.

Differential Diagnosis of Uveitic Entities

The differential diagnosis of uveitis is broad and includes infectious agents (viruses, bacteria, fungi, protozoa, and helminths), noninfectious entities of presumed immunologic or allergic origin, masquerade syndromes such as endophthalmitis and neoplastic disease, and unknown or idiopathic causes. Intraocular lymphoma, retinoblastoma, leukemia, and malignant melanoma may all be mistaken for uveitis. In addition, juvenile xanthogranuloma, pigment dispersion syndrome, retinal detachment, retinitis pigmentosa, and ocular ischemia syndrome all must be considered in the differential diagnosis of uveitis.

Although pattern recognition alone is frequently sufficient to establish a definitive diagnosis, accurate biomicroscopic and funduscopic descriptions of posterior segment inflammatory conditions are extremely helpful in forming the differential diagnosis and in distinguishing individual entities because the distribution and evolution of these findings may be quite characteristic. However, many patients do not present with the classic signs and symptoms of a particular disease. Some patients require ongoing monitoring, as the clinical appearance may be unclear or change with time and treatment. The presentation of a disease can also be modified by previous therapy or by a delay in evaluation by the physician.

Once a comprehensive history has been taken and physical examination performed, the most likely causes are ranked in a list based on how well the individual patient's uveitis "fits" with the various known uveitic entities. This *naming-meshing system* first classifies the type of uveitis based on anatomical criteria and associated factors (eg, acute versus chronic, unilateral versus bilateral) and then matches the pattern of uveitis exhibited by the patient with a list of potential uveitic entities that share similar characteristics. One such system for helping to identify a possible cause for a particular patient's uveitis is outlined in Table 5-4.

Epidemiology of Uveitis

Uveitis is responsible for 10% of all blindness cases in the United States, and the incidence of blindness attributable to uveitis is approximately 15 new cases/100,000 persons per year. Prevalence varies by geographic location, age of study population, academic center, and study date. For example, sarcoidosis has replaced Behçet disease as the most common identifiable cause of uveitis in Japan. An epidemiologic study of uveitis in northern California suggests an incidence of 52.4/100,000 person-years, threefold higher than previously reported in studies from the United States. In addition, the incidence and prevalence were lowest in the pediatric age groups (prevalence of 30/100,000) and highest in those over age 65 years (prevalence of 151.3/100,000). Females are slightly more commonly affected. Most cases are chronic and bilateral and carry significant complication rates. Table 5-11 summarizes the data from several surveys, providing a comparison of the prevalence of various types of uveitis in university/referral-based and community-based populations from around the world. This distribution is generally similar: anterior involvement is most common, followed by panuveitis, then posterior uveitis, and finally intermediate uveitis. Most university/referral-based studies probably overestimate the prevalence of intermediate and posterior uveitis actually present in the community.

Acharya NR, Tham VM, Esterberg E, et al. Incidence and prevalence of uveitis: results from the Pacific Ocular Inflammation Study. *JAMA Ophthalmol.* 2013;131(11):1405–1412.

Barisani-Asenbauer T, Maca SM, Mejdoubi L, Emminger W, Machold K, Auer H. Uveitis—a rare disease often associated with systemic diseases and infections: a systematic review of 2619 patients. *Orphanet J Rare Dis.* 2012;7:57.

Grégoire MA, Kodjikian L, Varron L, Grange JD, Broussolle C, Seve P. Characteristics of uveitis presenting for the first time in the elderly: analysis of 91 patients in a tertiary center. *Ocul Immunol Inflamm.* 2011;19(4):219–226.

Gritz DC, Wong IG. Incidence and prevalence of uveitis in Northern California; the Northern California Epidemiology of Uveitis Study. *Ophthalmology.* 2004;111(3):491–500.

Hwang DK, Chou YJ, Pu CY, Chou P. Epidemiology of uveitis among the Chinese population in Taiwan: a population-based study. *Ophthalmology.* 2012;119(11):2371–2376.

Jakob E, Reuland MS, Mackensen F, et al. Uveitis subtypes in a German interdisciplinary uveitis center—analysis of 1916 patients. *J Rheumatol.* 2009;36(1):127–136.

McCannel CA, Holland GN, Helm CJ, Cornell PJ, Winston JV, Rimmer TG. Causes of uveitis in the general practice of ophthalmology. UCLA Community-Based Uveitis Study Group. *Am J Ophthalmol.* 1996;121(1):35–46.

Nagpal A, Leigh JF, Acharya NR. Epidemiology of uveitis in children. *Int Ophthalmol Clin.* 2008;48(3):1–7.

Rathinam SR, Namperumalsamy P. Global variation and pattern changes in epidemiology of uveitis. *Indian J Ophthalmol.* 2007;55(3):173–183.

Sengün A, Karadağ R, Karakurt A, Saricaoğlu MS, Abdik O, Hasiripi H. Causes of uveitis in a referral hospital in Ankara, Turkey. *Ocul Immunol Inflamm.* 2005;13(1):45–50.

Smith JA, Mackensen F, Sen HN, et al. Epidemiology and course of disease in childhood uveitis. *Ophthalmology.* 2009;116(8):1544–1551.

Suhler EB, Lloyd MJ, Choi D, Rosenbaum JT, Austin DF. Incidence and prevalence of uveitis in Veterans Affairs Medical Centers of the Pacific Northwest. *Am J Ophthalmol.* 2008;146(6):890–896.

Table 5-11 Epidemiology of Uveitis

Study	Study Population	Anatomical Distribution of Uveitis, %*				
		Anterior	Intermediate	Posterior	Panuveitis	Indeterminate
McCannel et al (1996) United States (n = 213)	Community-based	90.6	1.4	4.7	1.4	–
Gritz and Wong (2004) United States (n = 382; new cases only)	Health maintenance organization	70.2	2.9	2.1	5	18
Sengun et al (2005) Turkey (n = 300)	Tertiary care	43.6	9	26.6	20.6	–
Rathinam and Namperumalsamy (2007) India (n = 8759)	Community-based eye hospital	57.4	9.5	10.6	22.4	–
Suhler et al (2008) United States (n = 105; incident and prevalent cases)	Veterans hospital	79	4.8	9.5	5.7	1
Smith et al (2009) United States (n = 527; pediatric only)	Tertiary care	44.6	28.1	14.4	12.9	–
Jakob et al (2009) Germany (n = 1916)	Tertiary care	45.4	22.9	13.5	6.2	–
Gregoire et al (2011) France (n = 91; ≥60 years of age only)	Tertiary care	22	8.8	20.9	41.7	–
Hwang et al (2012) Taiwan (n = 5866)	Population-based	77.7	0.4	6.7	15.2	–
Barisani et al (2012) Austria (n = 2619)	Tertiary care	59.9	14.8	13.5	7	–
Acharya et al (2013) United States (n = 224; incident and prevalent cases)	Health maintenance organization	72.3	6.3	13.4	8	–

*The variability of data is due to nomenclature, referral bias, geographic location, and the year when the study was performed. The SUN classification system has been more widely used since 2005 and should result in more standardized comparisons from these types of studies.

Laboratory and Medical Evaluation

Medical history, review of systems, thorough ophthalmologic and general physical examination, and formulation of a working differential diagnosis are cornerstones of the workup of a patient with uveitis and should precede any laboratory testing. Laboratory testing is not a substitute for a thorough, hands-on clinical evaluation.

Identification of the underlying cause of the disease may require laboratory and medical evaluation guided by the history and physical examination. *There is no one standardized battery of tests that needs to be ordered for all patients with uveitis.* Rather, a tailored approach should be taken based on the most likely causes for each patient. Once a list of differential diagnoses is compiled based on the anatomical location and clinical characteristics of the inflammation, appropriate laboratory tests can be ordered. Many patients require only a few diagnostic tests. At a minimum, most uveitis specialists will employ a few studies—purified protein derivative (PPD) skin test or interferon-gamma release assay, syphilis serologic testing, and chest radiograph—as part of their initial evaluation of uveitis. Tables 5-4 and 5-12 list some of the laboratory tests and their indications. These tests are discussed further in later chapters, which cover the various types of uveitis.

Table 5-12 Laboratory Tests and Imaging Studies Used in Uveitis Evaluations

Test	Indications and/or Potential Diagnoses
Hematologic tests	
Complete blood count	Immunomodulatory therapy (IMT), leukemia, lymphoma, immune status (neutropenia, etc)
Erythrocyte sedimentation rate	Giant cell arteritis
Interferon-gamma release assay	Latent and active tuberculosis
T-cell subsets	Opportunistic infection, HIV
Serologic tests	
Liver function tests (ALT, AST)	IMT, sarcoidosis, hepatitis
Serum urea nitrogen, creatinine	IMT (cyclosporine, sirolimus), glomerulonephritis
Angiotensin-converting enzyme	Sarcoidosis
Calcium	Sarcoidosis
Antinuclear antibody	Connective tissue disease, juvenile idiopathic arthritis
Antiphospholipid antibodies	Vascular occlusion
Rheumatoid factor, anticitrullinated protein antibody	Rheumatoid arthritis, juvenile idiopathic arthritis
HLA testing	
HLA-B27	Seronegative spondyloarthropathy
HLA-A29	Birdshot uveitis
HLA-B51 (rarely obtained and of limited value)	Behçet disease
ANCA testing—c-ANCA (proteinase 3) and p-ANCA (myeloperoxidase)	Systemic vasculitides
VDRL/RPR (nontreponemal tests)	Syphilis
Syphilis IgG/FTA-ABS/MHA-TP (treponomal-specific tests)	Syphilis
Lyme disease serology	Lyme disease
Brucella species serology	Brucellosis

Table 5-12 *(continued)*

Test	Indications and/or Potential Diagnoses
Toxoplasma gondii serology	Toxoplasmosis
Fungal serology (complement fixation)	Histoplasmosis, coccidioidomycosis
Bartonella quintana and *B henselae* serology	Cat-scratch disease
EBV, HSV, VZV, CMV serology	Viral uveitis (little benefit unless negative)
HIV serology/Western blot	HIV/AIDS, opportunistic infections
Cerebrospinal fluid (CSF) studies	
Protein, glucose, CSF VDRL cytology, cultures, Gram stain	APMPPE, VKH syndrome, infection, malignancy, syphilis, lymphoma
Urinalysis	Vasculitis, IMT (cyclophosphamide toxicity)
Radiographic studies	
Chest radiograph	Tuberculosis, sarcoidosis, granulomatosis with polyangiitis
Sacroiliac joint x-rays	HLA-B27–associated ankylosing spondylitis
Computed tomography (CT) of chest	Sarcoidosis
CT/magnetic resonance imaging—brain and orbits	Sarcoidosis, central nervous system lymphoma, toxoplasmosis, multiple sclerosis
Intraocular fluid analysis and tissue biopsy	
Intraocular fluid analysis (aqueous/vitreous tap)	
Local antibody production	Local antibody production: HSV, VZV, CMV, *Toxoplasma* organisms
Polymerase chain reaction (PCR)	PCR available for: Viridae: HSV-1, HSV-2, VZV, CMV, EBV Bacteria: *Staphylococcus, Bacillus, Streptococcus, Pseudomonas,* and *Neisseria* species *Mycobacterium tuberculosis* and nontuberculous mycobacteria (65-kDA sAg) *Borrelia burgdorferi* (41-kDa flagellin gene) *Bartonella henselae* *Propionibacterium* (Pa1, rPa2, rPa3 antigens) *Tropheryma whipplei* (16S rRNA gene) *Treponema pallidum* Protozoa: *Toxoplasma gondii, Onchocerca volvulus* Fungi: *Candida albicans, Aspergillus* species (28S rRNA gene) Intraocular lymphoma (IgH gene)
Endoretinal, subretinal, choroidal biopsy	Necrotizing retinitis, neoplasia (central nervous system lymphoma)
Skin, conjunctival, lacrimal biopsy	Sarcoidosis, infection
Stool for ova and parasites	Parasitic diseases

ALT = alanine aminotransferase; APMPPE = acute posterior multifocal placoid pigment epitheliopathy; AST = aspartate aminotransferase; c-ANCA = cytoplasmic antineutrophil cytoplasmic antibody; CMV = cytomegalovirus; EBV = Epstein-Barr virus; FTA-ABS = fluorescent treponemal antibody absorption; HIV = human immunodeficiency virus; HSV = herpes simplex virus; MHA-TP = microhemagglutination assay–*Treponema pallidum;* p-ANCA = perinuclear ANCA; RPR = rapid plasma reagin; VDRL = Venereal Disease Research Laboratory; VKH = Vogt-Koyanagi-Harada; VZV = varicella-zoster virus.

In the evaluation of patients with certain types of uveitis, ancillary testing can also be extremely helpful:

- *Fluorescein angiography* (FA) is an essential imaging modality for evaluating eyes with chorioretinal disease and structural complications caused by posterior uveitis. FA frequently provides crucial information not obtainable from biomicroscopic or fundus examination and is useful both diagnostically and in monitoring the patient's response to therapy. CME (Fig 5-6); retinal vasculitis; secondary choroidal or retinal neovascularization; and areas of optic nerve, retinal, and choroidal inflammation can all be detected angiographically. Several of the retinochoroidopathies, or white dot syndromes, have characteristic appearances on FA.
- *Fundus autofluorescence imaging* is a noninvasive modality that utilizes the fluorescent properties of lipofuscin to assess the viability of the retinal pigment epithelium (RPE)–photoreceptor complex in inflammatory chorioretinopathies that involve the outer retina, RPE, and inner choroid.
- *Indocyanine green angiography* may show 2 patterns of hypofluorescence in the presence of inflammatory choroidal vasculopathies. Type 1, which represents more selective inflammatory choriocapillaropathies, demonstrates early and late multifocal areas of hypofluorescence and may be observed in multiple evanescent white dot syndrome (MEWDS). Type 2 represents stromal inflammatory vasculopathies of the choroid and demonstrates areas of early hypofluorescence and late hyperfluorescence; it may be observed in sarcoidosis, sympathetic ophthalmia, birdshot uveitis, and VKH syndrome.
- *Ultrasonography* can be useful in demonstrating vitreous opacities, choroidal thickening, retinal detachment, and cyclitic membrane formation, as well as for ruling out occult foreign bodies, particularly if media opacities preclude a view of the posterior segment.
- *Electroretinography* can be used along with visual field studies to monitor progression of birdshot uveitis and, occasionally, to rule out retinitis pigmentosa as a uveitis masquerade.
- *Optical coherence tomography* (OCT) and *spectral-domain OCT* (SD-OCT) are cross-sectional imaging methods using coherent light to develop a low-coherence

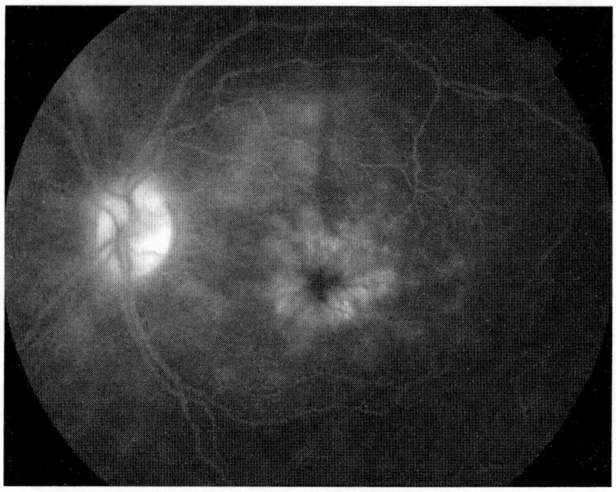

Figure 5-6 Late transit phase fluorescein angiogram of the left eye of a patient with sarcoid-associated anterior uveitis showing a petalloid pattern typical of cystoid macular edema (CME). *(Courtesy of Ramana S. Moorthy, MD.)*

interferometric image. Though primarily used in uveitis to image the posterior segment, anterior segment OCT may be useful to evaluate an eye for retained lens fragments or IOL chaffing in persistent postoperative uveitis and someday may provide an objective means of grading anterior segment cells. OCT has become the standard-of-care method for the objective measurement of uveitic CME (Fig 5-7), retinal thickening, subretinal fluid associated with choroidal neovascularization, and serous retinal detachments. It can be useful in eyes with smaller pupils but can be limited by media opacities. OCT can be valuable in monitoring patients with uveitic glaucoma. SD-OCT provides a high-resolution image of the retina that is helpful in elucidating morphologic changes in many posterior uveitic and panuveitic entities.

- *Anterior chamber paracentesis:* Aqueous humor may be analyzed for diagnostic purposes following anterior chamber paracentesis, which is performed using sterile technique at the slit lamp or with the patient supine on a treatment gurney or chair. Topical anesthetic drops are instilled; the eye is prepared with topical povidone-iodine solution; and a lid speculum is put in place. A tuberculin (1-mL) syringe is attached to a sterile 30-gauge needle, which is then advanced under direct or slit-lamp visualization into the anterior chamber through the temporal limbus or clear cornea parallel to the iris plane. As much aqueous is aspirated as is safely possible (usually 0.1–0.2 mL), avoiding the iris and lens. The needle is withdrawn. Compared with diagnostic vitrectomy, this procedure is much simpler to perform in an office setting. If infection is suspected, the aqueous specimen should be processed for microbiologic evaluation, such as with a Gram stain. Histologic evaluation may be useful if leukemia or lymphoma is suspected, as in the case of a hypopyon–hyphema combination that may occur in acute myelogenous leukemic infiltration of the uveal tract. Polymerase chain reaction (PCR) evaluation may be useful if infection with specific entities such as herpes simplex virus types 1 or 2 (HSV-1 or -2), varicella-zoster virus (VZV), cytomegalovirus (CMV), or *Toxoplasma* species is suspected. Recent studies suggest similar diagnostic sensitivity (81%) and specificity (97%) of aqueous and vitreous samples, particularly in uveitis caused by HSV-1 and -2, VZV, and CMV. Evaluation of aqueous antibody production based on the Goldmann-Witmer (GW) coefficient is considered the gold standard for the diagnosis of toxoplasmosis in Europe. (Chapter 2 explains calculation of the GW.) Diagnostic yield is increased when results of PCR and the GW coefficient are used together, especially in viral infections. Complications of aqueous paracentesis may include anterior chamber hemorrhage, endophthalmitis, and damage to the iris or

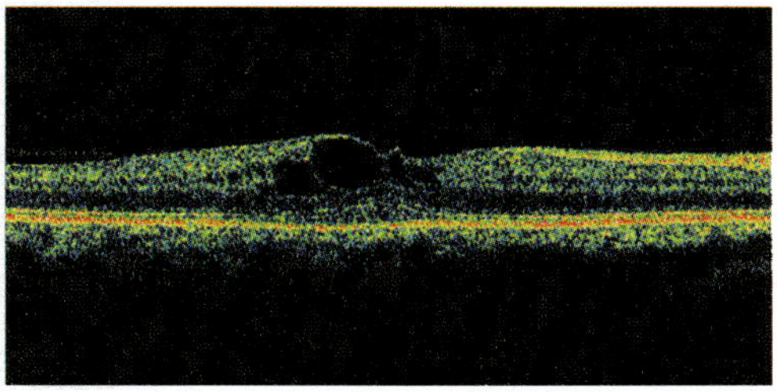

Figure 5-7 Optical coherence tomography image of the macula of the same eye as in Figure 5-6, showing cystoid spaces in the parafoveal outer plexiform layer. *(Courtesy of Ramana S. Moorthy, MD.)*

lens. When the differential diagnosis of the uveitic entity is broader and a larger ocular fluid sample is required, vitreous biopsy should be considered.

- *Vitreous biopsy* in selected patients, with carefully planned cytologic, cytofluorographic, and microbiologic examination of vitreous fluid, can be an effective means of confirming a clinical diagnosis. The procedure is performed via a standard 3-port pars plana vitrectomy (see BCSC Section 12, *Retina and Vitreous*). If the results of diagnostic vitrectomy (vitreous biopsy) could potentially alter management of the uveitis, it must be considered. The most common indications include suspected endophthalmitis, primary intraocular lymphoma or other intraocular malignancy, and infectious etiologies of posterior uveitis or panuveitis. (Endophthalmitis is discussed in detail in Chapter 8, and intraocular lymphoma in Chapter 9.) In addition, chronic uveitis that has an atypical presentation or an inadequate response to conventional therapy may warrant diagnostic vitrectomy. In all these scenarios, undiluted vitreous specimens are typically required for testing. It is possible to obtain 0.5–1.0 mL of undiluted vitreous for evaluation using standard vitrectomy techniques. PCR studies may also be performed on undiluted vitreous if an infectious posterior uveitis or panuveitis is suspected, but the differential diagnosis must be narrowed to a few causes because "global" PCR testing, even if it were available, would be of little value. However, many different infectious agents may be detected by PCR (see Table 5-12). Specific primers for *Toxoplasma gondii,* HSV, VZV, and CMV are readily available. Combined with the clinical picture, the presence of DNA from specific pathogens can be very sensitive and specific in establishing an etiology. Complications of diagnostic vitrectomy in uveitic eyes can include retinal tears or detachment, suprachoroidal or vitreous hemorrhage, and worsening of cataract or inflammation. Although vitreous surgery can be therapeutic and diagnostic in cases of uveitis, the pharmacokinetics of delivered intravitreal drugs are markedly altered in eyes that have undergone pars plana vitrectomy; the half-life of intravitreal corticosteroids, for example, is markedly reduced in vitrectomized eyes.
- *Chorioretinal biopsy,* a more technically challenging procedure, may be useful when the diagnosis cannot be confirmed on the basis of clinical appearance or other laboratory investigations. Rapidly progressive posterior uveitic or panuveitic entities, such as a necrotizing retinitis for which the etiology is unknown and the therapeutic regimen undetermined, may require chorioretinal biopsy. Suspected intraocular lymphoma confined to the subretinal space is also an indication for a chorioretinal biopsy. This procedure is performed only after all other less-invasive measures, such as serologic, radiologic, and aqueous and vitreous sample testing, have failed to confirm the diagnosis. It is associated with a high rate of complications and must be performed only by vitreoretinal surgeons with extensive experience using these techniques. Although full details of these methods are beyond the scope of this text (see BCSC Section 12, *Retina and Vitreous,* for additional discussion), an example video is included (Video 5-1).

VIDEO 5-1 Chorioretinal biopsy (04:35).
Courtesy of P. Kumar Rao, MD.
Scan the QR code or access the video at www.aao.org/bcscvideo_section09.

Davis JL, Miller DM, Ruiz P. Diagnostic testing of vitrectomy specimens. *Am J Ophthalmol.* 2005;140(5):822–829.

de Groot-Mijnes JD, Rothova A, van Loon AM, et al. Polymerase chain reaction and Goldmann-Witmer coefficient analysis are complementary for the diagnosis of infectious uveitis. *Am J Ophthalmol.* 2006;141(2):313–318.

Eliott D, Rao PK. *Surgical Management of Intraocular Inflammation and Infection.* London: JP Medical; 2013.

Harper TW, Miller D, Schiffman JC, Davis JL. Polymerase chain reaction analysis of aqueous and vitreous specimens in the diagnosis of posterior segment infectious uveitis. *Am J Ophthalmol.* 2009;147(1):140–147.

Matos K, Muccioli C, Belfort Júnior R, Rizzo LV. Correlation between clinical diagnosis and PCR analysis of serum, aqueous, and vitreous samples in patients with inflammatory eye disease. *Arq Bras Oftalmol.* 2007;70(1):109–114.

Quentin CD, Reiber H. Fuchs heterochromic cyclitis: rubella virus antibodies and genome in aqueous humor. *Am J Ophthalmol.* 2004;138(1):46–54.

Sowmya P, Madhavan HN. Diagnostic utility of polymerase chain reaction on intraocular specimens to establish the etiology of infectious endophthalmitis. *Eur J Ophthalmol.* 2009;19(5):812–817.

Van Gelder RN. Diagnostic testing in uveitis. *Focal Points: Clinical Modules for Ophthalmologists.* San Francisco: American Academy of Ophthalmology; 2013, module 4.

Therapy

Therapy for uveitis ranges from simple observation to complex medical or surgical intervention. Many patients with mild, self-limiting anterior uveitis need no referral to a uveitis specialist. However, in uveitis that is chronic or difficult to treat, early referral to a uveitis specialist may be helpful, not only in eliciting the cause and determining a therapeutic regimen but also in reassuring the patient that all avenues are being explored. Treatment may require coordination with other medical or surgical consultants and detailed informed consent. Discussion with the patient and other specialists about the prognosis and complications of uveitis helps determine the appropriate therapy.

Medical Management of Uveitis

The goal of medical management of uveitis is to effectively control inflammation so as to eliminate or reduce the risk of vision loss from structural and functional complications that result from uncontrolled inflammation—cataracts, glaucoma, CME, and hypotony. Generally, initial medical therapy includes topical cycloplegics, topical or systemic nonsteroidal anti-inflammatory drugs, and topical or systemic corticosteroids. Corticosteroids are the best drugs to control inflammation as quickly as possible. Route and dose are tailored as specifically as possible to each patient, taking into account the systemic involvement and other factors such as age, immune status, tolerance of adverse effects, and response to treatment. As these initial drugs are tapered, the dosage at which disease recrudescence occurs determines which, if any, second-line immunomodulatory drugs are then used. The choice of a second-line drug also requires consideration of numerous patient factors. If second-line therapy fails, there are few treatment guidelines, and combination therapy with multiple second-line drugs may be considered.

Mydriatic and Cycloplegic Drugs

Topical mydriatic and cycloplegic drugs are beneficial for breaking or preventing the formation of posterior synechiae and for relieving photophobia secondary to ciliary spasm. The stronger the inflammatory reaction, the stronger or more frequent the dosage of the cycloplegic drug. Short-acting drops such as cyclopentolate hydrochloride, 1%, or long-acting drops such as atropine may be used. Most cases of acute anterior uveitis require only short-acting cycloplegics such as cyclopentolate hydrochloride, 1%; these agents allow the pupil to remain mobile and permit rapid recovery when discontinued.

Nonsteroidal Anti-Inflammatory Drugs

Nonsteroidal anti-inflammatory drugs (NSAIDs) work by inhibiting cyclooxygenase (COX) isoforms 1 and 2, or 2 alone, and they reduce the synthesis of prostaglandins that mediate inflammation. COX-1 is present in nearly all cells and appears to be involved in cellular metabolic events such as gastric cytoprotection, platelet aggregation, and renal function, whereas COX-2 seems to mediate inflammation. Selective COX-2 inhibitors were introduced in the late 1990s. They reduced the risk of secondary gastrointestinal damage compared with nonselective COX inhibitors; however, rofecoxib and valdecoxib were withdrawn from the US market because numerous studies identified increased risks of adverse cardiovascular events. Celecoxib was thought to have the same dangers, although it is still available in the United States and carries significant warnings on the package insert. Because of this cardiovascular risk and controversy, the use of COX-2 inhibitors in the treatment of ocular inflammatory diseases has been somewhat limited. Traditional NSAIDs are still utilized for the treatment of mild to moderate forms of nonnecrotizing anterior scleritis. Several studies have shown that systemic NSAIDs may be efficacious in the treatment of chronic anterior uveitis (eg, JIA-associated anterior uveitis) and possibly CME, and they may allow the patient to be maintained on a lower dose of topical corticosteroids. Potential complications of prolonged systemic NSAID use include myocardial infarction, hypertension, and stroke (especially with selective COX-2 inhibitors); gastric ulceration; gastrointestinal bleeding; nephrotoxicity; and hepatotoxicity. COX-2 inhibitors should be used with caution, if no alternative medications are effective; detailed informed consent must be obtained. See also BCSC Section 1, *Update on General Medicine,* for more information.

Topical NSAIDs play an even smaller role in ocular inflammatory disease. They may be used in the treatment of very mild cases of diffuse episcleritis as well as in postoperative pseudophakic CME. They are not useful for treating noninfectious anterior uveitis. Ketorolac, bromfenac, and nepafenac may be used for the treatment of CME. In rare cases, severe corneal complications such as keratitis and corneal perforations may occur with the use of topical NSAIDs. Although most cases occurred with a generic formulation of diclofenac that is no longer available, all topical NSAIDs have been implicated. Patients who have severe dry eye and/or rheumatoid arthritis may be more prone to such complications. For further discussion of NSAIDs and corneal complications, refer to BCSC Section 8, *External Disease and Cornea.*

Finckh A, Aronson MD. Cardiovascular risks of cyclooxygenase-2 inhibitors: where we stand now. *Ann Intern Med.* 2005;142(3):212–214.

Topol EJ. Arthritis medicines and cardiovascular events—"house of coxibs." *JAMA.* 2005; 293(3):366–368.

Corticosteroids

Corticosteroids are the mainstay of uveitis therapy. Because of their potential adverse effects, however, they should be reserved for specific indications:

- treatment of active inflammation in the eye
- prevention or treatment of complications such as CME
- reduction of inflammatory infiltration of the retina, choroid, or optic nerve

Complications of corticosteroid therapy are numerous and can occur with any mode of administration. Therefore, these drugs should be used only when the benefits of therapy outweigh the risks of the medications themselves. Corticosteroids are not indicated in patients with chronic flare or for the therapy of specific diseases such as Fuchs heterochromic uveitis or pars planitis not accompanied by macular edema.

The dose and duration of corticosteroid therapy must be individualized. It is generally preferable to begin therapy with a high dose of corticosteroids (topical or systemic) and taper the dose as the inflammation subsides, rather than to begin with a low dose that may have to be progressively increased to control the inflammation. To reduce the complications of therapy, patients should be maintained on the minimum dosage needed to control the inflammation. Corticosteroids must be tapered gradually (over days to weeks) and not stopped abruptly if utilized for longer than 2–3 weeks to prevent cortisol deficiency resulting from hypothalamic-pituitary-adrenal (HPA) axis suppression. If surgical intervention to treat uveitis or its complications is required, the dosage may need to be increased to prevent postoperative exacerbation of the uveitis.

Topical administration

Topical corticosteroid drops are effective primarily for anterior uveitis, although they may have beneficial effects on vitritis or macular edema in some eyes. These drops are given at intervals ranging from once daily to hourly. The drugs can also be administered in ointment form for nighttime use or when preservatives in the eyedrops are not well tolerated. Difluprednate, 0.05%, a fluorinated corticosteroid, is highly potent; dosing at 4 times daily is considered the equivalent of 8 or more total drops per day of prednisolone acetate, 1%. Clinical studies suggest difluprednate has a similar adverse effect profile to prednisolone but is associated with potentially higher rises in IOP. Of the topical preparations, rimexolone, loteprednol, and fluorometholone have been shown to produce a smaller ocular hypertensive effect than that of other medications. However, these drugs are not as effective as prednisolone in controlling uveitis that is more intense than mild to moderate. Some generic forms of prednisolone may have less of an anti-inflammatory effect than that of the brand-name products; this difference should be considered when the uveitis does not respond adequately to topical corticosteroid therapy. Differences in efficacy may be a result of differences in particle size among various suspensions and may necessitate more vigorous agitation of the drug before instillation.

Slabaugh MA, Herlihy E, Ongchin S, van Gelder RN. Efficacy and potential complications of difluprednate use for pediatric uveitis. *Am J Ophthalmol.* 2012;153(5):932–938.

Periocular administration

Periocular corticosteroids are generally given as depot injections when a more posterior effect is needed or a patient is nonadherent or unresponsive to topical or systemic administration. These injections are often preferred for patients with intermediate or posterior uveitis or CME because they deliver a therapeutic dose of medication close to the site of inflammation. Periocular corticosteroids can cause systemic adverse effects similar to those of oral corticosteroids. Triamcinolone acetonide (40 mg) and methylprednisolone acetate (40–80 mg) are the most commonly used drugs.

Periocular injections can be performed using either a transseptal or a sub-Tenon (Nozik technique) approach (Fig 5-8). With a sub-Tenon injection, a 25-gauge, ⅝-inch needle is used in the original description by Nozik. If the injection is given in the superotemporal quadrant (the preferred location), the upper eyelid is retracted and the patient is instructed to look down and nasally. After anesthesia is applied with a cotton swab soaked in proparacaine or tetracaine, the needle is placed bevel-down against the sclera and advanced through the conjunctiva and Tenon capsule using a side-to-side movement, which allows the physician to determine whether or not the needle has entered the sclera. As long as the globe does not torque with the side-to-side movement of the needle, the physician can be reasonably sure that the needle has not penetrated the sclera. Once the needle has been advanced to the hub, the corticosteroid is injected into the sub-Tenon space.

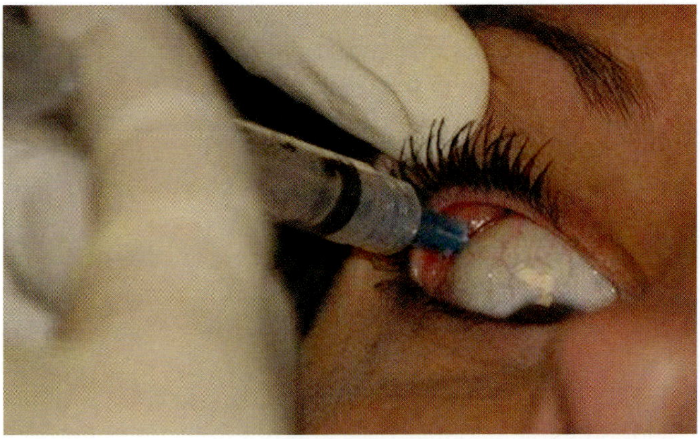

Figure 5-8 Posterior sub-Tenon injection of triamcinolone acetonide demonstrating correct position of the clinician's hands and the needle. The needle is advanced to the hub with a side-to-side motion to detect any scleral engagement and directed caudad and nasally prior to injection of the corticosteroid. The positioning of the tip of the needle in its ideal location is between the Tenon capsule and the sclera. *(Courtesy of Ramana S. Moorthy, MD.)*

Complications of the superotemporal approach include upper eyelid ptosis, periorbital hemorrhage, and globe perforation.

Although sub-Tenon injections are typically given in the superotemporal quadrant, the inferotemporal approach can also be performed in a similar fashion. However, the inferior approach using the Nozik technique can be awkward to perform. The transseptal route of delivery is preferred for the inferior approach and is performed by using a short 27-gauge needle, usually on a 3-mL syringe containing the drug (Fig 5-9). The index finger may be used to push the temporal lower eyelid posteriorly and locate the equator of the globe. The needle is inserted inferior to the globe through the skin of the eyelid and directed straight back through the orbital septum into the orbital fat to the hub of the needle. The needle is aspirated, and if there is no blood reflux, the corticosteroid is injected. Complications of the inferior approach can include periorbital and retrobulbar hemorrhage, lower eyelid retractor ptosis, orbital fat prolapse with periorbital festoon formation, orbital fat atrophy, and skin discoloration. This transseptal approach can be more painful than the sub-Tenon injection if a 25-gauge needle is used; pain can be reduced by using a 27-gauge needle.

Periocular injections should not be used in cases of infectious uveitis (eg, toxoplasmosis) and should be avoided in patients with necrotizing scleritis because scleral thinning and perforation may result. The physician should be aware that periocular corticosteroid injections have the potential to raise the IOP precipitously or for a long time, particularly with the longer-acting drugs (triamcinolone or methylprednisolone). If this effect occurs, the periocular steroid should be removed surgically, especially if it had been given anterior to the septum or in a subconjunctival space, although subconjunctival administration is generally not performed because of the risk of subconjunctival migration of the steroid vehicle.

Leder HA, Jabs DA, Galor A, Dunn JP, Thorne JE. Periocular triamcinolone acetonide injections for cystoid macular edema complicating noninfectious uveitis. *Am J Ophthalmol.* 2011;152(3):441–448.

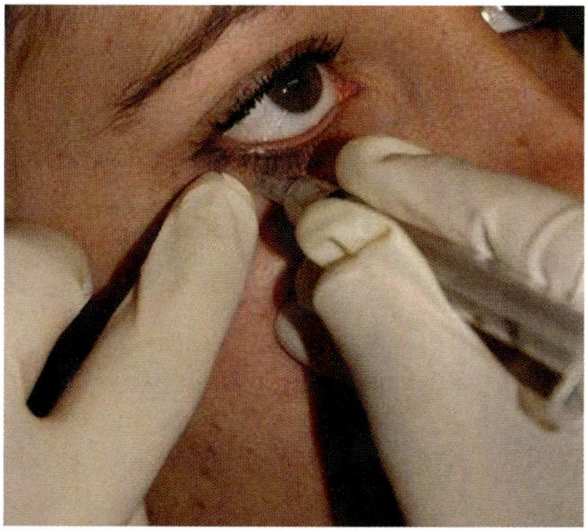

Figure 5-9 Inferior transseptal injection of triamcinolone acetonide in the right eye. A 27-gauge, ½-inch needle on a 3-mL syringe is inserted through the skin of the lower eyelid and the inferior orbital septum. By using the index finger of the opposite hand, the physician can determine the location of the equator of the globe to prevent perforation and to place the depot corticosteroid as posteriorly as possible. *(Courtesy of Ramana S. Moorthy, MD.)*

Intravitreal administration

Intravitreal injections of triamcinolone acetonide have been used extensively in the treatment of uveitic conditions. Published literature on intravitreal triamcinolone administration suggests a definite treatment benefit, although of limited duration, for recalcitrant uveitic CME.

Single trans–pars plana intravitreal injections of triamcinolone (4 mg; 0.1 mL) may produce sustained visual acuity improvements for 3–6 months in nonvitrectomized eyes. CME may recur after 3–6 months. Repeated injections increase the risk of cataract formation in phakic eyes, and IOP elevation may occur transiently in more than one-half of patients. Up to 25% of patients may require topical medications to control IOP, and 1%–2% may require filtering surgery. Complications such as "sterile endophthalmitis" may occur in 1%–6% of patients, but the incidence has dramatically declined since the introduction of a US Food and Drug Administration (FDA)–approved, preservative-free intravitreal triamcinolone. Infectious endophthalmitis and rhegmatogenous retinal detachment may occur, but these complications are rare when proper technique is used. This method of treatment is not curative of chronic uveitic conditions and should be used judiciously, as its effects are relatively short-lived.

The sustained-release fluocinolone implant was approved by the FDA in 2005 for the treatment of chronic noninfectious uveitis affecting the posterior segment; it is not approved in Europe. The implant is inserted through a small pars plana incision and sutured to the sclera (Video 5-2). Multicenter, controlled clinical studies have shown that the 0.59-mg implant is effective for a median of 30 months, with a mean time of 38 months to first recurrence. At 34 weeks after implantation, inflammation was well controlled in nearly all eyes, and recurrence rates decreased by 90%, with 77% of patients able to discontinue systemic therapy and 96% able to discontinue local corticosteroid injections. However, nearly all phakic eyes developed cataract within 2 years after implantation. Elevated IOP necessitating topical therapy developed in nearly 75% of patients after 3 years, and 37% required filtering surgery. Postoperative complications such as endophthalmitis, wound leaks, hypotony, vitreous hemorrhage, and retinal detachments have been reported. Reimplantation may be performed. The fluocinolone implant was compared with standard systemic therapy in the Multicenter Uveitis Steroid Treatment (MUST) trial, which enrolled 255 patients over 3 years. Corrected distance visual acuity (also called *best-corrected visual acuity*) was not significantly different between the 2 treatment groups at the 2-year primary endpoint.

VIDEO 5-2 Fluocinolone acetonide implant surgery (10:32).
Courtesy of P. Kumar Rao, MD.
Scan the QR code or access the video at www.aao.org/bcscvideo_section09.

A biodegradable intraocular implant containing 700 μg of dexamethasone is approved by the FDA and in Europe for the treatment of uveitis affecting the posterior segment of the eye and retinal vein occlusion. This implant is injected through the pars plana into the vitreous cavity using the provided injector. Relative contraindications to using this implant are aphakia, vitrectomy, and having a decentered intraocular lens because of the risk of implant migration into the anterior chamber.

Androudi S, Letko E, Meniconi M, Papadaki T, Ahmed M, Foster CS. Safety and efficacy of intravitreal triamcinolone acetonide for uveitic macular edema. *Ocul Immunol Inflamm.* 2005;13(2–3):205–212.

Goldstein DA, Godfrey DG, Hall A, et al. Intraocular pressure in patients with uveitis treated with fluocinolone acetonide implants. *Arch Ophthalmol.* 2007;125(11):1478–1485.

Jaffe GJ. Reimplantation of a fluocinolone acetonide sustained drug delivery implant for chronic uveitis. *Am J Ophthalmol.* 2008;145(4):667–675.

Jaffe GJ, Martin D, Callanan D, Pearson PA, Levy B, Comstock T; Fluocinolone Acetonide Uveitis Study Group. Fluocinolone acetonide implant (Retisert) for noninfectious posterior uveitis: thirty-four-week results of a multicenter randomized clinical study. *Ophthalmology.* 2006;113(6):1020–1027.

Jaffe GJ, McCallum RM, Branchaud B, Skalak C, Butuner Z, Ashton P. Long-term follow-up results of a pilot trial of a fluocinolone acetonide implant to treat posterior uveitis. *Ophthalmology.* 2005;112(7):1192–1198.

Lowder C, Belfort R Jr, Lightman S, et al; HURON Study Group. Dexamethasone intravitreal implant for noninfectious intermediate or posterior uveitis. *Arch Ophthalmol.* 2011:129(5): 545–553.

Multicenter Uveitis Steroid Treatment (MUST) Trial Research Group; Kempen JH, Altaweel MM, Holbrook JT, et al. Randomized comparison of systemic anti-inflammatory therapy versus fluocinolone acetonide implant for intermediate, posterior, and panuveitis: the multicenter uveitis steroid treatment trial. *Ophthalmology.* 2011;118(10):1916–1926.

Stepien KE, Eaton AM, Jaffe GJ, Davis JL, Raja J, Feuer W. Increased incidence of sterile endophthalmitis after intravitreal triamcinolone acetonide in Spring 2006. *Retina.* 2009; 29(2):207–213.

Systemic administration

Oral or intravenous therapy may supplement or replace other routes of administration. Systemic corticosteroids are used for vision-threatening chronic uveitis when topical corticosteroids are insufficient or when systemic disease also requires therapy; if systemic drugs are used, the dosing and taper should be individualized to the patient. Many oral corticosteroid formulations are available; prednisone is the most commonly used. The readily available blister packages of methylprednisolone that contain predetermined taper schedules have no role in the treatment of uveitis. Most patients require 1–2 mg/kg/day of oral prednisone, usually no higher than 60–80 mg daily, which is gradually tapered every 1–2 weeks. The lowest possible dose that will control the ocular inflammation and minimize adverse effects is desired. Treatment with corticosteroids may last for 3 months or, in some cases, longer. If corticosteroid therapy at a level of 10 mg or more per day is required for longer than 3 months, immunomodulatory therapy (IMT) is indicated.

In cases of an explosive onset of severe noninfectious posterior uveitis or panuveitis, therapy with intravenous, high-dose, pulse methylprednisolone (1 g/day infused over 1 hour) may be administered for 3 days, followed by a gradual taper of oral prednisone starting at 1–1.5 mg/kg/day. Although this approach may control intraocular inflammation, adverse effects are numerous and can be life-threatening. These effects can include psychological disturbances, hypertension, and elevated glucose levels. This therapy should be performed only in a hospital setting by personnel experienced with this approach and its potential adverse effects.

The many adverse effects of both short-term and long-term use of systemic corticosteroids must be discussed with patients, and their general health must be closely monitored, often with the assistance of an internist. Patients at high risk for corticosteroid-induced exacerbations of their conditions are those with a propensity toward or manifest diabetes mellitus; patients with hypertension, peptic ulcer, or gastroesophageal reflux disease; those who are immunocompromised (from acquired or congenital causes); and patients with psychiatric conditions. Corticosteroids should be avoided, if at all possible, in these patients.

Patients taking systemic corticosteroids and NSAIDs concomitantly have a higher risk of gastric ulcers, so this combination is best avoided; if necessary, these patients should receive a histamine-2 receptor blocker or proton-pump inhibitor. Patients receiving long-term corticosteroid maintenance therapy should supplement their diets with calcium and vitamin D to lessen the risk of osteoporosis. The following tests may be used to evaluate patients at risk for corticosteroid-induced bone loss:

- serial height measurements
- serum calcium and phosphorus levels
- serum 25-hydroxycholecalciferol levels (if vitamin D stores are uncertain)
- follicle-stimulating hormone and testosterone levels (if gonadal status is uncertain)
- bone-mineral-density screening (for anyone receiving corticosteroid therapy for more than 3 months)

The FDA has approved several drugs for prevention and treatment of corticosteroid-induced osteoporosis in men and women. These medications may be administered to at-risk patients receiving the equivalent of 7.5 mg or more of daily prednisone.

Involvement of the patient's internist and/or rheumatologist is often very helpful in the treatment of individuals taking systemic corticosteroids so the complications of therapy may be quickly identified and treated.

Jabs DA, Rosenbaum JT, Foster CS, et al. Guidelines for the use of immunosuppressive drugs in patients with ocular inflammatory disorders: recommendations of an expert panel. *Am J Ophthalmol.* 2000;130(4):492–513.

Immunomodulatory Medications

The addition of immunomodulatory (sometimes referred to as *immunosuppressive*) medications may greatly benefit patients with severe, sight-threatening uveitis or patients who are resistant to or cannot tolerate corticosteroids. These drugs are capable of modifying or regulating one or more immune functions and are thought to work by different mechanisms, depending on the class of the medication (see Part I, Ocular Immunology). As more evidence accumulates about the complications associated with long-term systemic corticosteroid use, IMT is being used with increasing frequency to permit corticosteroid sparing. Although the early use of IMT is indicated in certain diseases (see the following section), these drugs should also be considered in patients who require long-term corticosteroid therapy (longer than 3 months) at doses greater than 5–10 mg/day. The use of

IMT can also be considered in patients with long-term topical corticosteroid dependence and in patients requiring repeat corticosteroid injections. Currently, the use of IMT for treating uveitis is considered off-label in the United States.

Indications

The use of IMT in uveitis is warranted for consideration in the following settings:

- vision-threatening intraocular inflammation
- disease process that is likely reversible
- inadequate response to corticosteroid treatment
- failure of therapy
- corticosteroids contraindicated because of systemic problems or intolerable adverse effects
- unacceptable corticosteroid adverse effects
- long-term corticosteroid dependence

Certain uveitic entities warrant the early use of IMT, including ocular cicatricial pemphigoid, serpiginous choroiditis, Behçet disease, sympathetic ophthalmia, VKH syndrome, and necrotizing scleritis associated with systemic vasculitis. Although these disorders may initially respond well to corticosteroids, the initial treatment of these entities with IMT has been shown to improve long-term prognosis and lessen visual morbidity.

Relative indications for these drugs include conditions that do not respond adequately to initial corticosteroid treatment and cases in which patients incur serious corticosteroid-induced adverse effects. Examples include intermediate uveitis (pars planitis), retinal vasculitis, panuveitis, and chronic anterior uveitis.

Treatment

Before initiating IMT, the physician should ensure that there is

- an absence of infection
- an absence of hepatic and hematologic contraindications
- meticulous follow-up available from a physician who is, by virtue of training and experience, qualified to prescribe and safely monitor such medications and personally manage their potential toxicities
- objective longitudinal evaluation of the disease process
- informed consent

Several classes of immunomodulatory medications exist, including antimetabolites, inhibitors of T-cell signaling, alkylating agents, and biologic response modifiers. There may be a delay in therapeutic response for weeks to months after initiation of IMT; therefore, most patients need to be maintained on corticosteroids until the immunomodulatory agent begins to take effect, at which time the corticosteroid dose may be gradually tapered.

Because of the potentially serious complications associated with the use of IMT, patients must be monitored closely by a practitioner experienced with IMT. Blood monitoring, including complete blood count and liver and renal function tests, should be performed regularly. Serious complications include renal and hepatic toxicity, bone marrow suppression, and increased susceptibility to infection. In addition, alkylating agents may cause sterility and were associated in earlier studies with an increased risk of future malignancies such as leukemia or lymphoma. A recent retrospective study of 7957 patients (66,802 patient-years) with noninfectious uveitis treated with IMT showed, however, that patients who took azathioprine, methotrexate, mycophenolate mofetil, cyclosporine, systemic corticosteroids, or dapsone had overall cancer mortality rates similar to those who never took those medications. Conversely, tumor necrosis factor inhibitors were associated with increased overall (twofold) and cancer (3.8-fold) risk of mortality. Trimethoprim-sulfamethoxazole prophylaxis against *Pneumocystis jirovecii* (previously known as *Pneumocystis carinii*) infection should be considered in patients receiving alkylating agents. The physician should obtain thorough informed consent prior to initiating IMT. All of these medications are potentially teratogenic, and women should be advised to avoid becoming pregnant while taking them.

Jabs DA, Rosenbaum JT, Foster CS, et al. Guidelines for the use of immunosuppressive drugs in patients with ocular inflammatory disorders: recommendations of an expert panel. *Am J Ophthalmol.* 2000;130(4):492–513.

Kempen JH, Daniel E, Dunn JP, et al. Overall and cancer related mortality among patients with ocular inflammation treated with immunosuppressive drugs: retrospective cohort study. *BMJ.* 2009;339:b2480.

Antimetabolites

The antimetabolites include azathioprine, methotrexate, mycophenolate mofetil, and leflunomide. Clinical trials are lacking, but retrospective series report that compared with the other antimetabolites, azathioprine has a slightly higher incidence of adverse effects and mycophenolate mofetil has a significantly shorter time to treatment success. Antimetabolites are often the first immunomodulatory therapies used when corticosteroid sparing is desired.

Azathioprine, a purine nucleoside analogue, interferes with DNA replication and RNA transcription. It is administered at a dose of up to 2 mg/kg/day in adults. It is well absorbed orally and, in a randomized, placebo-controlled trial in patients with Behçet disease, it was shown to be effective in preventing ocular involvement among patients without eye disease and in decreasing the occurrence of contralateral eye involvement among patients with unilateral Behçet uveitis. Azathioprine has also been found beneficial in patients with intermediate uveitis, VKH syndrome, sympathetic ophthalmia, and necrotizing scleritis. Overall, nearly 50% of patients treated with azathioprine achieve inflammatory control and are able to taper prednisone dosage to 10 mg/day or less. Many clinicians start administering azathioprine at 50 mg/day for 1 week to watch for development of any gastrointestinal adverse effects (nausea, upset stomach, and vomiting) before escalating the dose. These symptoms are common and may occur in up to 25% of patients, necessitating discontinuation. Bone marrow suppression is unusual at the doses of azathioprine used to treat uveitis. However, patients taking allopurinol and azathioprine concomitantly are at higher risk for bone marrow suppression. Reversible hepatic toxicity occurs in less than 2% of patients, and dose reduction may remedy mild hepatotoxicity. Complete blood counts and liver function tests must be closely monitored. The variability of clinical response to azathioprine among patients is probably caused by genetic variability in the activity of thiopurine S-methyltransferase (TPMT), an enzyme responsible for the metabolism of 6-mercaptopurine (6-MP). A genotypic test is available that can help determine patient candidacy for azathioprine therapy before treatment and can help clinicians individualize patient doses. Evaluation of TPMT activity has revealed 3 groups of patients:

- low/no TPMT activity (0.3% of patients); azathioprine therapy not recommended
- intermediate TPMT activity (11% of patients); azathioprine therapy at reduced dosage
- normal/high TPMT activity (89% of patients); azathioprine therapy at higher doses than in patients with intermediate TPMT activity

Methotrexate is a folic acid analogue and inhibitor of dihydrofolate reductase; it inhibits DNA replication, but its anti-inflammatory effects result from extracellular release of adenosine. Numerous studies have shown methotrexate to be effective in treating various types of uveitis, including JIA-associated anterior uveitis, sarcoidosis, panuveitis, and scleritis. Treatment with this medication is unique in that it is given as a *weekly* dose, usually starting at 10–15 mg/week and gradually increasing to a maintenance dose of 15–25 mg/week in adults. The dosing is variable in children and depends on body surface area. Methotrexate can be given orally, subcutaneously, intramuscularly, or intravenously and is usually well tolerated. It has greater bioavailability when given parenterally. Folate is given concurrently at a dose of 1 mg/day to reduce adverse effects. Methotrexate may take up to 6 months to produce its full effect in controlling intraocular inflammation. Gastrointestinal distress and anorexia may occur in 10% of patients. Reversible hepatotoxicity occurs in up to 15% of patients, and cirrhosis occurs in less than 0.1% of patients receiving methotrexate long-term. Methotrexate is teratogenic, and complete blood counts and liver function tests should be conducted regularly. The drug has a long record of success in the treatment of children with JIA. For that reason, it has been a first-line choice for IMT in children. Uncontrolled clinical trials have shown that it can enable corticosteroid sparing in two-thirds of patients with chronic ocular inflammatory disorders. Recently, a prospective study of intravitreal injections of methotrexate (400 μg) for the treatment of refractory uveitis and uveitic CME demonstrated a reduction of inflammation and CME and well as a reduced need for systemic IMT.

Mycophenolate mofetil inhibits both inosine monophosphate dehydrogenase and DNA replication. It has good oral bioavailability and is given at a dose of 1–1.5 g twice daily in adults. It tends to work rapidly; median time to successful control of ocular inflammation (in combination with less than 10 mg/day of prednisone) is approximately 4 months. Less than 20% of patients receiving mycophenolate mofetil have adverse effects—reversible gastrointestinal distress and diarrhea are common—and these can usually be managed by dose reduction. Very few patients find the drug intolerable. Regular laboratory monitoring is required to check for adverse effects. Two large, retrospective studies found mycophenolate mofetil to be an effective corticosteroid-sparing agent in up to 85% of patients with chronic uveitis. It has similar efficacy in children (88%) and can be a safe alternative to methotrexate in patients with pediatric uveitis.

Doycheva D, Deuter C, Stuebiger N, Biester S, Zierhut M. Mycophenolate mofetil in the treatment of uveitis in children. *Br J Ophthalmol.* 2007;91(2):180–184.

Galor A, Jabs DA, Leder H, et al. Comparison of antimetabolite drugs as corticosteroid-sparing therapy for noninfectious ocular inflammation. *Ophthalmology.* 2008;115(10): 1826–1832.

Gangaputra S, Newcomb CW, Liesegang TL, et al; Systemic Immunosuppressive Therapy for Eye Diseases Cohort Study. Methotrexate for ocular inflammatory diseases. *Ophthalmology.* 2009:116(11):2188–2198.

Malik AR, Pavesio C. The use of low dose methotrexate in children with chronic anterior and intermediate uveitis. *Br J Ophthalmol.* 2005;89(7):806–808.

Pasadhika S, Kempen JH, Newcomb CW, et al. Azathioprine for ocular inflammatory diseases. *Am J Ophthalmol.* 2009;148(4):500–509.

Siepmann K, Huber M, Stübiger N, Deuter C, Zierhut M. Mycophenolate mofetil is a highly effective and safe immunosuppressive agent for the treatment of uveitis: a retrospective analysis of 106 patients. *Graefes Arch Clin Exp Ophthalmol.* 2006;244(7):788–794.

Taylor SR, Habot-Wilner Z, Pacheco P, Lightman SL. Intraocular methotrexate in the treatment of uveitis and uveitic cystoid macular edema. *Ophthalmology.* 2009;116(4): 797–801.

Teoh SC, Hogan AC, Dick AD, Lee RW. Mycophenolate mofetil for the treatment of uveitis. *Am J Ophthalmol.* 2008;146(5):752–760.

Thorne JE, Jabs DA, Qazi FA, Nguyen QD, Kempen JH, Dunn JP. Mycophenolate mofetil therapy for inflammatory eye disease. *Ophthalmology.* 2005;112(8):1472–1477.

Inhibitors of T-cell signaling

Agents that inhibit T-cell signaling include cyclosporine, tacrolimus, and sirolimus. Cyclosporine, a macrolide product of the fungus *Beauveria nivea,* and tacrolimus, a product of *Streptomyces tsukubaensis,* are calcineurin inhibitors that eliminate T-cell receptor signal transduction and downregulate interleukin-2 (IL-2) gene transcription and receptor expression of $CD4^+$ T lymphocytes. Sirolimus, an antifungal product of *Streptomyces hygroscopicus,* is a noncalcineurin inhibitor of T-cell signaling that inhibits antibody production and B lymphocytes.

Cyclosporine is available in 2 oral preparations. One is a microemulsion (Neoral, Novartis, Basel, Switzerland) and has better bioavailability than the other formulation (Sandimmune, Novartis). These 2 formulations are not bioequivalent. Neoral is initiated at 2 mg/kg/day and Sandimmune at 2.5 mg/kg/day in adults. The dose is adjusted based on toxicity and clinical response to 1–5 mg/kg/day. The most common adverse effects with cyclosporine are systemic hypertension and nephrotoxicity. Additional adverse effects include paresthesia, gastrointestinal upset, fatigue, hypertrichosis, and gingival hyperplasia. Blood pressure, serum creatinine levels, and complete blood counts must be assessed regularly. If serum creatinine level rises by 30%, dose adjustment is required. Sustained elevation of serum creatinine levels will require a cessation of medication until levels return to baseline. It is usually not necessary to monitor drug levels unless there is a concern about patient adherence or drug absorption. Patients with psoriasis treated with cyclosporine appear to be at greater risk of primary skin cancers. Cyclosporine was shown to be effective in a randomized, controlled clinical trial for the treatment of Behçet uveitis, with control of inflammation in 50% of patients. However, the dose used in this study was 10 mg/kg/day—substantially higher than current dosing (5 mg/kg/day)—and led to substantial nephrotoxicity. Cyclosporine has also been shown to be effective in the treatment of intermediate uveitis and several types of posterior uveitis, including VKH syndrome. Overall, cyclosporine combined with corticosteroids has been shown to be modestly effective in controlling ocular inflammation (in up to 33% of patients), but toxicity necessitating cessation of therapy is more common in patients over the age of 55 years.

Tacrolimus is given orally at 0.10–0.15 mg/kg/day in adults. Because of its lower dose and increased potency, its main adverse effect, nephrotoxicity, is less common than with cyclosporine. Serum creatinine level and complete blood counts are monitored regularly. A prospective trial of cyclosporine and tacrolimus suggested equal efficacy in controlling chronic posterior and intermediate uveitis, with tacrolimus demonstrating greater safety (lower risk of hypertension and hyperlipidemia). Long-term tolerability and efficacy are excellent as well, with an 85% chance of reducing prednisone dosage to less than 10 mg/day.

Hogan AC, McAvoy CE, Dick AD, Lee RW. Long-term efficacy and tolerance of tacrolimus for the treatment of uveitis. *Ophthalmology.* 2007;114(5):1000–1006.

Kaçmaz RO, Kempen JH, Newcomb C, et al. Cyclosporine for ocular inflammatory diseases. *Ophthalmology.* 2010;117(3):576–584.

Murphy CC, Greiner K, Plskova J, et al. Cyclosporine vs tacrolimus therapy for posterior and intermediate uveitis. *Arch Ophthalmol.* 2005;123(5):634–641.

Alkylating agents

Alkylating agents include cyclophosphamide and chlorambucil. These drugs are generally used only if other immunomodulators fail to control uveitis; they are also used as first-line therapy for necrotizing scleritis associated with systemic vasculitides such as granulomatosis with polyangiitis (formerly, Wegener granulomatosis) or relapsing polychondritis. They have been found beneficial as well in patients with intermediate uveitis, VKH syndrome, sympathetic ophthalmia, and Behçet disease. The most worrisome adverse effect of alkylating agents is an increased risk of malignancy. With the doses and durations used for the treatment of uveitis, the risk is probably low. Patients with polycythemia rubra vera treated with chlorambucil had a 13.5-fold greater risk of leukemia. Patients with granulomatosis with polyangiitis treated with cyclophosphamide had a 2.4-fold increased risk of cancer and a 33-fold increased risk of bladder cancer. Therefore, these drugs should be used with great caution and only by clinicians experienced in the management of their dosing and potential toxicity. Patients may wish to consider sperm or embryo banking before beginning cyclophosphamide or chlorambucil therapy because of the high rate of sterility if the cumulative dose exceeds certain limits.

Cyclophosphamide is an alkylating agent whose active metabolites alkylate purines in DNA and RNA, resulting in impaired DNA replication and cell death. Cyclophosphamide is cytotoxic to resting and actively dividing lymphocytes. It is absorbed orally and metabolized in the liver into its active metabolites. It is probably more effective in controlling ocular inflammation when given orally at a dose of 2 mg/kg/day in adults than when administered as intermittent intravenous pulses. Most patients are treated for 1 year, and the dose is adjusted to maintain leukocyte counts between 3000 and 4000 cells/µL after the patient has been tapered off corticosteroids. Inflammation control is achieved in three-fourths of patients within 12 months; disease remission occurs in two-thirds of patients within 2 years; and one-third of patients discontinue therapy within 1 year because of reversible adverse effects. Myelosuppression and hemorrhagic cystitis are the most common adverse effects. Hemorrhagic cystitis is more common when cyclophosphamide is administered orally. Patients must be encouraged to drink more than 2 liters of fluid per day while on this regimen. Complete blood counts and urinalysis are monitored weekly to monthly. Microscopic hematuria is a warning for the patient to increase hydration, and gross hematuria is an indication to discontinue therapy. If the leukocyte count falls below 2500 cells/µL, cyclophosphamide should be discontinued until the cell count recovers. Other toxicities include teratogenicity, sterility, and reversible alopecia. Opportunistic infections such as *Pneumocystis jirovecii* pneumonia occur more commonly in patients receiving cyclophosphamide; trimethoprim-sulfamethoxazole prophylaxis is recommended for these patients. Cyclophosphamide has been shown to be effective in treating necrotizing scleritis, retinal vasculitis, mucous membrane pemphigoid, and other uveitic conditions in uncontrolled case series.

Chlorambucil is a very long-acting alkylating agent that also interferes with DNA replication. It is absorbed well when administered orally. The drug is traditionally given as a single daily dose of 0.1–0.2 mg/kg in adults. It may also be administered as short-term high-dose therapy. Because chlorambucil is myelosuppressive, complete blood counts should be monitored closely. It is also teratogenic and causes sterility. Uncontrolled case series suggest that chlorambucil is effective, providing long-term, drug-free remissions in 66%–75% of patients with sympathetic ophthalmia, Behçet disease, and other sight-threatening uveitic syndromes.

Faurschou M, Sorensen IJ, Mellemkjaer L, et al. Malignancies in Wegener's granulomatosis: incidence and relation to cyclophosphamide therapy in a cohort of 293 patients. *J Rheumatol.* 2008;35(1):100–105.

Patel SS, Dodds EM, Echandi LV, et al. Long-term, drug-free remission of sympathetic ophthalmia with high-dose, short-term chlorambucil therapy. *Ophthalmology.* 2014; 121(2):596–602.

Pujari SS, Kempen JH, Newcomb CW, et al. Cyclophosphamide for ocular inflammatory diseases. *Ophthalmology.* 2010;117(2):356–365.

Biologic response modifiers

Inflammation is driven by a complex series of cell–cell and cell–cytokine interactions. Inhibitors of various cytokines have been labeled *biologic response modifiers.* They play an important role in the treatment of uveitis, as these drugs result in targeted immunomodulation, thereby theoretically reducing the systemic adverse effects that are common with the previously discussed immunomodulatory drugs. Biologic response modifiers are considerably more expensive than traditional IMT and are reserved for specific conditions, such as Behçet disease, or situations in which traditional IMT has failed. Infliximab and adalimumab are biologics that inhibit the action of tumor necrosis factor α (TNF-α) and have changed the management of some uveitic entities. TNF-α is believed to play a major role in the pathogenesis of JIA, ankylosing spondylitis, and other spondyloarthropathies. These drugs are generally prescribed and administered by uveitis specialists and rheumatologists experienced with their use, adverse effects, and toxicities.

Etanercept, a TNF receptor blocker, has proven effective in controlling joint inflammation in polyarticular JIA and adult rheumatoid arthritis but showed no effect in controlling active intraocular inflammation or in allowing for the taper of other immunomodulators in previously well-controlled cases. It is generally less effective than infliximab and is not a preferred biologic for uveitis treatment. There are also some reports of paradoxical inflammation with etanercept.

Infliximab, a chimeric, immunoglobulin G1 kappa (IgG1κ) monoclonal antibody directed against TNF-α, is effective in controlling current inflammation and decreasing the likelihood of future attacks in Behçet uveitis, idiopathic uveitis, sarcoidosis, VKH syndrome, and many other entities in more than 75% of patients. It is administered through infusions. It has a corticosteroid-sparing effect and appears to improve the visual prognosis of patients with recalcitrant Behçet uveitis. Similar favorable effects have been reported in patients with HLA-B27–associated anterior uveitis treated with infliximab. However, in a recent study, although 78% of patients achieved successful control of inflammation at 10 weeks, nearly one-half could not complete the 50 weeks of therapy because of drug-induced toxicity, which included drug-induced lupus, systemic vascular thrombosis, congestive heart failure, new malignancy, demyelinating disease, and vitreous hemorrhage. As many as 75% of patients receiving more than 3 infusions developed antinuclear antibodies. Low-dose methotrexate (5–7.5 mg/week) may be administered concomitantly to reduce the risk of drug-induced lupus syndrome and the formation of human antichimeric antibodies, which can lead to reduced efficacy of infliximab. Also, reports have clearly shown that some patients with unknown, inactive, postprimary tuberculosis treated with infliximab subsequently developed disseminated tuberculosis. Thus, a PPD test or interferon-gamma release assay to assess for tuberculosis (TB) exposure is mandatory before starting infliximab. In the case of TB exposure, treatment with TNF inhibitors may be possible with concurrent TB therapy. More recent reports of infliximab suggest a lower frequency of adverse effects than that reported in earlier studies.

Adalimumab, a fully human monoclonal IgG1 antibody directed against TNF-α, has been shown to be as effective as infliximab in controlling inflammation, with success rates of up to 88% without relapse in pediatric patients with uveitis and 100% in adult patients with Behçet uveitis, posterior uveitis, and panuveitis. However, uveitis relapses requiring local corticosteroid injections occurred in 42% of adult patients taking adalimumab. Adverse effects, including development of antidrug antibodies, appear to be less common than with infliximab. As for infliximab, patients must be tested for TB exposure before starting therapy. Adalimumab is less expensive than infliximab and can be self-administered by subcutaneous injection every 2 weeks, without the need for the intravenous infusions required by infliximab. Several other TNF-α inhibitors are currently in use, including golimumab and certolizumab, but there is limited information about their utility for uveitis.

Rituximab, a chimeric monoclonal antibody directed against $CD20^+$ cells (mainly B lymphocytes) may also be useful in the treatment of Behçet retinal vasculitis, granulomatosis with polyangiitis–associated necrotizing scleritis, and mucous membrane pemphigoid.

Anakinra is a recombinant IL-1 receptor antagonist that holds some promise as a biologic treatment alternative for JIA-associated uveitis. It also successfully treats neonatal-onset multisystem inflammatory disease (NOMID), which can cause uveitis.

Tocilizumab is a humanized monoclonal antibody against the IL-6 receptor. There are case reports of successful treatment of JIA-associated uveitis and other types of uveitis that have been refractory to other treatments.

Intravenous immunoglobulin (IVIG) has been reported to be effective in some patients with uveitis that is otherwise refractory to immunosuppressive therapy, as well as in patients with mucous membrane pemphigoid.

Interferon alfa-2a/2b (IFN-α2a/b) has been reported to be beneficial in some patients with uveitis. IFN-α2a seems to be an alternative to anti-TNF drugs. It has antiviral, immunomodulatory, and antiangiogenic effects. Reports in the European literature seem to indicate that IFN-α2a is efficacious and well tolerated in patients with Behçet uveitis, controlling inflammation in almost 90%; it is somewhat less effective in non-Behçet uveitis, with inflammation control in 60%. There are also reports of IFN-α2b successfully treating uveitic CME. Prior to initiation of IFN-α2a therapy, patients discontinue any other immunosuppressive drugs. A flulike syndrome has been observed, most frequently during the first weeks of therapy, but symptoms may be reduced through prophylactic administration of acetaminophen. Despite the use of low interferon doses, leukopenia or thrombocytopenia may occur. Depression is another important adverse effect of interferon therapy.

Biester S, Deuter C, Michels H, et al. Adalimumab in the therapy of uveitis in childhood. *Br J Ophthalmol.* 2007;91(3):319–324.

Bodaghi B, Gendron G, Wechsler B, et al. Efficacy of interferon alpha in the treatment of refractory and sight threatening uveitis: a retrospective monocentric study of 45 patients. *Br J Ophthalmol.* 2007;91(3):335–339.

Braun J, Baraliakos X, Listing J, Sieper J. Decreased incidence of anterior uveitis in patients with ankylosing spondylitis treated with the anti–tumor necrosis factor agents infliximab and etanercept. *Arthritis Rheum.* 2005;52(8):2447–2451.

Butler NJ, Suhler EB, Rosenbaum JT. Interferon alpha 2b in the treatment of uveitic cystoid macular edema. *Ocul Immunol Inflamm.* 2012;20(2):86–90.

Díaz-Llopis M, Salom D, Garcia-de-Vicuña C, et al. Treatment of refractory uveitis with adalimumab: a prospective multicenter study of 131 patients. *Ophthalmology.* 2012;119(8): 1575–1581.

Gueudry J, Wechsler B, Terrada C, et al. Long-term efficacy and safety of low-dose interferon alpha2a therapy in severe uveitis associated with Behçet disease. *Am J Ophthalmol.* 2008; 146(6):837–844.

Kötter I, Zierhut M, Eckstein AK, et al. Human recombinant interferon alfa-2a for the treatment of Behçet's disease with sight threatening posterior or panuveitis. *Br J Ophthalmol.* 2003; 87(4):423–431.

Levy-Clarke G, Jabs DA, Read RW, Rosenbaum JT, Vitale A, Van Gelder RN. Expert panel recommendations for the use of anti-tumor necrosis factor biologic agents in patients with ocular inflammatory disorders. *Ophthalmology.* 2014;121(3):785–796.

Schmeling H, Horneff G. Etanercept and uveitis in patients with juvenile idiopathic arthritis. *Rheumatology (Oxford)*. 2005;44(8):1008–1011.

Sfikakis PP, Markomichelakis N, Alpsoy E, et al. Anti-TNF therapy in the management of Behçet's disease—review and basis for recommendations. *Rheumatology (Oxford)*. 2007; 46(5):736–741.

Smith JA, Thompson DJ, Whitcup SM, et al. A randomized, placebo-controlled, double-masked clinical trial of etanercept for the treatment of uveitis associated with juvenile idiopathic arthritis. *Arthritis Rheum*. 2005;53(1):18–23.

Suhler EB, Smith JR, Wertheim MS, et al. A prospective trial of infliximab therapy for refractory uveitis: preliminary safety and efficacy outcomes. *Arch Ophthalmol*. 2005; 123(7):903–912.

Tugal-Tutkun I, Mudun A, Urgancioglu M, et al. Efficacy of infliximab in the treatment of uveitis that is resistant to treatment with the combination of azathioprine, cyclosporine, and corticosteroids in Behçet's disease: an open-label trial. *Arthritis Rheum*. 2005;52(8): 2478–2484.

Surgical Management of Uveitis

Surgery is performed in patients with uveitis for diagnostic and/or therapeutic reasons. Therapeutic surgical procedures for uveitis and its complications are discussed in Chapter 10.

CHAPTER 6

Noninfectious Ocular Inflammatory Diseases

Ocular inflammatory diseases are either infectious or noninfectious. Noninfectious disease can be further subdivided into masquerade syndromes, drug-induced, traumatic, and autoimmune ocular inflammatory conditions. Masquerade syndromes are covered in Chapter 9, and the remaining noninfectious entities are the focus of this chapter.

Noninfectious Scleritis

Scleritis, inflammation of the sclera, is a typically painful, destructive condition that carries a potential risk of permanent ocular structural damage with visual compromise. Scleritis may be classified similarly to uveitis, both anatomically and etiologically. Thus, scleritis may be anterior or posterior; its etiologies include infection, autoimmunity, trauma, or drug induced. Approximately 40% of scleritis cases are associated with a systemic disease, especially rheumatoid arthritis. See BCSC Section 8, *External Disease and Cornea,* for a discussion of the epidemiology and classification of scleritis.

Treatment of Noninfectious Scleritis

Nonsteroidal anti-inflammatory drugs

Nonsteroidal anti-inflammatory drugs (NSAIDs) may be effective in the treatment of nonnecrotizing scleritis. These drugs serve to relieve pain and reduce inflammation, although they are useful primarily in milder cases. No one drug has proved more effective than another, but indomethacin, flurbiprofen, and naproxen have all been used successfully. If the initial NSAID fails, a second can be tried before switching to corticosteroids.

Corticosteroids

Topical corticosteroids such as difluprednate and prednisolone acetate are potentially useful in mild cases of scleritis or as adjunctive therapy. Subconjunctival injections of corticosteroid have been shown to be effective in anterior nonnecrotizing scleritis, although controversy remains surrounding this route of administration because of the theoretical complication of localized necrotizing disease following injection. Systemic corticosteroids may be administered orally or as a high-dose intravenous pulse when rapid control is required.

Immunomodulatory therapy

Scleritis that is nonresponsive to corticosteroids or that requires doses of corticosteroids too high for long-term use should be transitioned to steroid-sparing immunomodulatory therapy (IMT). Antimetabolites such as methotrexate, azathioprine, and mycophenolate mofetil have been used successfully, and calcineurin inhibitors are also an option. Scleritis associated with granulomatosis with polyangiitis (formerly, Wegener granulomatosis) and polyarteritis nodosa typically require more aggressive therapy with rituximab or cyclophosphamide. Biologic agents such as the tumor necrosis factor (TNF) inhibitors and rituximab have been reported to be useful in the treatment of many forms of recalcitrant scleritis.

Pain management

Because scleritis can be excruciatingly painful, attention to pain control is necessary. Oral NSAIDs may be of benefit, but their use in combination with oral corticosteroids or other systemic therapies should be avoided or—at a minimum—monitored carefully. The judicious use of oral narcotics may be appropriate for brief periods while anti-inflammatory therapy is instituted. Topical cycloplegia may also be of benefit.

Surgery

Scleral reinforcement surgery may be needed to address scleral thinning and to avoid the complications of globe rupture, which can occur with minimal trauma in patients with this disorder. Materials used for grafting include cadaveric donor sclera, but the scleral graft may melt, and some authors have recommended use of autogenous periosteum.

Doctor P, Sultan A, Syed S, Christen W, Bhat P, Foster CS. Infliximab for the treatment of refractory scleritis. *Br J Ophthalmol.* 2010;94(5):579–583.

Raiji VR, Palestine AG, Parver DL. Scleritis and systemic disease association in a community-based referral practice. *Am J Ophthalmol.* 2009;148(6):946–950.

Anterior Uveitis

Anterior uveitis is the most common form of uveitis, accounting for more than 90% of cases in a community-based practice. Incidence in the United States varies by age, from approximately 7 cases per 100,000 person-years in persons aged 14 years and younger up to approximately 220 per 100,000 persons aged 65 years and older.

Because uveitis may occur secondary to inflammation of the cornea and/or sclera, the physician should evaluate these structures carefully to rule out a primary keratitis or scleritis. Inflammation of the sclera and the cornea is covered in depth in BCSC Section 8, *External Disease and Cornea;* see also the section on scleritis in this chapter.

Gritz DC, Wong IG. Incidence and prevalence of uveitis in Northern California; the Northern California Epidemiology of Uveitis Study. *Ophthalmology.* 2004;111(3):491–500.

Reeves SW, Sloan FA, Lee PP, Jaffe GJ. Uveitis in the elderly: epidemiological data from the National Long-term Care Survey Medicare Cohort. *Ophthalmology.* 2006;113(2):307–321.

Acute Nongranulomatous Anterior Uveitis

The classic presentation of acute anterior uveitis is the sudden onset of pain, redness, and photophobia that can be associated with decreased vision. Fine keratic precipitates (KPs) dust the corneal endothelium in most cases. The anterior chamber shows an intense cellular response and variable flare. Severe cases may show a protein coagulum in the aqueous or, less commonly, a hypopyon (Fig 6-1). Occasionally, a fibrin net forms across the pupillary margin (Fig 6-2), potentially producing a seclusion membrane and iris bombé. Iris vessels may be dilated, and, on rare occasions, a spontaneous hyphema occurs. Cells may also be present in the anterior vitreous. Fundus lesions are not characteristic, although cystoid macular edema (CME) and disc edema may be noted. Occasionally, intraocular pressure (IOP) may be elevated because of trabeculitis, blockage of the trabecular meshwork by debris and cells, or pupillary block.

The inflammation usually lasts several days to weeks, up to 3 months. Two patterns may occur. In the first type, the attack is acute and unilateral, with a history of episodes alternating between the 2 eyes; this pattern is typical for HLA-B27–associated anterior uveitis. Either eye may be affected, but recurrence is rarely bilateral. The second pattern is acute and bilateral.

Corticosteroids are the mainstay of treatment to eliminate inflammation, prevent cicatrization, and minimize damage to the uveal vasculature. Topical corticosteroids are the first line of treatment, and administration every 1–2 hours is often needed. If necessary, periocular or oral corticosteroids may be used for severe episodes. Initial attacks may require all 3 routes of administration, particularly in severe cases.

Severely damaged vessels may leak continuously, transforming the typical course from acute and limited to chronic. The risk of chronicity can be reduced by timely diagnosis, aggressive initial therapy, and patient adherence. In cases with a recurrent course, maintenance therapy with low-dose topical corticosteroids may be needed.

Corticosteroid-sparing drugs, such as antimetabolites, sulfasalazine, NSAIDs, and others may be needed for long-term therapy in chronic or frequently recurrent anterior uveitis. Anti-TNF therapy has been effective in recalcitrant anterior uveitis, particularly in HLA-B27–positive patients. Cycloplegic agents are used to relieve pain and to break and prevent formation of synechiae. They may be given topically or with conjunctival cotton pledgets soaked in tropicamide, cyclopentolate, or phenylephrine hydrochloride (Fig 6-3).

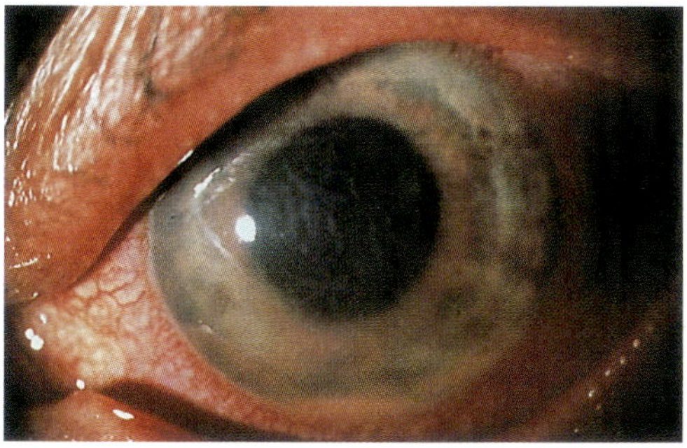

Figure 6-1 Acute HLA-B27–positive anterior uveitis that was accompanied by pain, photophobia, marked injection, fixed pupil, loss of iris detail from corneal edema, and hypopyon. *(Courtesy of David Meisler, MD.)*

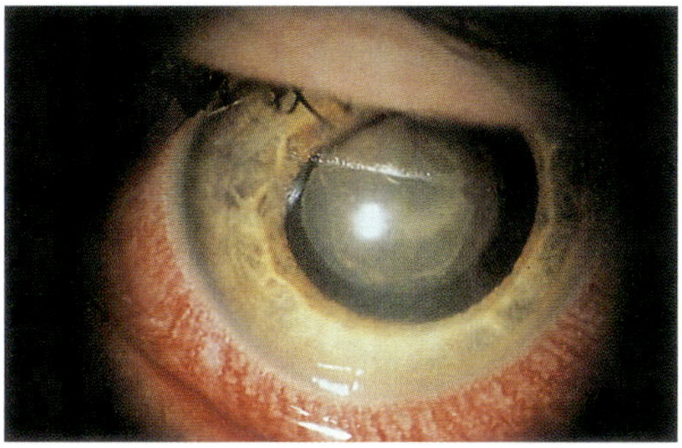

Figure 6-2 Ankylosing spondylitis: acute unilateral anterior uveitis with severe anterior chamber reaction, central fibrinous exudate contracting anterior to the lens capsule, and posterior synechiae from 10 o'clock to 12 o'clock. *(Courtesy of David Meisler, MD.)*

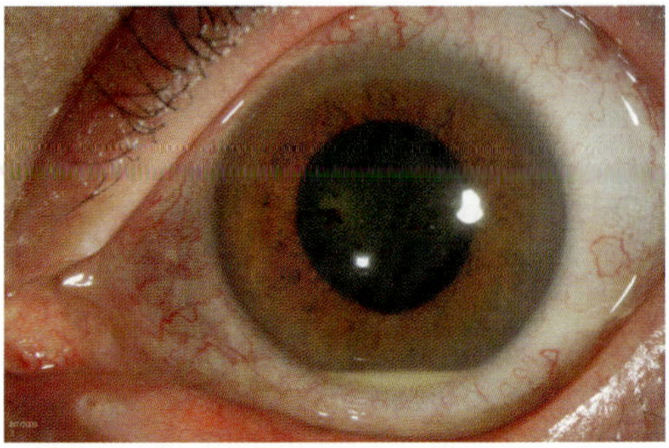

Figure 6-3 Acute nongranulomatous anterior uveitis: hypopyon and anterior capsular ring of pigment following posterior synechiolysis after intensive treatment with dilating agents. *(Courtesy of H. Nida Sen, MD.)*

HLA-B27 is a major histocompatibility complex (MHC) class I antigen present in approximately 6.1% of the US general population: 7.5% among non-Hispanic whites, 6.3% among Hispanics, and 1.1% among African Americans. Approximately one-half of patients with acute anterior uveitis are HLA-B27 positive. Thus, although patients with recurrent anterior nongranulomatous uveitis should be tested for HLA-B27, the presence of HLA-B27 does not provide an absolute diagnosis. Further, the precise trigger for acute anterior uveitis in HLA-B27–positive persons is not clear.

Several autoimmune diseases known collectively as the seronegative spondyloarthropathies are strongly associated with both acute anterior uveitis and HLA-B27. Patients with these diseases, by definition, do not test positive for rheumatoid factor. The seronegative spondyloarthropathies include

- ankylosing spondylitis
- reactive arthritis syndrome
- inflammatory bowel disease
- psoriatic arthritis

These entities are sometimes clinically indistinguishable, and all may be associated with spondylitis and sacroiliitis. Women are more likely than men to experience atypical spondyloarthropathies.

Cunningham ET Jr. Diagnosis and management of anterior uveitis. *Focal Points: Clinical Modules for Ophthalmologists.* San Francisco: American Academy of Ophthalmology; 2002, module 1.

Wakefield D, Chang JH, Amjadi S, Maconochie Z, Abu El-Asrar A, McCluskey P. What is new HLA-B27 acute anterior uveitis? *Ocul Immunol Inflamm.* 2011;19(2):139–144.

HLA-B27–related diseases

Ankylosing spondylitis Ankylosing spondylitis (AS) ranges in severity from asymptomatic to crippling. Symptoms of this disorder include lower back pain and morning stiffness. Up to 90% of patients with AS test positive for HLA-B27, although most HLA-B27–positive individuals do not develop the disease. The chance that an HLA-B27–positive patient will develop spondyloarthritis or eye disease is 1 in 4. Family members may also have AS or anterior uveitis. Often, persons with anterior uveitis lack symptoms of back disease.

The ophthalmologist may be the first physician to suspect AS in an individual patient. Symptoms or family history of back problems together with HLA-B27 positivity suggest the diagnosis. Sacroiliac imaging studies should be obtained when indicated by a suggestive history of morning lower back stiffness that improves with exertion. Patients should be informed of the risk of deformity and referred to a rheumatologist. Pulmonary apical fibrosis and cardiovascular disease (aortic valvular insufficiency) may also develop.

NSAIDs are the mainstay of medical treatment. Sulfasalazine may be used in patients whose joint disease is not controlled with NSAIDs, and it may reduce the frequency of recurrences of uveitis. However, anti-TNF drugs are gaining favor for second-line treatment in recalcitrant cases given their rapid therapeutic effect and overall efficacy. Ophthalmologists should also recognize that early diagnosis is important because nonpharmacologic interventions such as exercise, physical therapy, and smoking cessation may help slow disease progression.

Braun J, Baraliakos X, Listing J, Sieper J. Decreased incidence of anterior uveitis in patients with ankylosing spondylitis treated with the anti-tumor necrosis factor agents infliximab and etanercept. *Arthritis Rheum.* 2005;52(8):2447–2451.

Monnet D, Breban M, Hudry C, Dougados M, Brézin AP. Ophthalmic findings and frequency of extraocular manifestations in patients with HLA-B27 uveitis: a study of 175 cases. *Ophthalmology.* 2004;111(4):802–809.

Reactive arthritis syndrome Reactive arthritis syndrome, formerly known as *Reiter syndrome,* consists of the classic diagnostic triad of nonspecific urethritis, polyarthritis, and conjunctival inflammation, often accompanied by nongranulomatous anterior uveitis. The HLA-B27 marker is found in up to 95% of patients. The condition constitutes less than 2% of all spondyloarthropathies and occurs most frequently in young adult men, although 10% of patients are female.

Reactive arthritis syndrome may be triggered by episodes of diarrhea or dysentery without urethritis. *Ureaplasma urealyticum* as well as *Chlamydia, Shigella, Salmonella,* and *Yersinia* species have all been implicated as triggering infections, although pathogens cannot be isolated from affected joints. Arthritis begins within 30 days of infection in 80% of patients. The knees, ankles, feet, and wrists are affected asymmetrically and in an oligoarticular (4 or fewer joints) distribution. Sacroiliitis is present in as many as 70% of patients.

In addition to the classic triad, 2 other conditions are considered major diagnostic criteria:

1. *keratoderma blennorrhagicum:* a scaly, erythematous, irritating disorder of the palms and soles of the feet (Fig 6-4)
2. *circinate balanitis:* a persistent, scaly, erythematous, circumferential rash of the distal penis

Extraarticular findings such as nail bed pitting, oral ulcers, conjunctivitis, uveitis, and constitutional symptoms help establish a diagnosis of reactive arthritis syndrome, according to criteria established by the Assessment of SpondyloArthritis International Society (ASAS). Eye involvement occurs in approximately 20%. Conjunctivitis is the most common eye finding associated with this disease, and it is usually mucopurulent and papillary. Punctate and subepithelial keratitis may also occur, occasionally leaving permanent corneal scars. Acute nongranulomatous anterior uveitis occurs in up to 10% of patients and may become bilateral and chronic.

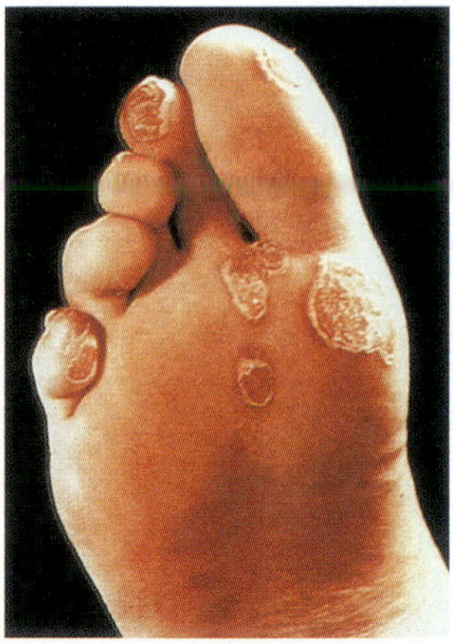

Figure 6-4 Reactive arthritis syndrome with pedal discoid keratoderma blennorrhagicum. *(Courtesy of John D. Sheppard, Jr, MD.)*

Inflammatory bowel disease Ulcerative colitis and Crohn disease (granulomatous ileocolitis) are both associated with acute anterior uveitis. Up to 12% of patients with ulcerative colitis and 2.4% of patients with Crohn disease develop acute anterior uveitis. Occasionally, bowel disease is asymptomatic and follows the onset of uveitis. Twenty percent of patients with inflammatory bowel disease (IBD) have sacroiliitis; of these, 60% are HLA-B27 positive. Patients with both acute anterior uveitis and IBD are more likely to be HLA-B27 positive and have sacroiliitis. Patients with IBD may also develop sclerouveitis, but these individuals are more commonly HLA-B27 negative, have symptoms resembling rheumatoid arthritis, and usually do not develop sacroiliitis. HLA-B27–negative IBD patients may also be more likely to develop intermediate uveitis.

Psoriatic arthritis Diagnosis of psoriatic arthritis is made according to findings of typical cutaneous changes (Fig 6-5), terminal phalangeal joint inflammation (Fig 6-6), and ungual involvement. Twenty percent of patients may have sacroiliitis, and IBD occurs more frequently than would be expected by chance. Up to 25% of patients develop anterior uveitis, which tends to be insidious and bilateral; it is also more likely to be chronic than is the uveitis associated with other spondyloarthropathies. Uveitis may be more severe in

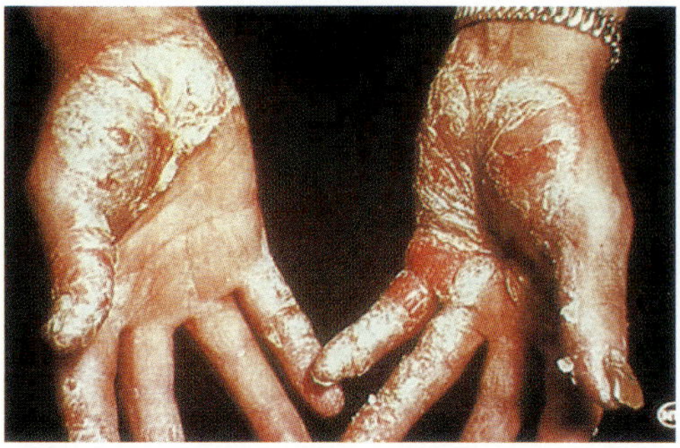

Figure 6-5 Psoriatic arthritis with classic erythematous, hyperkeratotic rash. *(Courtesy of John D. Sheppard, Jr, MD.)*

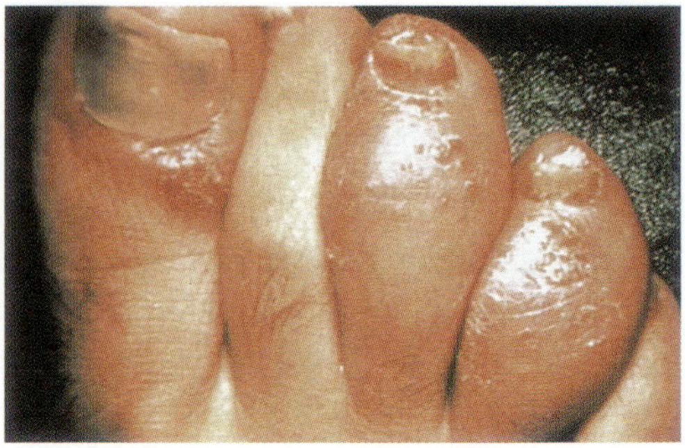

Figure 6-6 Psoriatic arthritis with sausage digits resulting from tissue swelling and distal interphalangeal joint inflammation. *(Courtesy of John D. Sheppard, Jr, MD.)*

HLA-B27–positive patients. Treatment consists of cycloplegic and mydriatic agents and corticosteroids, which are usually given topically. In severe cases, periocular or systemic corticosteroids may be required, and chronic cases may need immunomodulatory therapy.

Anterior uveitis in patients with psoriasis without arthritis has distinct clinical features. The mean age of onset is older than in idiopathic or HLA-B27–associated uveitis and may be bilateral and of longer duration. Posterior segment involvement can be present.

Durrani K, Foster CS. Psoriatic uveitis: a distinct clinical entity? *Am J Ophthalmol.* 2005; 139(1):106–111.

Fraga NA, Oliveira Mde F, Follador I, Rocha Bde O, Rêgo VR. Psoriasis and uveitis: a literature review. *An Bras Dermatol.* 2012;87(6):877–883.

Sampaio-Barros PD, Pereira IA, Hernández-Cuevas C, et al; Respondia Group. An analysis of 372 patients with anterior uveitis in a large Ibero-American cohort of spondyloarthritis: the RESPONDIA Group. *Clin Exp Rheumatol.* 2013;(4):484–489.

Tubulointerstitial nephritis and uveitis syndrome

Tubulointerstitial nephritis and uveitis (TINU) syndrome occurs predominantly in adolescent girls and women up to their early 30s; the mean age of onset is 21 years. Uveitis is typically a bilateral, nongranulomatous, anterior uveitis. Ocular symptoms and findings are more severe in patients with recurrent disease, with development of fibrin, posterior synechiae, larger KPs, and, rarely, hypopyon. Posterior segment involvement is atypical but may include mild vitritis as well as optic nerve and macular edema.

Patients may present with ophthalmic findings before systemic symptoms and tubulointerstitial nephritis develop. More commonly, however, patients present with systemic symptoms before the development of uveitis. The following criteria are required for a clinical diagnosis of TINU syndrome:

- abnormal serum creatinine level or decreased creatinine clearance
- abnormal urinalysis findings, with increased β2-microglobulin level, proteinuria, presence of eosinophils, pyuria or hematuria, urinary white cell casts, and normoglycemic glycosuria
- associated systemic illness, consisting of fever, weight loss, anorexia, fatigue, arthralgias, and myalgias; there may also be abnormal liver function, eosinophilia, and an elevated erythrocyte sedimentation rate

The etiology remains unclear. Seroreactivity against retinal and renal antigens has been demonstrated. The syndrome has a genetic susceptibility and has been reported to be strongly associated with HLA-DRB1*0102. The predominance of activated $CD4^+$ (helper) T lymphocytes in the kidney interstitium suggests a role for cellular immunity. Renal biopsies have shown severe interstitial fibrosis. TINU syndrome is very responsive to treatment with high-dose oral corticosteroids. A small proportion of patients with a prolonged course may require immunomodulatory therapy.

Mackensen F, Billing H. Tubulointerstitial nephritis and uveitis syndrome. *Curr Opin Ophthalmol.* 2009;20(6):525–531.

Mandeville JT, Levinson RD, Holland GN. The tubulointerstitial nephritis and uveitis syndrome. *Surv Ophthalmol.* 2001;46(3):195–208.

Glaucomatocyclitic crisis

Glaucomatocyclitic crisis, also known as *Posner-Schlossman syndrome,* usually manifests as a recurrent unilateral, mild, acute nongranulomatous anterior uveitis. Symptoms are vague discomfort, blurred vision, and halos. Signs include markedly elevated IOP, corneal edema, KPs that may vary in size and/or distribution, low-grade cell and flare, and a slightly dilated pupil. Episodes last from several hours to several days, and recurrences are common over many years. Treatment is with topical corticosteroids and antiglaucoma medication, including, if necessary, systemic carbonic anhydrase inhibitors. Recent studies link infection with herpetic viruses such as cytomegalovirus (CMV) with glaucomatocyclitic crisis, indicating a possible role for antiviral therapy.

Chee SP, Jap A. Presumed Fuchs heterochromic iridocyclitis and Posner-Schlossman syndrome: comparison of cytomegalovirus-positive and negative eyes. *Am J Ophthalmol.* 2008;146(6):883–889.

Lens-associated uveitis

An immune reaction to lens material may result in ocular inflammatory disease. This reaction may follow disruption of the lens capsule (traumatic or surgical), termed *phacoantigenic uveitis,* or leakage of lens protein through the intact lens capsule in mature or hypermature cataracts, termed *phacolytic uveitis* (Figs 6-7, 6-8).

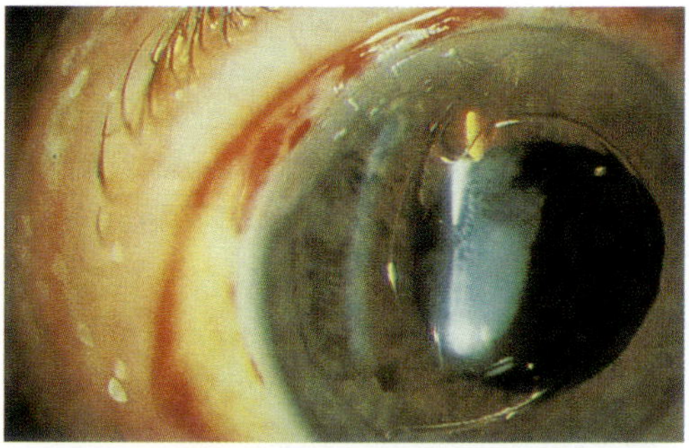

Figure 6-7 Low-grade postoperative uveitis in this patient could be secondary to retained lens cortex or to the anterior chamber intraocular lens (IOL). *(Courtesy of John D. Sheppard, Jr, MD.)*

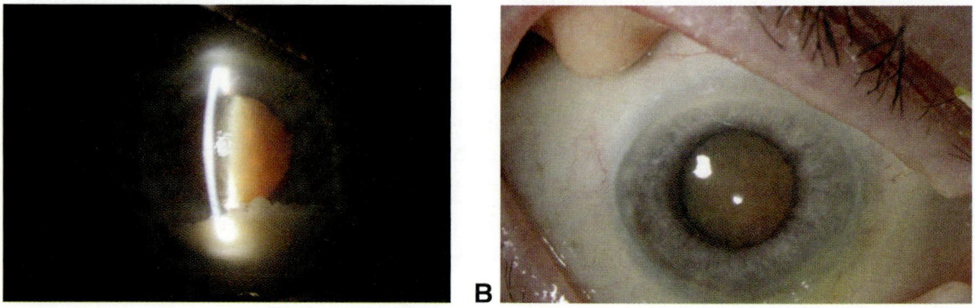

A B

Figure 6-8 A, Phacolytic uveitis with glaucoma, corneal edema, granulomatous anterior uveitis, and pseudohypopyon in a patient with hypermature cataract. **B,** Resolution of anterior chamber inflammation with intense topical corticosteroid use; treatment eventually necessitated cataract surgery. *(Courtesy of H. Nida Sen, MD.)*

The exact mechanism of lens-induced uveitis, although unknown, is thought to represent an immune reaction to lens protein. Experimental animal studies suggest that altered tolerance to lens protein leads to the inflammation, which usually has an abrupt onset but may occasionally occur insidiously. Patients previously sensitized to lens protein (eg, after cataract extraction in the fellow eye) can experience inflammation within 24 hours after capsular rupture.

Phacoantigenic uveitis Phacoantigenic uveitis was previously termed *phacoanaphylactic endophthalmitis,* an incorrect nomenclature because anaphylaxis involves immunoglobulin E (IgE), mast cells, and basophils, none of which is present in the more appropriately termed phacoantigenic uveitis. Clinically, patients exhibit an anterior uveitis that may be granulomatous or nongranulomatous. KPs are usually present and may be small or large. Anterior chamber reaction varies from mild (eg, postoperative inflammation involving a small amount of retained cortex) to severe (eg, traumatic lens capsule disruption); hypopyon may be present. Posterior synechiae are common, and IOP is often elevated. Inflammation in the anterior vitreous cavity is common, but fundus lesions do not occur.

Histologically, a zonal granulomatous inflammation is centered at the site of lens injury. Neutrophils are present around the lens material with surrounding lymphocytes, plasma cells, epithelioid cells, and occasional giant cells.

Treatment consists of topical and, in severe cases, systemic corticosteroids, as well as cycloplegic and mydriatic agents. Surgical removal of all lens material is usually curative. When small amounts of lens material remain, corticosteroid therapy alone may be sufficient to allow resorption of the inciting material.

Phacolytic uveitis Phacolytic uveitis (or *phacolytic glaucoma,* as it is frequently referred to) involves an acute increase in IOP caused by clogging of the trabecular meshwork by macrophages engorged with lens proteins leaking through the intact capsule of a hypermature cataract. The diagnosis is suggested by the presence of elevated IOP, refractile bodies in the aqueous (representing lipid-laden macrophages), and a lack of KPs and synechiae. Therapy includes pressure reduction, often through use of osmotic agents and topical medications, followed quickly by cataract extraction. An aqueous tap may reveal swollen macrophages.

Kalogeropoulos CD, Malamou-Mitsi VD, Asproudis I, Psilas K. The contribution of aqueous humor cytology in the differential diagnosis of anterior uvea inflammations. *Ocul Immunol Inflamm.* 2004;12(3):215–225.

Postoperative inflammation: infectious endophthalmitis

Infectious endophthalmitis must be included in the differential diagnosis of postoperative inflammation and hypopyon. Infection with low-virulence organisms such as *Propionibacterium acnes* and *Staphylococcus epidermidis* as well as fungal species can cause delayed or late-onset endophthalmitis after cataract surgery. Infectious endophthalmitis is discussed in more detail in Chapter 8.

Postoperative inflammation: IOL-associated uveitis

Intraocular lens (IOL)–associated uveitis may range from mild inflammation to the uveitis-glaucoma-hyphema (UGH) syndrome. Surgical manipulation results in breakdown of the blood–aqueous barrier, leading to vulnerability in the early postoperative period. IOL implantation can activate complement cascades and promote neutrophil chemotaxis, leading to cellular deposits on the IOL, synechiae formation, capsular opacification, and anterior capsule phimosis. Retained lens material from extracapsular cataract extraction may exacerbate the usual transient postoperative inflammation. Iris chafing caused by the edges or loops of IOLs on either the anterior or the posterior surface of the iris can result in mechanical irritation and inflammation, although incidence of this type of complication using modern lenses is less than 1%. The motion of an iris-supported or anterior chamber IOL may cause intermittent corneal touch and lead to corneal endothelial damage or decompensation, low-grade anterior uveitis, peripheral anterior synechiae, recalcitrant glaucoma, and CME (Figs 6-9, 6-10). These lenses should be removed and exchanged when penetrating keratoplasty is performed.

UGH syndrome may be caused by irritation of the iris root by any intraocular implant. Flexible anterior chamber IOLs (ACIOLs) are less likely than older rigid ACIOLs to cause UGH syndrome. Because ACIOL use is rare, UGH syndrome is encountered most commonly with sulcus placement of a single-piece acrylic IOL (something that should never be intentionally done). UGH syndrome may also occur even with the appropriate placement of a 3-piece IOL in the sulcus. Ultrasound biomicroscopy or anterior segment optical coherence tomography (OCT) can be helpful in evaluating lens position in cases of chronic pseudophakic uveitis. Many cases can be managed with topical corticosteroids only, although some may require IOL explantation or repositioning. UGH syndrome and chronic uveitis are also discussed in BCSC Section 11, *Lens and Cataract.*

As a general rule, the more biocompatible the IOL material, the less likely it is to incite an inflammatory response. Irregular or damaged IOL surfaces as well as polypropylene haptics have been associated with enhanced bacterial and leukocyte binding and probably should be avoided in patients with uveitis. Several attempts have been made to modify the IOL surface to increase its biocompatibility. These modifications have had little clinical impact on postoperative inflammation and have been abandoned with the advent of acrylic IOLs.

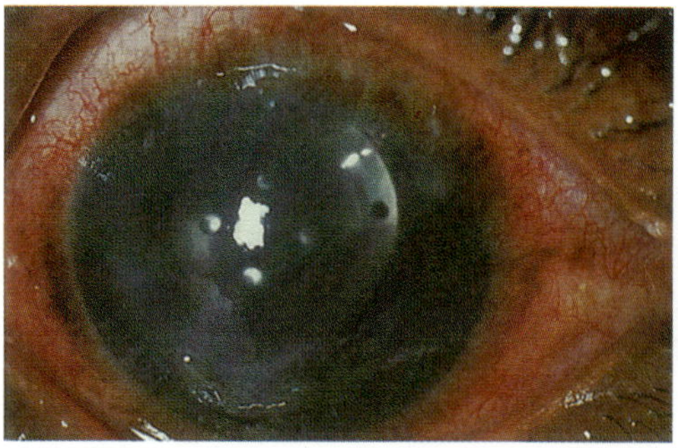

Figure 6-9 Pseudophakic bullous keratopathy and chronic anterior uveitis caused by an iris-fixated anterior chamber IOL, with corneal touch, iris stromal erosion, and chronic recalcitrant cystoid macular edema. *(Courtesy of John D. Sheppard, Jr, MD.)*

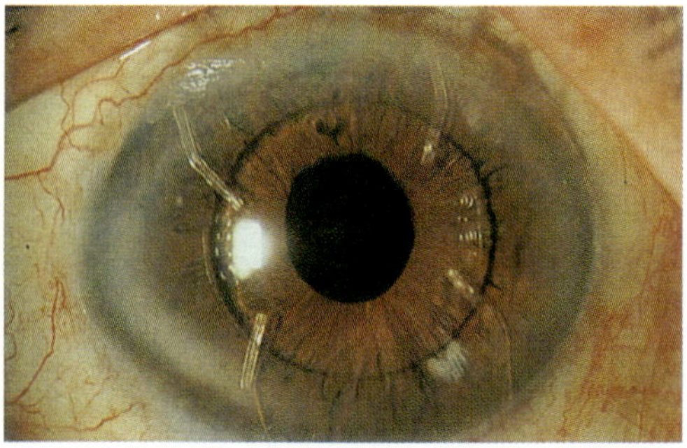

Figure 6-10 Fixed-haptic anterior chamber IOL associated with peripheral and superior corneal edema, chronic low-grade anterior uveitis, peripheral anterior synechiae, globe tenderness, and intermittent microhyphema. *(Courtesy of John D. Sheppard, Jr, MD.)*

Foldable implant materials have also been found to be well tolerated in many patients with uveitis. Some studies have shown increased cellular deposition on silicone optics compared with acrylic or hydrogel optics, but others have shown no difference. In general, acrylic IOLs appear to have excellent biocompatibility, with low rates of cellular deposits and capsular opacification.

One of the most important factors in the success of cataract surgery in patients with uveitis is aggressive control of intraocular inflammation in the preoperative and postoperative periods. For further discussion and illustrations, see Chapter 10 in this book and BCSC Section 11, *Lens and Cataract.*

Ozdal PC, Mansour M, Deschênes J. Ultrasound biomicroscopy of pseudophakic eyes with chronic postoperative inflammation. *J Cataract Refract Surg.* 2003;29(6):1185–1191.

Roesel M, Heinz C, Heimes B, Koch JM, Heiligenhaus A. Uveal and capsular biocompatibility of two foldable acrylic intraocular lenses in patients with endogenous uveitis—a prospective randomized study. *Graefes Arch Clin Exp Ophthalmol.* 2008;246(11): 1609–1615.

Taravati P, Lam DL, Leveque T, Van Gelder RN. Postcataract surgical inflammation. *Curr Opin Ophthalmol.* 2012;23(1):12–18.

Drug-induced uveitis

Use of certain medications has been associated with the development of intraocular inflammation; these drugs include rifabutin (an antibiotic used in the treatment of *Mycobacterium avium-intracellulare* infection), systemic fluoroquinolones (especially moxifloxacin, which may induce iris depigmentation and uveitis), bisphosphonates, sulfonamides, diethylcarbamazine (an antifilarial drug), and oral contraceptives. Paradoxically, certain anti-TNF drugs (eg, etanercept) have also been associated with new-onset uveitis and a systemic sarcoid-like syndrome. Vaccines such as BCG vaccine and influenza vaccines, as well as the purified protein derivative (PPD) used in the tuberculin skin test, have also been implicated in the development of uveitis. Intravesical BCG vaccine (used in the treatment of bladder cancer) can result in an infectious uveitis.

Numerous topical antiglaucoma medications have been associated with uveitis: metipranolol (a nonselective beta-blocking drug used in the treatment of glaucoma), anticholinesterase inhibitors, and prostaglandin $F_{2\alpha}$ analogues. Drugs that are injected directly into the eye have also been associated with uveitis. These medications include antibiotics, urokinase (a plasminogen activator), cidofovir (a cytosine analogue effective against CMV) and vascular endothelial growth factor (VEGF) inhibitors. Treatment generally involves topical corticosteroids and cycloplegic drugs, if necessary. Recalcitrant cases may require cessation or tapering of the offending medication.

Cunningham ET Jr, Pasadhika S, Suhler EB, Zierhut M. Drug-induced inflammation in patients on TNF-α inhibitors. *Ocul Immunol Inflamm.* 2012;20(1):2–5.

Moorthy RS, London NJ, Garg SJ, Cunningham ET Jr. Drug-induced uveitis. *Curr Opin Ophthalmol.* 2013;24(6):589–597.

Chronic Anterior Uveitis

Inflammation of the anterior segment that is persistent and relapses less than 3 months after discontinuation of therapy is termed *chronic anterior uveitis;* it may persist for years.

This type of inflammation usually starts insidiously, with variable amounts of redness, discomfort, and photophobia. Some patients have no symptoms. The disease can be unilateral or bilateral, and the amount of inflammatory activity is variable. CME is common.

Juvenile idiopathic arthritis

In 1997 the International League of Associations of Rheumatologists (ILAR) adopted the term *juvenile idiopathic arthritis* (JIA) to replace the previously used terms *juvenile chronic arthritis* and *juvenile rheumatoid arthritis.* JIA is the most common systemic disorder associated with anterior uveitis in the pediatric age group; it is characterized by arthritis beginning before age 16 years and lasting for at least 6 weeks.

Ocular involvement in JIA JIA can be classified into 3 types according to medical history and other presenting factors:

1. *Systemic onset (Still disease).* This type, usually observed in children under age 5 years, accounts for approximately 10%–15% of all cases of JIA. It is characterized by fever, rash, lymphadenopathy, and hepatosplenomegaly. Joint involvement may be minimal or absent initially. Ocular involvement is rare; fewer than 6% of patients have uveitis.
2. *Polyarticular onset.* Patients with this type show involvement of more than 4 joints in the first 6 months of the disease; it represents 40% of JIA cases overall but only about 10% of cases of JIA-associated anterior uveitis. Patients who are positive for rheumatoid factor may not develop uveitis.
3. *Oligoarticular onset.* This type, also known as *pauciarticular onset,* constitutes 40%–50% of all cases of JIA and includes the vast majority (80%–90%) of patients with JIA-associated uveitis. Four or fewer joints may be involved during the first 6 months of disease, and patients may have no joint symptoms. Oligoarticular-onset JIA is further subdivided: type 1 disease is observed in girls under age 5 years who are typically positive for antinuclear antibody (ANA); chronic anterior uveitis occurs in up to 25% of these patients. Type 2 disease is found in older boys, many of whom develop evidence of seronegative spondyloarthropathy (75% are HLA-B27 positive). The uveitis in these patients is more likely to be acute and recurrent rather than chronic, unlike in type 1 disease.

The average age of onset of uveitis in patients with JIA is 6 years. Uveitis generally develops within 5–7 years of the onset of joint disease but may occur as long as 28 years after the development of arthritis. There is usually little or no correlation between ocular and joint inflammation. Risk factors for the development of chronic uveitis in patients with JIA include female sex, oligoarticular onset, and the presence of circulating ANA. Most patients test negative for rheumatoid factor.

The eye is frequently white, without redness. Symptoms may include mild to moderate pain, photophobia, and blurring, although some patients are asymptomatic. Often, the eye disease is found incidentally during a routine school physical examination. The signs of inflammation include fine KPs, band keratopathy, flare and cells, posterior synechiae, and cataract (Figs 6-11, 6-12). Patients in whom JIA is suspected should undergo ANA

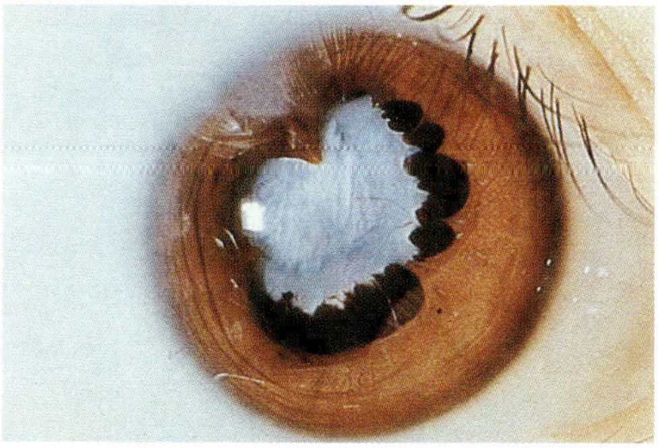

Figure 6-11 Juvenile idiopathic arthritis with chronic anterior uveitis and cataract.

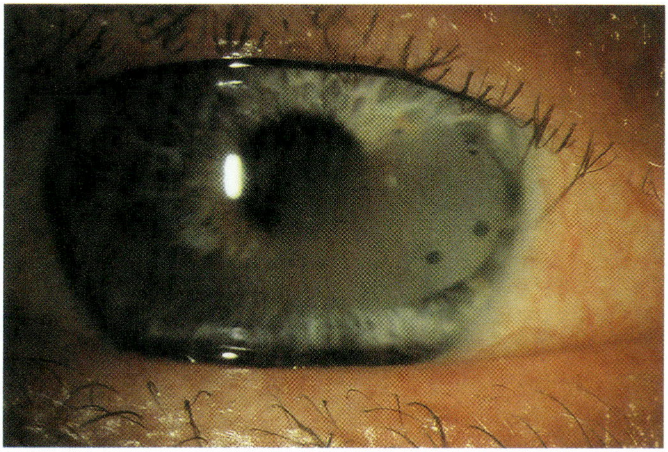

Figure 6-12 Juvenile idiopathic arthritis with chronic calcific band keratopathy.

testing and be evaluated by a pediatric rheumatologist because the joint disease may be minimal or absent at the time the uveitis is diagnosed. The differential diagnosis includes TINU, Fuchs heterochromic uveitis, sarcoidosis, Behçet disease, the seronegative spondyloarthropathies, herpetic uveitis, and Lyme disease.

Prognosis Because of the frequently asymptomatic nature of the uveitis, profound silent ocular damage can occur, and the long-term prognosis often depends on the extent of structural complications at the time of first diagnosis. Complications are frequent and often severe; they include band keratopathy, cataract, glaucoma, macular edema, chronic hypotony, and phthisis. Children with JIA, especially those who are ANA positive or have oligoarticular disease, should undergo regular slit-lamp examinations. Table 6-1 outlines the recommended schedule for screening patients with JIA for uveitis, as developed by the American Academy of Pediatrics.

Treatment The initial treatment for patients with JIA who have uveitis consists of topical corticosteroids. More severe cases may require use of systemic corticosteroids or IMT. The goal of treatment is to eliminate active inflammation (anterior chamber cells) and

Table 6-1 Frequency of Ophthalmologic Examination in Patients With JIA

Type	ANA	Age at Onset, y	Duration of Disease, y	Risk Category	Eye Examination Frequency, mo
Oligoarthritis or polyarthritis	+	≤6	≤4	High	3
	+	≤6	>4	Moderate	6
	+	≤6	>7	Low	12
	+	>6	≤4	Moderate	6
	+	>6	>4	Low	12
	–	≤6	≤4	Moderate	6
	–	≤6	>4	Low	12
	–	>6	NA	Low	12
Systemic disease (fever, rash)	NA	NA	NA	Low	12

JIA = juvenile idiopathic arthritis; ANA = antinuclear antibodies; NA = not applicable.
Recommendations for follow-up continue through childhood and adolescence.

Reprinted with permission from Cassidy J, Kivlin J, Lindsley C, Nocton J; Section on Rheumatology; Section on Ophthalmology. Ophthalmologic examinations in children with juvenile rheumatoid arthritis. *Pediatrics.* 2006;117(5):1844.

prevent new complications. Short-acting mydriatic drugs may be useful in patients with chronic flare to keep the pupil mobile and to prevent posterior synechiae formation. Use of systemic NSAIDs may permit a lower dose of corticosteroids.

Because of the chronic nature of the inflammation, corticosteroid-induced complications are common. The long-term use of systemic corticosteroids in children presents numerous problems, including growth retardation from premature closure of the epiphyses. Also, prolonged use of topical corticosteroids leads to cataracts and glaucoma. Because long-term use of topical corticosteroids at doses ≥3 times daily can increase the risk of cataract formation, systemic IMT should be considered for such cases. In addition, there is evidence that even low-grade inflammation, if present for a prolonged period, can result in unacceptable ocular morbidity and loss of vision. For these reasons, many of these children are treated with weekly low-dose methotrexate. Numerous studies have shown that this treatment regimen can effectively control the uveitis, is generally well tolerated, and can spare patients the complications of long-term corticosteroid use. In addition, several studies have demonstrated a benefit from TNF inhibitors and other biologic agents.

Treatment of cataracts in patients with JIA remains a challenge, and the use of IOLs remains controversial. Children who are left aphakic may develop amblyopia. Cataract surgery in patients with JIA-associated anterior uveitis has a high complication rate due to the difficulty in controlling the more aggressive inflammatory response present in these children. Lensectomy and vitrectomy via the pars plana have been advocated.

There have been reports, however, of more successful cataract surgery with IOL implants in patients with JIA. These reports highlight the importance of well-controlled uveitis through systemic IMT and the use of perioperative corticosteroids.

The following guidelines are useful when selecting patients with JIA for cataract surgery with IOL implants:

- The patient's intraocular inflammation must be well controlled with systemic IMT for at least 3 months before surgery and must not require frequent instillation of topical corticosteroids.
- Only acrylic lenses should be implanted.
- Patients must be monitored frequently after cataract surgery to watch for any inflammation, and inflammation that occurs must be aggressively treated.
- IMT must be used preoperatively and postoperatively, not just perioperatively.
- Because long-term results are not available, patients must be strongly advised about the need for careful, regular, lifelong follow-up to detect late complications that may lead to loss of the eye.
- The ophthalmologist must have a low threshold for IOL explantation in patients who have persistent postoperative inflammation and recurrent cyclitic membranes.

Patients with band keratopathy should be treated (eg, using chelation with sodium ethylenediaminetetraacetic acid [EDTA]) and allowed to heal well before cataract surgery is attempted. See also Chapter 10 and BCSC Section 6, *Pediatric Ophthalmology and Strabismus,* Chapter 24.

Glaucoma should be treated with medical therapy initially, although surgical intervention is often necessary in severe cases. Standard filtering procedures are usually unsuccessful, and the use of antifibrotic drugs or aqueous drainage devices is usually required for successful control of the glaucoma.

Angeles-Han S, Yeh S. Prevention and management of cataracts in children with juvenile idiopathic arthritis–associated uveitis. *Curr Rheumatol Rep.* 2012;14(2):142–149.

Grajewski RS, Zurek-Imhoff B, Roesel M, Heinz C, Heiligenhaus A. Favourable outcome after cataract surgery with IOL implantation in uveitis associated with juvenile idiopathic arthritis. *Acta Ophthalmol.* 2012;90(7):657–662.

Gregory AC 2nd, Kempen JH, Daniel E, Kaçmaz RO, et al; Systemic Immunosuppressive Therapy for Eye Diseases Cohort Study Research Group. Risk factors for loss of visual acuity among patients with uveitis associated with juvenile idiopathic arthritis: the Systemic Immunosuppressive Therapy for Eye Diseases Study. *Ophthalmology.* 2013;120(1):186–192.

Holland GN, Denove CS, Yu F. Chronic anterior uveitis in children: clinical characteristics and complications. *Am J Ophthalmol.* 2009;147(4):667–678.

Mehta PJ, Alexander JL, Sen HN. Pediatric uveitis: new and future treatments. *Curr Opin Ophthalmol.* 2013;24(5):453–462.

Paroli MP, Spinucci G, Fabiani C, Pivetti-Pezzi P. Retinal complications of juvenile idiopathic arthritis–related uveitis: a microperimetry and optical coherence tomography study. *Ocul Immunol Inflamm.* 2010;18(1):54–59.

Simonini G, Taddio A, Cattalini M, et al. Superior efficacy of adalimumab in treating childhood refractory chronic uveitis when used as first biologic modifier drug: adalimumab as starting anti-TNF-alpha therapy in childhood chronic uveitis. *Pediatr Rheumatol Online J.* 2013;11(1):16.

Thorne JE, Woreta FA, Dunn JP, Jabs DA. Risk of cataract development among children with juvenile idiopathic arthritis–related uveitis treated with topical corticosteroids. *Ophthalmology.* 2010;117(7):1436–1441.

Zannin ME, Birolo C, Gerloni VM, et al. Safety and efficacy of infliximab and adalimumab for refractory uveitis in juvenile idiopathic arthritis: 1-year followup data from the Italian Registry. *J Rheumatol.* 2013;40(1):74–79.

Fuchs heterochromic uveitis

Fuchs heterochromic uveitis (also sometimes called *Fuchs heterochromic iridocyclitis* or *Fuchs uveitis syndrome*), is an entity that is frequently overlooked. Between 2% and 3% of patients referred to uveitis clinics have Fuchs heterochromic uveitis. This condition is usually unilateral, and its symptoms vary from none to mild blurring and discomfort. Signs include

- diffuse iris stromal atrophy with variable pigment epithelial layer atrophy (Fig 6-13)
- small, white, stellate KPs scattered diffusely over the entire endothelium (Fig 6-14)
- cells in the anterior chamber as well as in the anterior vitreous
- glaucoma and cataracts, which occur frequently
- macular edema, which is seldomly present
- synechiae, fundus scars, and retinal periphlebitis, all of which are rare or absent

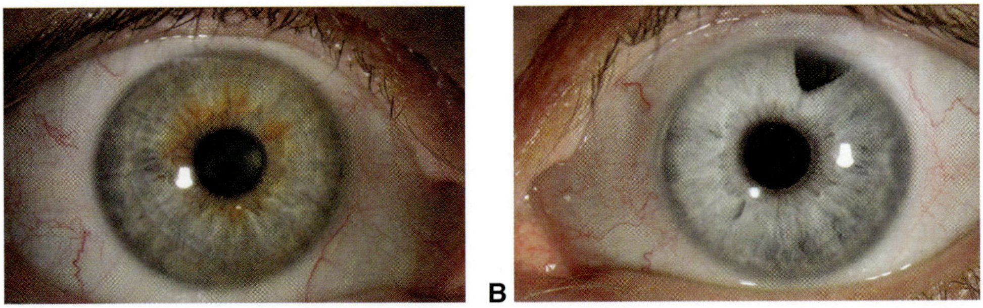

A B

Figure 6-13 Heterochromia in Fuchs heterochromic uveitis. **A,** Right (unaffected) eye. **B,** Left (affected) eye in the same patient. Note the lighter iris color and stromal atrophy ("moth-eaten appearance") in the affected eye, which underwent surgical iridectomy at the same time as cataract surgery. *(Courtesy of H. Nida Sen, MD.)*

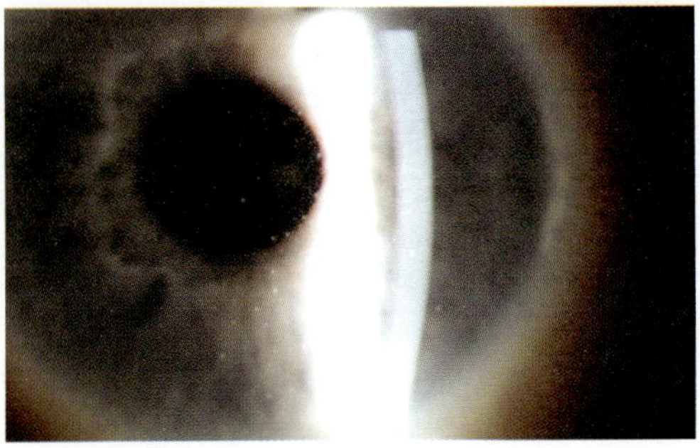

Figure 6-14 Diffusely distributed stellate keratic precipitates in a patient with Fuchs heterochromic uveitis. *(Courtesy of H. Nida Sen, MD.)*

The diagnosis is made according to the distribution of KPs, presence of heterochromia, lack of synechiae, and lack of symptoms. Heterochromia may be subtle in a brown-eyed patient, and the clinician must look carefully for signs of iris stromal atrophy. Often, the inflammation is discovered during a routine examination, such as when a unilateral cataract develops. Usually, but not invariably, a lighter-colored iris indicates the involved eye. In blue-eyed persons, however, the affected eye may become darker as the stromal atrophy progresses and the darker iris pigment epithelium shows through.

The etiology of Fuchs heterochromic uveitis remains unclear. Associations with ocular toxoplasmosis, herpes simplex virus infection, rubella, and CMV infection have been suggested.

Patients generally do well with cataract surgery, and IOLs can usually be implanted successfully. However, some patients may experience substantial visual disability as a result of extensive vitreous opacification. Pars plana vitrectomy should be carefully considered in such instances. Glaucoma control can be difficult. Abnormal vessels bridging the angle can be seen on gonioscopy. These vessels may bleed during surgery, resulting in postoperative hyphema.

Few cases require therapy for inflammation. The prognosis is good in most cases even when the inflammation persists for decades. Because topical corticosteroids can lessen the inflammation but typically do not resolve it, aggressive treatment to eradicate the cellular reaction is not indicated. Cycloplegia is seldom necessary. Histologic examination shows plasma cells in the ciliary body, indicating that true inflammation occurs. See BCSC Section 10, *Glaucoma,* for further discussion of Fuchs heterochromic uveitis.

Birnbaum AD, Tessler HH, Schultz KL, et al. Epidemiologic relationship between Fuchs heterochromic iridocyclitis and the United States rubella vaccination program. *Am J Ophthalmol.* 2007;144(3):424–428.

de Groot-Mijnes JD, de Visser L, Rothova A, Schuller M, van Loon AM, Weersink AJ. Rubella virus is associated with Fuchs heterochromic iridocyclitis. *Am J Ophthalmol.* 2006;141(1):212–214.

Idiopathic anterior uveitis

Inability to positively identify a diagnosis, as is the case in many patients with chronic anterior uveitis, does not preclude treatment with topical steroids and/or cycloplegics, assuming infectious causes have been ruled out. In some cases initially labeled idiopathic, repeat diagnostic testing at a later date may reveal an underlying systemic condition.

Intermediate Uveitis

The Standardization of Uveitis Nomenclature (SUN) Working Group defines *intermediate uveitis* as the subset in which the predominant site of inflammation is in the vitreous; this subset accounts for up to 15% of all cases of uveitis. Intermediate uveitis is characterized by ocular inflammation concentrated in the vitreous and the vitreous base overlying the ciliary body and peripheral retina–pars plana complex. Inflammatory cells may aggregate in the vitreous ("snowballs"), where some coalesce. In some patients, inflammatory exudative accumulation on the inferior pars plana ("snowbanking") seems to correlate with a more severe disease process. There may be associated peripheral retinal phlebitis. Anterior chamber reaction of varying severity may also occur.

Intermediate uveitis can be associated with various conditions, including sarcoidosis, multiple sclerosis (MS), Lyme disease, peripheral toxocariasis, syphilis, tuberculosis, primary Sjögren syndrome, and infection with human T-cell lymphotropic virus type 1 (HTLV-1).

Pars Planitis

The term *pars planitis* refers to the subset of intermediate uveitis in which snowbank or snowball formation occurs in the absence of an associated infection or systemic disease. It is the most common form of intermediate uveitis, constituting approximately 85%–90% of cases. Previously also known as *chronic cyclitis* and *peripheral uveitis,* the condition most commonly affects persons aged 5–40 years. It has a bimodal distribution, concentrating in younger (5–15 years) and older (20–40 years) groups. No overall sex predilection is apparent. The pathogenesis of pars planitis is not well understood but is thought to involve autoimmune reactions against the vitreous, peripheral retina, and ciliary body.

Clinical characteristics

Approximately 80% of cases of pars planitis are bilateral, which can often be asymmetric in severity. In children, the initial presentation may consist of significant anterior chamber inflammation accompanied by redness, photophobia, and discomfort. The onset in teenagers and young adults may be more insidious, with the presenting complaint generally being floaters. Ocular manifestations include a variable number of anterior chamber inflammatory cells, vitreous cells, snowballs (Fig 6-15), and pars plana exudates. Inferior peripheral retinal phlebitis with retinal venous sheathing is common. With long-standing inflammation, CME often develops; this condition becomes chronic and refractory in approximately 10% of patients and is the major cause of vision loss. Ischemia from retinal phlebitis, combined with angiogenic stimuli from intraocular inflammation, can lead to neovascularization along the inferior snowbank in up to 10% of cases. These neovascular

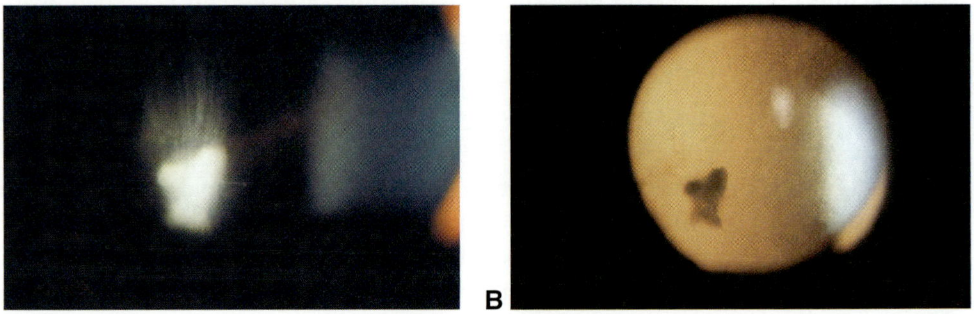

A B

Figure 6-15 Pars planitis. **A,** Vitreous "snowball" opacity in the anterior, inferior retrolental vitreous. **B,** Same vitreous snowball opacity shown in retroillumination, revealing its location with respect to the lens as well as evidence of vitreous cellularity. *(Courtesy of Ramana S. Moorthy, MD.)*

complexes can result in vitreous hemorrhages, more common in children than adults; they also may contract, leading to peripheral tractional and rhegmatogenous retinal detachments. In rare cases, the complexes evolve into secondary peripheral retinal vasoproliferative tumors—vascular masses with exudative retinopathy and minimally dilated vessels—years after the initial diagnosis. Retinal detachments occur in 10% of patients with pars planitis. With chronicity, posterior synechiae and band keratopathy may also develop. Other possible causes of loss of vision include cataracts, epiretinal membrane, and vitreous opacification.

Differential diagnosis

The differential diagnosis of pars planitis includes syphilis, tuberculosis, Lyme uveitis, sarcoidosis, intermediate uveitis associated with MS, and toxocariasis. Lyme and syphilitic uveitis may simulate any anatomical subtype of uveitis. Measurement of Lyme antibody titers may be particularly useful in regions where the disease is endemic, especially in the presence of cutaneous and articular disease. Anterior and intermediate uveitis may occur in up to 20% of patients with MS. Sarcoidosis-associated uveitis presents as an intermediate disease in 7% of cases. A peripheral granuloma such as that seen in toxocariasis can mimic the unilateral pars plana snowbank in a child and should be ruled out. Serologic testing can be helpful in these cases.

Vitritis without other ocular findings can be suggestive of primary central nervous system (CNS) lymphoma. These patients are generally much older at presentation than patients with pars planitis, usually in their sixth decade of life or older. Fuchs heterochromic uveitis can produce mild to dense vitritis but has characteristic KPs and iris heterochromia.

Ancillary tests and histologic findings

Diagnosis of pars planitis is made according to classic clinical findings. Laboratory workup to exclude other causes of intermediate uveitis, including sarcoidosis, Lyme disease, and syphilis, is important. Measurement of serum angiotensin converting enzyme (ACE) and Lyme antibody titers, chest imaging, and syphilis serology testing can be considered. Fluorescein angiography (FA) may show diffuse peripheral venous leakage, disc leakage, and CME. Ultrasound biomicroscopy may be used in the case of a small pupil or dense cataract to demonstrate peripheral exudates or membranes over the pars plana.

Histologic examination of eyes with pars planitis shows vitreous condensation and cellular infiltration in the vitreous base. The inflammatory cells consist mostly of macrophages, lymphocytes, and a few plasma cells. Pars planitis is also characterized by peripheral lymphocytic cuffing of venules and a loose fibrovascular membrane over the pars plana.

Prognosis

The clinical course of pars planitis may be divided into 3 types. Approximately 10% of cases have a self-limiting, benign course; 30% have a smoldering course with remissions and exacerbations; and 60% have a prolonged course without exacerbations. Pars planitis may remain active for many years. In some cases, the disease "burns out" after a few years. If CME is treated until resolution and kept from returning by adequate control of inflammation, the long-term visual prognosis can be good, with nearly 75% of patients maintaining visual acuity of 20/40 or better after 10 years.

Treatment

Therapy should be directed toward treating the underlying cause of the inflammation, if possible. For example, infectious causes such as Lyme disease, tuberculosis, and syphilis should be treated with appropriate antimicrobial drugs. If an underlying condition is not identified, as in pars planitis, or if therapy of an associated condition consists of nonspecific control of inflammation, as in sarcoidosis, anti-inflammatory therapy should be implemented.

Corticosteroids, oral or periocular, usually constitute the first line of therapy. Periocular depot corticosteroid injections of triamcinolone or methylprednisolone may be given using the posterior sub-Tenon (see Chapter 5, Fig 5-8) or orbital floor route. These can be repeated as frequently as every 3–4 weeks. In the majority of cases, the inflammation responds and the CME improves; however, some cases prove recalcitrant and CME may recur. Patients, especially those with a history of glaucoma, must be carefully monitored for corticosteroid-induced IOP elevation. Other complications of periocular corticosteroids include aponeurotic ptosis, fat prolapse, enophthalmos, and, in rare instances, globe perforation. Cataract formation can occur with any form of corticosteroid therapy.

Intravitreal triamcinolone injections may be an alternative to periocular injections in refractory cases. These injections carry risks of sustained IOP elevation and glaucoma and very small risks of retinal detachment, vitreous hemorrhage, and endophthalmitis. Injections should be administered away from areas of snowbanking and areas with peripheral retinal pathology. Local treatment with corticosteroid injections is a particularly appealing approach in unilateral cases.

Systemic corticosteroid therapy may also be used, especially in severe or bilateral cases. Patients may be treated with an initial dosage of 1–1.5 mg/kg/day, with gradual tapering every 1–2 weeks to dosages of less than 10 mg/day.

As with all autoimmune uveitis, if corticosteroid therapy fails or long-term use of high doses of corticosteroids are needed to control the inflammation, immunomodulatory treatment is indicated. Systemic immunomodulatory drugs such as antimetabolites (eg, methotrexate, azathioprine, mycophenolate mofetil), T-cell inhibitors (eg, cyclosporine, tacrolimus), biologic agents (eg, TNF inhibitors, interferon), and alkylating drugs (eg, cyclophosphamide, chlorambucil) can be considered. Several reports from the *S*ystemic *I*mmunosuppressive *T*herapy for *E*ye Diseases (SITE) cohort study indicated that cyclosporine, azathioprine, and mycophenolate mofetil were effective in achieving sustained control of inflammation in 70%–80% of patients with intermediate uveitis. It should be remembered that anti-TNF therapy can exacerbate MS and therefore should be avoided in patients with MS-associated intermediate uveitis.

Alternative therapies for pars planitis include peripheral ablation of the pars plana snowbank with cryotherapy and/or indirect laser photocoagulation to the peripheral retina. Cryotherapy is rarely used at present because of concerns about further inducing inflammation. Laser photocoagulation can be used in cases of retinal ischemia and neovascularization to prevent vitreous hemorrhage; it does not seem to increase the risk of rhegmatogenous retinal detachment. Intravitreal anti-VEGF treatment can also be used for retinal or choroidal neovascularization in pars planitis in otherwise quiet eyes.

Pars plana vitrectomy, with or without laser photocoagulation, can also be helpful in treating complications of pars planitis or in cases recalcitrant to IMT. In such cases, a perioperative increase in systemic immunosuppression and/or corticosteroids should be considered. Pars plana vitrectomy may be necessary to treat severe vision loss caused by vitreous hemorrhage or traction, retinal detachment, or epiretinal membrane. It can also be considered for cases with significant vitreous opacities despite adequate IMT. In cases involving epiretinal membrane or vitreomacular traction, separation of the posterior hyaloid membrane during vitrectomy may have a beneficial effect in reducing CME. Potential complications include retinal detachment, endophthalmitis, and cataract formation.

Complications

Complications of pars planitis include cataract, glaucoma, CME, retinal neovascularization, vitreous hemorrhage, and tractional or rhegmatogenous retinal detachment. Cataracts occur in up to 60% of cases. Cataract surgery with IOL implantation may be complicated by smoldering low-grade inflammation; recurring opacification of the posterior capsule despite capsulotomy; recurrent retrolental membranes; and chronic CME, even in cases in which there is no active cellular inflammation. Combining pars plana vitrectomy with cataract extraction and IOL implantation may reduce the risk of these complications. Glaucoma—both angle-closure and open-angle—occurs in approximately 10% of patients with pars planitis. CME may occur in 50% of patients with intermediate uveitis and is a hallmark of pars planitis. Neovascularization of the retina, disc, and peripheral snowbank has been reported. Occasionally, vitreous hemorrhage is the presenting sign of pars planitis, especially in children; it can be treated effectively with pars plana vitrectomy. Tractional and rhegmatogenous retinal detachments occur in up to 15% of patients and require scleral buckling, sometimes combined with vitrectomy. Risk factors for rhegmatogenous retinal detachment include severe inflammation, use of cryotherapy at the time of a vitrectomy, and neovascularization of the pars plana snowbank.

Donaldson MJ, Pulido JS, Herman DC, Diehl N, Hodge D. Pars planitis: a 20-year study of incidence, clinical features, and outcomes. *Am J Ophthalmol.* 2007;144(6):812–817.

Lauer AK, Smith JR, Robertson JE, Rosenbaum JT. Vitreous hemorrhage is a common complication of pediatric pars planitis. *Ophthalmology.* 2002;109(1):95–98.

Leder HA, Jabs DA, Galor A, Dunn JP, Thorne JE. Periocular triamcinolone acetonide injections for cystoid macular edema complicating noninfectious uveitis. *Am J Ophthalmol.* 2011;152(3):441–448.

Mackensen F, Jakob E, Springer C, et al. Interferon versus methotrexate in intermediate uveitis with macular edema: results of a randomized controlled clinical trial. *Am J Ophthalmol.* 2013;156(3):478–486.

Pato E, Muñoz-Fernández S, Francisco F, et al; Uveitis Working Group from Spanish Society of Rheumatology. Systematic review on the effectiveness of immunosuppressants and biological therapies in the treatment of autoimmune posterior uveitis. *Semin Arthritis Rheum.* 2011;40(4):314–323.

Multiple Sclerosis

Uveitis is 10 times more common in MS patients than in the general population. The frequency of uveitis in patients with MS is reported to be as high as 30%, and the onset of uveitis may precede the diagnosis of MS in up to 25% of patients and by 5–10 years. MS usually affects white women 20–50 years of age, and intermediate uveitis is the most common manifestation of MS-associated uveitis. Up to 95% of cases are bilateral. Up to 15% of patients with pars planitis may eventually develop MS. Intermediate uveitis appears to be of milder severity in MS than in idiopathic cases. Macular edema is less common. Most patients develop mild vitritis with periphlebitis. Periphlebitis in MS is not clearly related to optic neuritis, systemic exacerbations, or disease severity.

The immunopathogenesis of MS is not well understood but appears to involve humoral, cellular, and immunogenetic components directed against myelin. HLA-DR15 appears to be associated with the combination of MS and uveitis. Immunocytologic studies have shown some cross-reactivity between myelin-associated glycoprotein and Müller cells.

It is unclear whether treatment of MS with interferon has any effect on intermediate uveitis; however, reports of macular edema associated with fingolimod therapy for MS are of interest. As biologic therapies for uveitis become more common, it is particularly important to consider the possibility of MS in any patient who presents with intermediate uveitis or pars planitis, as anti-TNF drugs have been associated with exacerbations of MS.

Chen L, Gordon LK. Ocular manifestations of multiple sclerosis. *Curr Opin Ophthalmol.* 2005;16(5):315–320.

Zein G, Berta A, Foster CS. Multiple sclerosis–associated uveitis. *Ocul Immunol Inflamm.* 2004;12(2):137–142.

Posterior Uveitis

Posterior uveitis is defined by the SUN classification system as intraocular inflammation that involves primarily the retina and/or choroid. Inflammatory cells may be observed diffusely throughout the vitreous cavity, overlying foci of active inflammation, or on the posterior vitreous face. Structural complications, such as macular edema, peripheral retinal vasculitis, optic disc edema, and retinal or choroidal neovascularization may occur in the posterior segment as the result of a number of uveitic entities. However, these complications are not considered when determining whether a patient has posterior uveitis. For instance, the presence of macular edema as part of an HLA-B27–associated anterior uveitis does not mean that the patient also has posterior uveitis. Noninfectious syndromes with primarily posterior segment involvement are included in this section; diagnoses routinely producing both anterior and posterior segment involvement are addressed in the Panuveitis section later in the chapter.

Collagen Vascular Diseases

Systemic lupus erythematosus

Systemic lupus erythematosus (SLE) is a connective tissue disorder with multisystem involvement that affects primarily women of childbearing age, with higher incidence rates among African Americans and Hispanic persons in the United States. The pathogenesis of SLE is incompletely understood. It is thought to be an autoimmune disorder characterized by B-lymphocyte hyperactivity, polyclonal B-lymphocyte activation, hypergammaglobulinemia, autoantibody formation, and T-lymphocyte autoreactivity with immune complex deposition, leading to end-organ damage. Autoantibodies arising in SLE include antinuclear antibodies (ANA), antibodies to both single- and double-stranded DNA (anti-ssDNA and anti-dsDNA), antibodies to cytoplasmic components (anti-Sm, anti-Ro, and anti-La), and antiphospholipid antibodies. The systemic manifestations of SLE are protean and include acute cutaneous diseases in approximately 70%–80% of patients (malar rash, discoid lupus, photosensitivity, and mucosal lesions); arthritis in 80%–85%; renal disease in approximately 50%–75%; Raynaud phenomenon in 30%–50%; and neurologic involvement in 35%. Cardiac, pulmonary, hepatic, and hematologic abnormalities can also occur. The diagnosis is essentially clinical and based on criteria enumerated by the American College of Rheumatology (American College of Rheumatology Criteria for Classification of Systemic Lupus Erythematosus http://www.ncbi.nlm.nih.gov/pubmedhealth/PMH0041704/).

Ocular manifestations occur in 50% of patients with SLE and include cutaneous lesions on the eyelids (discoid lupus erythematosus), secondary Sjögren syndrome in approximately 20% of patients (a concern in patients considering laser in situ keratomileusis), all subtypes of scleral inflammatory disease, neuro-ophthalmic lesions (cranial nerve palsies, optic neuropathy, and retrochiasmal and cerebral visual disorders), retinal vasculopathy, and, in rare cases, uveitis.

Lupus retinopathy, the most well-recognized posterior segment manifestation, is considered an important marker of systemic disease activity, with a prevalence ranging from 3% among outpatients with mild disease to 29% among those with more active disease. Its clinical spectrum varies from mild to severe and is characterized by the following signs:

- *Cotton-wool spots with or without intraretinal hemorrhages.* These lesions occur independently of hypertension and are thought to be due to the underlying microangiopathy of the disease (Fig 6-16).

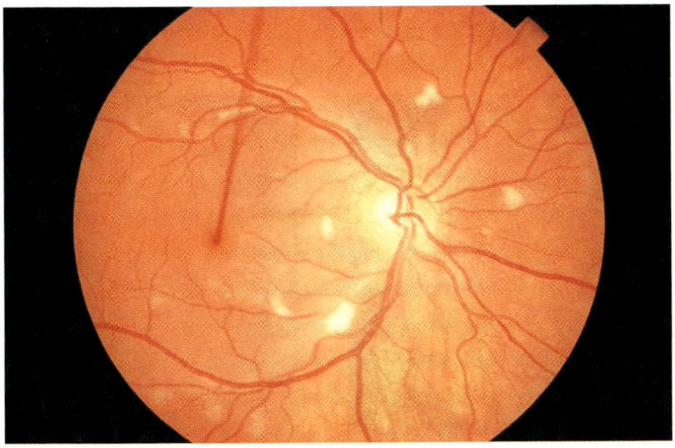

Figure 6-16 Systemic lupus erythematosus (SLE): fundus photograph showing multiple cotton-wool spots. *(Courtesy of E. Mitchel Opremcak, MD.)*

- *Severe retinal vascular occlusive disease (arterial and venous thrombosis).* Retinal vaso-occlusion results in retinal nonperfusion and ischemia, secondary retinal neovascularization, and vitreous hemorrhage (Fig 6-17). More severe retinal vascular occlusive disease in SLE appears to be associated with CNS lupus and the presence of antiphospholipid antibodies. Retinal vascular thrombosis is thought to be related to these autoantibodies and to the induction of a hypercoagulable state rather than to an inflammatory retinal vasculitis. See BCSC Section 1, *Update on General Medicine,* for a discussion of antiphospholipid antibodies.
- *Lupus choroidopathy.* This entity is characterized by serous elevations of the retina, retinal pigment epithelium (RPE), or both; choroidal infarction; and choroidal neovascularization (CNV). It may be observed with severe systemic vascular disease, due to either hypertension from lupus nephritis or systemic vasculitis (Fig 6-18). SLE-induced hypertension and nephritis may also result in arteriolar narrowing, retinal hemorrhage, and disc edema.

The typical types of uveitis, such as anterior or intermediate uveitis, are not commonly associated with SLE. Unfortunately, ANA testing is often done in patients with uveitis but no systemic or ocular findings to suggest SLE; under those circumstances, the test has a very high false-positive rate. ANA testing should be limited to use in patients

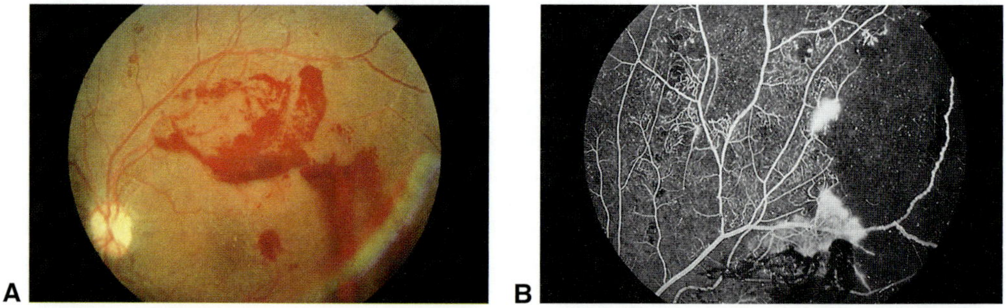

Figure 6-17 **A,** Fundus photograph showing ischemic retinal vasculitis and neovascularization in a patient with SLE. **B,** Fluorescein angiogram of the same patient as in **A,** showing capillary nonperfusion. *(Courtesy of E. Mitchel Opremcak, MD.)*

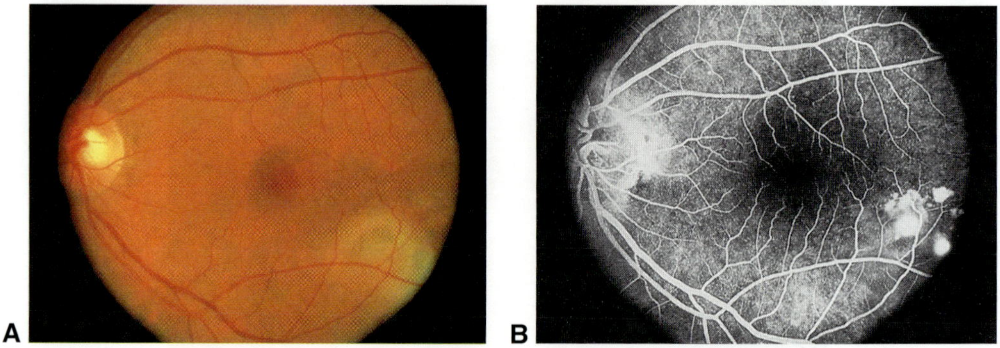

Figure 6-18 **A,** Fundus photograph of multifocal choroiditis in a patient with SLE. **B,** Fluorescein angiogram showing multifocal areas of hyperfluorescence. *(Courtesy of E. Mitchel Opremcak, MD.)*

with signs or symptoms suggestive of SLE or who have juvenile idiopathic arthritis, for which the test can help determine the level of risk for uveitis.

Treatment of ophthalmic disease in SLE is directed toward control of the underlying disease, using NSAIDs, corticosteroids, IMT, plasmapheresis, and systemic antihypertensive medications. Patients with severe vaso-occlusive disease or antiphospholipid antibodies may benefit from antiplatelet therapy or systemic anticoagulation. Ischemic complications, including proliferative retinopathy and vitreous hemorrhage, are managed with panretinal photocoagulation and vitrectomy surgery.

Some patients with SLE—even those without ophthalmic manifestations—may remain on glucocorticoids for extended periods and thus need monitoring for cataracts and glaucoma. In addition, hydroxychloroquine is often used to treat SLE because it can ameliorate skin, joint, and constitutional symptoms and prevent relapses; it may also help prevent nephritis and ANA-mediated thrombosis. Ophthalmologists should determine if SLE patients are receiving this drug so they can be sure patients and their primary care physicians are well informed about the ophthalmic risks and the need for regular screening examinations for retinal toxicity. For further information, see BCSC Section 12, *Retina and Vitreous.*

D'Cruz DP, Khamashta MA, Hughes GR. Systemic lupus erythematosus. *Lancet.* 2007;369(9561):587–596.

Jabs DA, Fine SL, Hochberg MC, Newman SA, Heiner GG, Stevens MB. Severe retinal vaso-occlusive disease in systemic lupus erythematosus. *Arch Ophthalmol.* 1986;104(4):558–563.

Marmor MF, Kellner U, Lai TY, Lyons JS, Mieler WF: American Academy of Ophthalmology. Revised recommendations on screening for chloroquine and hydroxychloroquine retinopathy. *Ophthalmology.* 2011;118(2):415–422.

Nguyen QD, Uy HS, Akpek EK, Harper SL, Zacks DN, Foster CS. Choroidopathy of systemic lupus erythematosus. *Lupus.* 2000;9(4):288–298.

Palejwala NV, Walia HS, Yeh S. Ocular manifestations of systemic lupus erythematosus: a review of the literature. *Autoimmune Dis.* 2012;2012:290898.

Polyarteritis nodosa

Polyarteritis nodosa (PAN) is an uncommon systemic vasculitis characterized by subacute or chronic, focal, episodic necrotizing inflammation of medium-sized and small muscular arteries. The disease presents in patients between the ages of 40 and 60 years and affects men 3 times more frequently than women; the annual incidence rate is approximately 0.7 per 100,000 individuals. Although there are no racial or geographic predisposing factors, 10% of patients test positive for hepatitis B surface antigen, implicating hepatitis B as an etiologic agent. Indeed, the demonstration of circulating immune complexes composed of hepatitis B antigen and antibodies to hepatitis B in vessel walls during the early stages of the disease strongly implicates immune-complex–mediated mechanisms in the pathogenesis of PAN.

Constitutional symptoms, including fatigue, fever, weight loss, and arthralgia, are present in up to 75% of patients; vasculitis-induced mononeuritis multiplex is the most common symptom, if not the initial presenting sign. (Mononeuritis multiplex is defined as nerve damage in 2 or more named nerves in separate parts of the body, such as a combination of wrist-drop due to infarction of the radial nerve and foot-drop due to peroneal nerve involvement.) Renal involvement, which is related to vasculitis, is common, as is secondary hypertension, which affects approximately one-third of patients. Gastrointestinal disease with small-bowel ischemia and infarction occurs less frequently but may lead to serious complications. Other systemic manifestations include cutaneous involvement (eg, subcutaneous nodules), purpura or Raynaud phenomenon, coronary arteritis, pericarditis, and hematologic abnormalities. CNS disease associated with PAN is rare. The American College of Rheumatology has developed specific criteria for the diagnosis of PAN (http://www.rheumatology.org/practice/clinical/classification/polyart.asp).

Ocular involvement is present in up to 20% of patients with PAN and arises as a consequence of the underlying vascular disease. In the posterior pole, involvement may manifest as hypertensive retinopathy replete with macular star formation, cotton-wool spots, and intraretinal hemorrhage in patients with renal disease; retinal arteriolar occlusive disease; or choroidal infarcts with exudative retinal detachment secondary to vasculitis involving the posterior ciliary arteries and choroidal vessels (Fig 6-19). Elschnig spots—focal areas of hyperpigmentation surrounded by hypopigmentation—may be observed in the posterior pole as a result of lobular choroidal ischemia (see BCSC Section 12, *Retina and Vitreous*). Neuro-ophthalmic manifestations include cranial nerve palsies, amaurosis fugax, homonymous hemianopia, Horner syndrome, and optic atrophy. Scleral inflammatory disease of all types, including necrotizing and posterior scleritis, has been reported. Peripheral ulcerative keratitis (PUK), typically accompanied by scleritis, may be the presenting manifestation of PAN.

Unlike granulomatosis with polyangiitis (discussed in the next section), PAN is not associated with antineutrophil cytoplasmic antibodies (ANCA). The 5-year mortality rate of untreated PAN is 90%. Although systemic corticosteroid use may reduce this rate to 50%, appropriate treatment mandates combination therapy with immunomodulatory

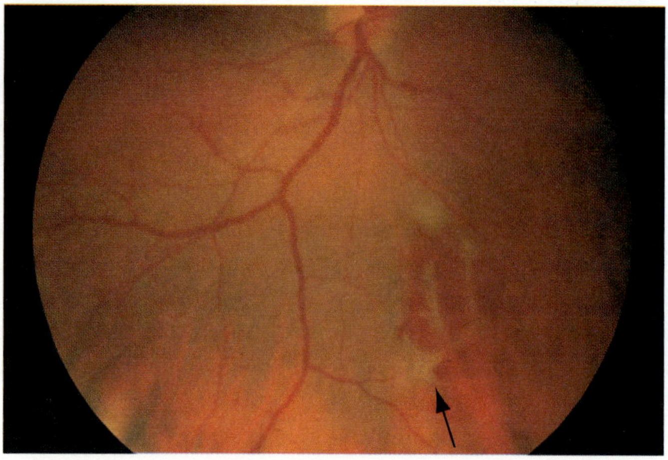

Figure 6-19 Polyarteritis nodosa: fundus photograph indicating retinal vasculitis associated with vascular sheathing *(arrow)* and intraretinal hemorrhage. *(Courtesy of E. Mitchel Opremcak, MD.)*

medications such as cyclophosphamide, which improves 5-year survival to 80% and may induce long-term remission of the disease. It is therefore important to consider PAN in the differential diagnosis of retinal vasculitis presenting in patients with multiple systemic effects in whom an underlying necrotizing vasculitis is suspected; appropriate diagnosis and management can be life-saving. Tissue biopsy confirms the diagnosis.

Gayraud M, Guillevin L, le Toumelin P, et al; French Vasculitis Study Group. Long-term followup of polyarteritis nodosa, microscopic polyangiitis, and Churg-Strauss syndrome: analysis of four prospective trials including 278 patients. *Arthritis Rheum.* 2001;44(3): 666–675.

Perez VL, Chavala SH, Ahmed M, et al. Ocular manifestations and concepts of systemic vasculitides. *Surv Ophthalmol.* 2004;49(4):399–418.

Rothschild PR, Pagnoux C, Seror R, Brézin AP, Delair E, Guillevin L. Ophthalmologic manifestations of systemic necrotizing vasculitides at diagnosis: a retrospective study of 1286 patients and review of the literature. *Semin Arthritis Rheum.* 2013;42(5):507–514.

Granulomatosis with polyangiitis

Granulomatosis with polyangiitis (GPA; formerly, Wegener granulomatosis), is a multisystem autoimmune disorder characterized by the classic triad of necrotizing granulomatous vasculitis of the upper and lower respiratory tract, focal segmental glomerulonephritis, and necrotizing vasculitis of small arteries and veins. Involvement of the paranasal sinuses is the most characteristic clinical feature of this disorder, followed by pulmonary and renal disease. Renal involvement may or may not be evident at presentation, but its early detection is important, as glomerulonephritis develops in up to 85% of patients during the course of the disease and carries significant mortality if left untreated. A limited form of this disease has also been described, consisting of granulomatous inflammation involving the respiratory tract without overt involvement of the kidneys.

Another entity believed to belong to the GPA spectrum is microscopic polyangiitis (MPA). Patients with MPA may have clinical features similar to those of GPA but lack granulomatous changes on biopsy. Patients with MPA are also more likely to have ANCA directed at myeloperoxidase (discussed further shortly). There is some degree of controversy in the rheumatologic literature about differentiating the 2 entities; however, ophthalmic involvement is much less common in MPA.

Patients with GPA may present with constitutional symptoms, sinusitis associated with bloody nasal discharge, pulmonary symptomatology, and arthritis. Dermatologic involvement is present in approximately one-half of patients, with purpura involving the lower extremities occurring most frequently; less common are ulcers and subcutaneous nodules. Nervous system involvement may occur in approximately one-third of patients with peripheral neuropathies; the most common are mononeuritis multiplex and less frequently observed are cranial neuropathies, seizures, stroke syndromes, and cerebral vasculitis.

Ocular or orbital involvement is found in 15% of patients at presentation and in up to 50% of patients during the course of the disease. Orbital involvement, one of the most frequently reported ocular findings, is usually secondary to contiguous extension of the granulomatous inflammatory process from the paranasal sinuses into the orbit. Orbital pseudotumor, distinct from the sinus inflammation; orbital cellulitis; and dacryocystitis may arise from the involved and secondarily infected nasal mucosa. Scleritis of any type, particularly diffuse anterior or necrotizing disease, with or without peripheral ulcerative keratitis, affects up to 40% of patients. Posterior scleritis has also been reported.

Approximately 10% of patients with GPA and ocular involvement have been reported to have an associated nonspecific, unilateral or bilateral anterior, intermediate, or posterior uveitis, with varying degrees of vitritis. Retinal involvement is relatively uncommon, occurring in up to 10% of patients. Retinal vascular manifestations range from relatively benign cotton-wool spots, with or without associated intraretinal hemorrhages, to more severe vaso-occlusive disease, including branch or central retinal artery or vein occlusion. Retinitis has been reported in up to 20% of patients; those with accompanying retinal vasculitis may incur retinal neovascularization, vitreous hemorrhage, and neovascular glaucoma (Fig 6-20). Orbital involvement can lead to compressive ischemic optic neuropathy. Vision loss in GPA may occur in up to 40% of patients, especially among those with longstanding or inadequately treated disease.

Tissue biopsy establishes the histologic diagnosis; chest x-ray may disclose nodular, diffuse, or cavitary lesions; and laboratory evaluation may note proteinuria or hematuria, elevated erythrocyte sedimentation rate (ESR) and C-reactive protein level as well as the presence of ANCA. ANCA are antibodies directed against cytoplasmic azurophilic granules of neutrophils and monocytes that are specific markers for a group of related systemic vasculitides, including GPA, MPA, eosinophilic granulomatosis with polyangiitis (Churg-Strauss syndrome), renal limited vasculitis, and pauci-immunoglomerulonephritis. Two main classes of ANCA have been described according to their immunofluorescence staining patterns. The cytoplasmic, or c-ANCA, pattern is both sensitive and specific for GPA and is present in up to 95% of patients; proteinase 3 is the most common target antigen (referred to as PR3-ANCA). The perinuclear, or p-ANCA, pattern is associated with MPA, renal limited vasculitis, and pauci-immunoglomerulonephritis. Myeloperoxidase is the

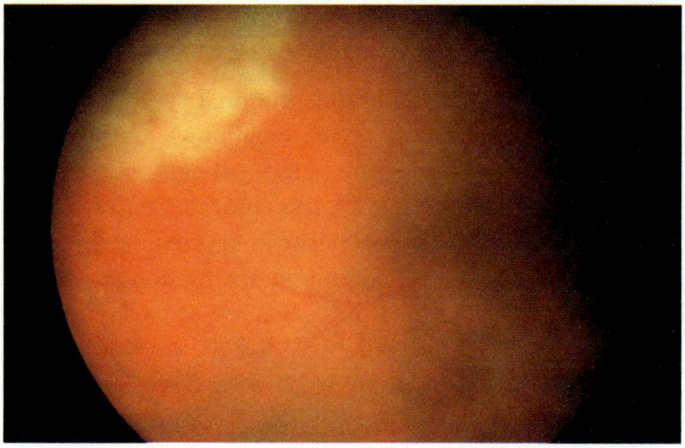

Figure 6-20 Granulomatosis with polyangiitis: fundus photograph of retinitis. *(Courtesy of E. Mitchel Opremcak, MD.)*

most common antigenic target (MPO-ANCA). Standardized testing for ANCA should include both immunofluorescence testing for c- and p-ANCA and specific antibody testing for PR3-ANCA and MPO-ANCA; the latter 2 are most specific.

As for PAN, appropriate treatment of GPA mandates combination therapy with oral corticosteroids and IMT medications such as rituximab and cyclophosphamide. Without therapy, the 1-year mortality rate is 80%. However, 93% of patients treated with cyclophosphamide and corticosteroids successfully achieve remission with resolution of ocular manifestations. As with PAN, ophthalmologists must be intimately familiar with GPA, as ocular inflammatory manifestations are frequently present, and timely diagnosis and treatment are essential in reducing not only ocular morbidity but also patient mortality.

Kubal AA, Perez VL. Ocular manifestations of ANCA-associated vasculitis. *Rheum Dis Clin North Am.* 2010;36(3):573–586.

Pakrou N, Selva D, Leibovitch I. Wegener's granulomatosis: ophthalmic manifestations and management. *Semin Arthritis Rheum.* 2006;35(5):284–292.

Susac Syndrome

Susac syndrome (also known as *SICRET syndrome,* for *s*mall *i*nfarctions of *c*ochlear, *r*etinal, and *e*ncephalic *t*issue) is a rare entity, initially reported in 1979 by Susac and colleagues; it consists of the clinically observed triad of encephalopathy, hearing loss, and retinal artery branch occlusions. The syndrome occurs mostly in young women but has been noted in patients aged 16–58 years. Differential diagnosis at presentation includes MS, herpetic encephalitis, acute disseminated encephalomyelitis, and Behçet disease. However, ocular findings are highly specific and allow prompt diagnostic confirmation with subsequent therapeutic adjustments. Ophthalmoscopy shows diffuse or localized narrowing of retinal arteries with a "boxcar" segmentation of the blood column at the level of peripheral retinal arteries. Vitreous haze or cells are absent. Retinal FA discloses focal nonperfused retinal arterioles with hyperfluorescent walls (Fig 6-21). There is

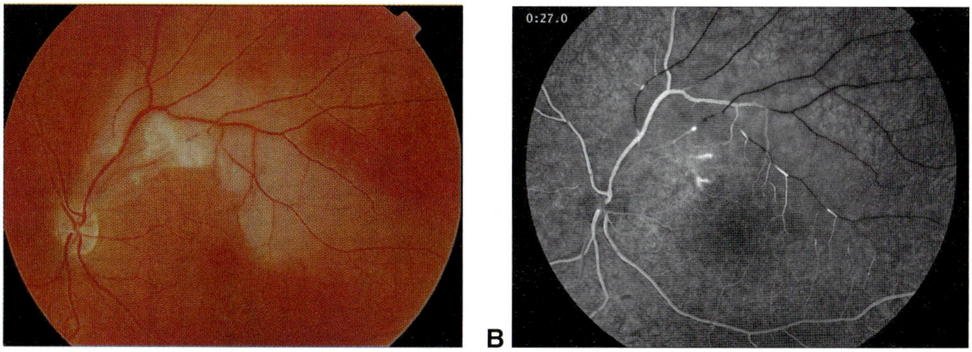

A B

Figure 6-21 Susac syndrome. **A,** Color fundus photograph revealing an area of intraretinal whitening corresponding to a supratemporal branch artery occlusion in the left eye. **B,** Fluorescein angiogram showing a supratemporal branch artery occlusion with multiple areas of segmental staining well away from sites of bifurcation. *(Courtesy of Albert T. Vitale, MD.)*

usually no evidence of embolic material or inflammatory reactions around the vessels. Magnetic resonance imaging (MRI) is another useful diagnostic tool and shows multifocal supratentorial white matter lesions; the corpus callosum may be involved. Audiometry should be performed in any patient being evaluated for this entity; sensorineural hearing loss is a common finding. Treatment remains controversial and includes high-dose intravenous corticosteroids, anticoagulants, and IMT. The course of Susac syndrome is not always self-limiting, and isolated retinal arteriolar involvement may occur as a very late manifestation.

Dörr J, Krautwald S, Wildemann B, et al. Characteristics of Susac syndrome: a review of all reported cases. *Nat Rev Neurol.* 2013;9(6):307–316.

Inflammatory Chorioretinopathies of Unknown Etiology

The inflammatory chorioretinopathies, or white dot syndromes, are a heterogeneous group of inflammatory disorders with overlapping clinical features that share in common the presence of discrete, multiple, well-circumscribed, yellow-white lesions at the level of the retina, outer retina, RPE, choriocapillaris, and/or choroid during some phase of their course. The white dot syndromes consist of the predominantly noninfectious ocular syndromes listed in Table 6-2. Their differential diagnosis includes systemic and ocular infectious entities such as syphilis, diffuse unilateral subacute neuroretinitis (DUSN), and ocular histoplasmosis syndrome (OHS), as well as noninfectious entities such as sarcoidosis, sympathetic ophthalmia, Vogt-Koyanagi-Harada (VKH) syndrome, and intraocular lymphoma. Common presenting symptoms include photopsias, blurred vision, nyctalopia, floaters, and visual field loss contiguous with the blind spot. In many cases, a prodromal viral syndrome can be identified. Bilateral involvement, albeit asymmetrically (with the exception of multiple evanescent white dot syndrome [MEWDS]), is the rule. Other than patients with birdshot uveitis or serpiginous choroiditis, the majority of individuals are younger than 50 years of age. A female predominance is observed in patients with MEWDS, birdshot uveitis, multifocal choroiditis and panuveitis, punctate inner choroiditis (PIC), subretinal fibrosis and uveitis syndrome, and acute zonal occult outer retinopathy.

The etiology of the white dot syndromes is unknown. Some investigators have postulated an infectious cause; others have suggested an autoimmune/inflammatory pathogenesis arising in individuals with common non–disease-specific genetics, triggered by some exogenous agent. An increased prevalence of systemic autoimmunity both in patients with white dot syndromes and their first- and second-degree relatives suggests that inflammatory chorioretinopathies may occur in families with inherited immune dysregulation that predisposes to autoimmunity. Whether the white dot syndromes represent a clinical spectrum of a single disease entity or are each discrete diseases awaits identification of the underlying mechanisms. Although they have similarities, the white dot syndromes can be differentiated by their variable lesion morphology and evolution, distinct natural histories, and appearance with multimodal imaging. This differentiation has important implications with respect to disease-specific treatments and visual prognosis.

Table 6-2 Inflammatory Chorioretinopathies

	Birdshot Uveitis	APMPPE	Serpiginous Choroiditis	MCP	PIC	SFU	MEWDS	ARPE	AZOOR
Age, y	Older (30–70)	Young (20–50)	Young, middle-age (20–60)	Young (9–69)	Young (18–40)	Young (14–34)	Young (10–47)	Young (16–40)	Young (13–63)
Sex	F>M	M=F	M=F	F (3:1)	F (90%)	F (>95%)	F (3:1)	M=F	F (3:1)
Laterality	Bilateral	Bilateral	Bilateral, asymmetric	Bilateral	Bilateral	Asymmetric	Unilateral	Unilateral (75%)	Unilateral (24%), bilateral (76%)
Systemic associations	80%–98% HLA-A29+, lymphocyte proliferation to retinal S-antigen	Viral prodrome, cerebrovasculitis, CSF abnormalities	HLA-B7, rule out TB-associated disease	None	None	None	Viral prodrome (50%)	None	Systemic autoimmune disease (28%)
Onset	Insidious	Acute	Variable	Insidious	Acute	Insidious	Acute	Acute	Insidious
Course	Chronic, recurrent	Self-limited	Chronic, recurrent	Chronic, recurrent	Self-limited	Chronic, recurrent	Self-limited	Self-limited	Chronic, recurrent (31%)
Symptoms	Blurred vision, floaters, photopsias, disturbed night and color vision	Blurred vision, scotomata, photopsias	Blurred vision, scotomata	Blurred vision, floaters, photopsias, metamorphopsia, scotomata	Paracentral scotomata, photopsias, metamorphopsia	Blurred vision, decreased vision	Blurred or decreased vision, scotomata, photopsias	Central metamorphopsia, scotomata	Photopsias, scotomata
Examination	Vitritis; ovoid, creamy, white-yellow, postequatorial lesions (50–1500 μm), do not pigment	Multifocal, flat, gray-white lesions, 1–2 disc areas, outer retina/RPE with evolving pigmentation	Geographic, yellow-gray, peripapillary, macular chorioretinal lesions with centrifugal extension; activity at leading, peripheral edge with RPE/choriocapillaris atrophy in its wake	Myopia, anterior uveitis (50%), vitritis (100%), active white-yellow chorioretinal lesions (50–200 μm) evolving to punched-out scars	Myopia, vitritis absent, white-yellow chorioretinal lesions	Moderate vitritis, 50–500 μm yellow-white lesions posterior pole to mid-periphery, RPE, hypertrophy, atrophy, large stellate zones of subretinal fibrosis	Myopia; mild anterior uveitis; vitritis; small white-orange, evanescent, perifoveal dots (100–200 μm) outer retina/RPE; macular granularity	Small, hyperpigmented lesions with yellow halo (100–200 μm), unassociated vitritis	Initially normal to subtle RPE changes, late pigment migration, focal perivenous sheathing
Structural complications	Retinal vasculitis, disc edema, CME, CNVM (6%)	Disc edema, pigment alterations	CNVM (25%), RPE mottling, scarring, loss of choriocapillaris	Optic disc edema, peripapillary pigment changes, CME (14%–44%), CNVM (33%)	CNVM (17%–40%), serous detachment over confluent lesions	Neurosensory retinal detachment, CME, CNVM	Disc edema, venous sheathing	None	RPE mottling, occasional CME

(Continued)

Table 6-2 *(continued)*

	Birdshot Uveitis	APMPPE	Serpiginous Choroiditis	MCP	PIC	SFU	MEWDS	ARPE	AZOOR
Fluorescein angiography (FA)	Early hypofluorescence vs silence, subtle late stain; leakage from disc, vessels, CME; delayed retinal circulation time	Acute lesions: early blockage, late staining; late window defects	Early hypofluorescence, late staining/leak of active border, leakage in presence of CNVM	Early blockage, late staining of lesions, leakage from CME, CNVM	Early blockage or hyperfluorescence, variable late leakage/staining of acute lesions, leakage in presence of CME, CNVM	Multiple areas of alternating hypo- and hyperfluorescence; early, late staining	Early punctate hyperfluorescence, wreathlike configuration, late staining of lesions, optic nerve	Early hyperfluorescence with surrounding halo of hyperfluorescence and late staining	In acute stage, normal with increased retinal circulation time; in late stage, diffuse hyperfluorescence, RPE atrophy
Indocyanine green angiography (ICG)	Corresponding hypofluorescent lesions more numerous than on exam, FA	Hypofluorescent spots corresponding to those seen on exam, FA	Early hypofluorescence, late staining, more widespread extent than seen on exam, FA	Multiple hypofluorescent lesions, confluence around optic nerve, more numerous than on exam, FA	Multiple hypofluorescent, peripapillary, posterior pole lesions, corresponding to those seen on exam, FA	Hypofluorescent lesions in one report	Multiple hypofluorescent spots, more numerous than on exam, FA	Early- and mid-phase patchy macular hyperfluorescence; late hyperfluorescent halo in the macula	Hypofluorescence in atrophic areas with late leakage in subacute areas
Fundus autofluorescence (FAF)	Hypoautofluorescent spots more numerous than clinically apparent lesions; placoid macular hypoautofluorescence with central vision loss	Hyperautofluorescent areas correspond to FA blockage; hypoautofluorescent areas correspond to areas of staining; FAF findings lag FA findings	Hyperfluorescent active lesions; hypofluorescent regressed lesions	Acute lesions variably hyper- to hypoautofluorescent; more may be seen with FAF than clinically	Similar to MCP	NI	Hyperfluorescent spots corresponding to lesions on clinical exam	NI	Lesions may have central hypoautofluorescence with peripheral hyperautofluorescence
Optical coherence tomography (OCT)	Macular edema; loss of inner/outer segment line (ellipsoid zone); suprachoroidal fluid	Outer retinal hyperreflectivity with intra- and subretinal fluid	Outer retinal hyperreflectivity in active lesions; retinal and RPE atrophy in regressed lesions	Sub-RPE deposits with overlying outer retinal disruption	Similar to MCP	Variable retinal edema; subretinal fluid and subretinal fibrosis	Abnormal reflectivity of the inner/outer segment line	Transient disruption of the inner/outer segment line (ellipsoid zone) and of the RPE inner band	Loss of the inner/outer segment line (ellipsoid zone)

	Birdshot Uveitis	APMPPE	Serpiginous Choroiditis	MCP	PIC	SFU	MEWDS	ARPE	AZOOR
Electrophysiology, visual fields (VF)	ERG: abnormal rod and cone responses	EOG: variably abnormal	ERG: normal	ERG: abnormal, extinguished responses	ERG: normal; VF: enlargement of blind spot (41%)	VF, ERG, and EOG markedly attenuated	ERG: diminished a wave, early receptor potentials (reversible); VF: enlarged blind spot, paracentral scotomata	ERG: normal EOG: abnormal	ERG, mfERG: abnormal; VF: temporal, superior defects, enlarged blind spot
Visual prognosis	Guarded without treatment	Good	Guarded	Guarded	Good in absence of CNVM	Guarded	Excellent	Excellent	Guarded
Treatment	Systemic or local corticosteroids, IMT	Observation; systemic corticosteroids with CNS involvement	Systemic or local corticosteroids, IMT. Anti-VEGF agents with or without laser for CNVM	Systemic or local corticosteroids, IMT. Anti-VEGF agents with or without laser for CNVM	Observation; systemic or local corticosteroids. Anti-VEGF agents with or without laser for CNVM	Corticosteroids for CME, IMT of equivocal efficacy long term	Observation	None	Corticosteroids, IMT, antivirals of equivocal efficacy

APMPPE = acute posterior multifocal placoid pigment epitheliopathy; ARPE = acute retinal pigment epitheliitis; AZOOR = acute zonal occult outer retinopathy; CME = cystoid macular edema; CNVM = choroidal neovascular membrane; CNS = central nervous system; EOG = electro-oculogram; ERG = electroretinogram; IMT = immunomodulatory therapy; MCP = multifocal choroiditis and panuveitis syndrome; MEWDS = multiple evanescent white dot syndrome; mfERG = multifocal electroretinogram; NI = no information; PIC = punctate inner choroiditis; RPE = retinal pigment epithelium; SFU = subretinal fibrosis and uveitis syndrome; TB = tuberculosis; VEGF = vascular endothelial growth factor.

Abu-Yaghi NE, Hartono SP, Hodge DO, Pulido JS, Bakri SJ. White dot syndromes: a 20-year study of incidence, clinical features, and outcomes. *Ocul Immunol Inflamm.* 2011;19(6):426–430.

Gass JD. Are acute zonal occult outer retinopathy and the white spot syndromes (AZOOR complex) specific autoimmune diseases? *Am J Ophthalmol.* 2003;135(3):380–381.

Jampol LM, Becker KG. White spot syndromes of the retina: a hypothesis based on the common genetic hypothesis of autoimmune/inflammatory disease. *Am J Ophthalmol.* 2003;135(3):376–379.

Pearlman RB, Golchet PR, Feldmann MG, et al. Increased prevalence of autoimmunity in patients with white spot syndromes and their family members. *Arch Ophthalmol.* 2009; 127(7):869–874.

Quillen DA, Davis JB, Gottlieb JL, et al. The white dot syndromes. *Am J Ophthalmol.* 2004; 137(3):538–550.

Birdshot uveitis

Birdshot uveitis (also known as *birdshot retinochoroidopathy, birdshot chorioretinopathy,* and *vitiliginous chorioretinitis*) is an uncommon disease presenting predominantly in white women of northern European descent past the fourth decade of life. Although no consistent systemic disease association has been identified, birdshot uveitis is highly correlated with the HLA-A29 gene, with a sensitivity of 96% and a specificity of 93%. The presence of the haplotype confers considerable increased relative risk (224-fold) for the development of this disease. HLA-A29 is confirmatory rather than diagnostic, as 7% of the general population carries this haplotype, and in the absence of characteristic clinical features, an alternative diagnosis should be considered.

Presenting symptoms include blurred vision, floaters, nyctalopia, and disturbance of color vision. Visual complaints can be out of proportion to the measured Snellen visual acuity, reflecting the diffuse retinal dysfunction that occurs in this entity. Patients may also report unusual peripheral visual phenomena, such as pinwheels, sparkles, or flickering lights, and these symptoms may be indicators of subtle disease activity. Anterior segment inflammation may be minimal or lacking; however, varying degrees of vitritis are commonly noted. Funduscopy reveals characteristic multifocal, hypopigmented, ovoid, cream-colored lesions (50–1500 μm) at the level of the choroid and RPE in the postequatorial fundus; typically these lesions show a nasal and radial distribution, emanating from the optic nerve, and frequently they follow the underlying choroidal vessels (Fig 6-22). The lesions do not become pigmented over time and are best appreciated by indirect ophthalmoscopy. The characteristic lesions may not be readily apparent at first, and the disorder may be misdiagnosed initially as idiopathic intermediate or posterior uveitis. Retinal vasculitis, CME, and optic nerve head inflammation are important components of active disease. Late complications include optic atrophy, epiretinal membrane (ERM) formation, and, rarely, CNV.

Fluorescein angiography reveals inconsistent findings depending on age, lesions, and phase of study. Although early birdshot uveitis lesions may show initial hypofluorescence with subtle late staining, in general, FA does not typically highlight the lesions themselves but rather is useful in identifying more subtle indices of active inflammation such as retinal vasculitis, CME, and optic nerve head leakage (Figs 6-23, 6-24).

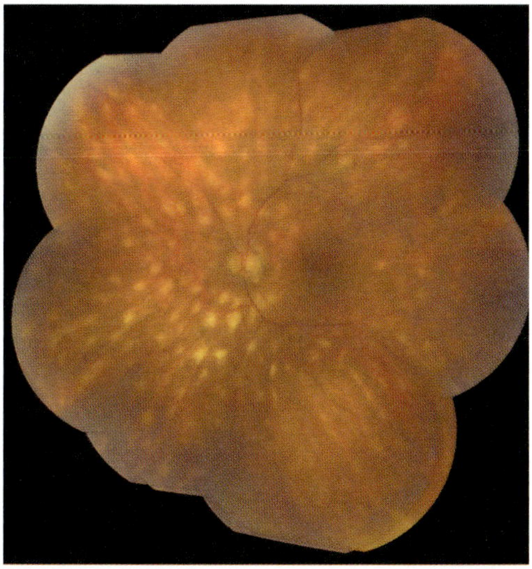

Figure 6-22 Birdshot uveitis: fundus photograph showing multiple postequatorial, cream-colored ovoid lesions. *(Courtesy of H. Nida Sen, MD.)*

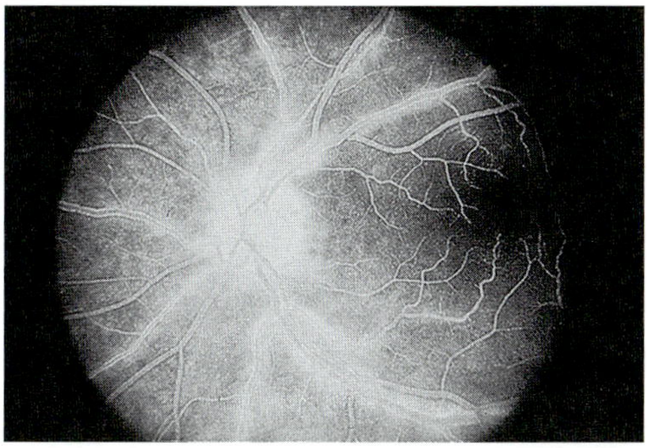

Figure 6-23 Birdshot uveitis: fluorescein angiogram showing diffuse retinal phlebitis. *(Courtesy of E. Mitchel Opremcak, MD.)*

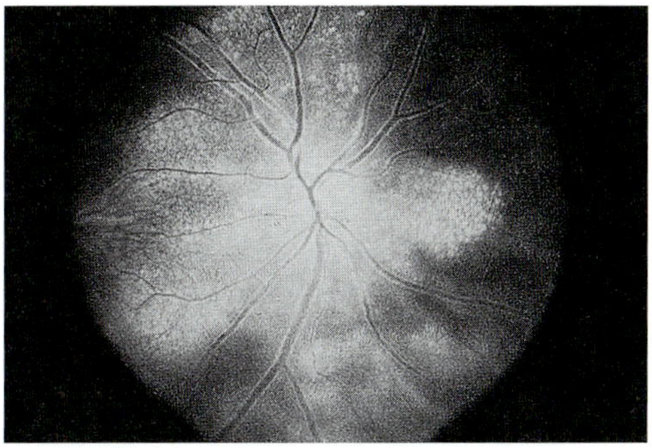

Figure 6-24 Birdshot uveitis: fluorescein angiogram showing cystoid retinal edema. *(Courtesy of E. Mitchel Opremcak, MD.)*

Late hypopigmented lesions typically do not show transmission defects, implying loss of pigment concurrent with loss of choriocapillaris. Indocyanine green (ICG) angiography discloses multiple hypofluorescent spots, which are typically more numerous than those apparent on clinical examination or FA (Fig 6-25). Fundus autofluorescence (FAF) imaging reveals hypoautofluorescence in areas of RPE atrophy that are more numerous and not uniformly correspondent with the birdshot uveitis lesions, suggesting that the choroid and RPE may be affected independently. Placoid macular hypoautofluorescence may be an important predictor of central vision loss (Fig 6-26). OCT imaging can show macular edema, if present. It can also demonstrate patchy or diffuse loss of photoreceptors (inner/outer segment line or ellipsoid zone) and macular thinning, especially with long-standing disease.

Important differential diagnostic considerations include pars planitis, VKH syndrome, sympathetic ophthalmia, OHS, intraocular lymphoma, and especially sarcoidosis,

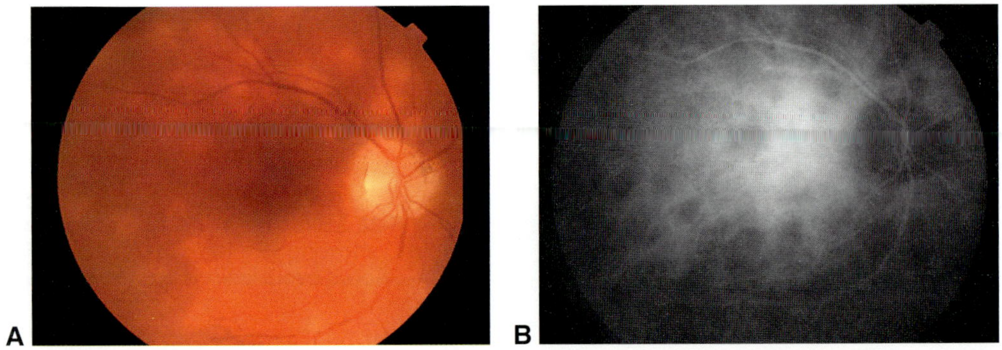

Figure 6-25 Birdshot uveitis: fundus photograph **(A)** and indocyanine green angiogram **(B)** showing numerous midphase hypofluorescent spots corresponding to fundus lesions. *(Courtesy of Albert T. Vitale, MD.)*

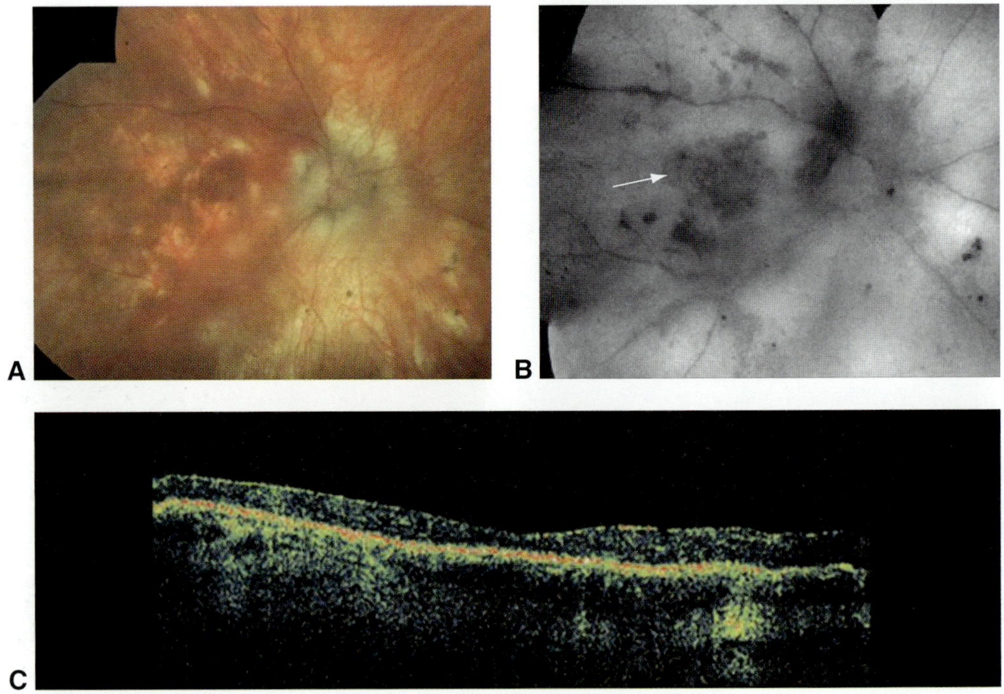

Figure 6-26 Birdshot uveitis. **A,** Color fundus photograph showing multifocal hypopigmented spots within the macula and outside the arcades. **B,** Autofluorescence photograph showing placoid hypoautofluorescence in the central macula *(arrow)*. **C,** Optical coherence tomography (OCT) image showing foveal thinning. *(Reprinted with permission from Koizumi H, Pozzoni MC, Spaide RF. Fundus autofluorescence in birdshot chorioretinopathy.* Ophthalmology. *2008:115(5):e15–20.)*

which may present with chorioretinal lesions of similar morphology and distribution as those present in birdshot uveitis.

It is crucial for clinicians to recognize that this entity can be insidious and understand that simply monitoring visual acuity and clinical examination findings is insufficient to protect patients from vision loss. Progressive worsening of the visual field and abnormal electroretinogram (ERG) results are commonly found with extended follow-up, suggesting a more diffuse retinal dysfunction not fully explained by the presence of CME or other structural abnormality. For this reason, full-field ERGs (with attention to the 30-Hz flicker implicit time and scotopic b-wave amplitudes) as well as Goldmann and automated visual field (30-2 with attention to the mean deviation) testing are more useful parameters for monitoring disease course and response to therapy than are changes in funduscopic examination results or visual acuity.

A subset of patients with birdshot uveitis may have self-limited disease and do well without treatment. However, there is no way to determine in advance which patients will have disease progression and which will not, so any patient who is not treated should be monitored closely using the modalities discussed above. It turns out that the majority of patients do require ongoing treatment. Although older studies demonstrated high rates of vision loss in patients who were either not treated or treated in a limited or intermittent fashion, a more recent study indicates that up to 88% of patients can maintain vision with aggressive, long-term control of inflammation.

Treatment consists of the initial administration of systemic corticosteroids, with early introduction of corticosteroid-sparing IMT. Birdshot uveitis is typically incompletely responsive to corticosteroids alone, and extended treatment is anticipated in most patients given the chronic nature of the disease. Corticosteroid-sparing immunomodulators include low-dose cyclosporine (2–5 mg/kg/day), mycophenolate mofetil, azathioprine, methotrexate, TNF-α inhibitors, and intravenous polyclonal immunoglobulin. This approach is effective in reducing intraocular inflammation, inflammatory recurrences, and the risk of developing CME, as well as in preserving visual acuity. Periocular or intravitreal corticosteroid injections are useful as adjunctive therapy in managing CME and inflammatory recurrences. The intravitreal fluocinolone acetonide implant is an option for patients who cannot tolerate systemic therapy or in whom systemic therapy has failed.

Gordon LK, Monnet D, Holland GN, Brézin AP, Yu F, Levinson RD. Longitudinal cohort study of patients with birdshot chorioretinopathy. IV. Visual field results at baseline. *Am J Ophthalmol.* 2007;144(6):829–837.

Holder GE, Robson AG, Pavesio C, Graham EM. Electrophysiological characterisation and monitoring in the management of birdshot chorioretinopathy. *Br J Ophthalmol.* 2005;89(6):709–718.

Kiss S, Ahmed M, Letko E, Foster CS. Long-term follow-up of patients with birdshot retinochoroidopathy treated with corticosteroid-sparing systemic immunomodulatory therapy. *Ophthalmology.* 2005;112(6):1066–1071.

Menezo V, Taylor SR. Birdshot uveitis: current and emerging treatment options. *Clin Ophthalmol.* 2014;8:73–81.

Piffer AL, Boissonnot M, Gobert F, et al. Relevance of wide-field autofluorescence imaging in birdshot retinochoroidopathy: descriptive analysis of 76 eyes. *Acta Ophthalmol.* 2014;92(6):e463–469.

Thorne JE, Jabs DA, Peters GB, Hair D, Dunn JP, Kempen JH. Birdshot retinochoroidopathy: ocular complications and visual impairment. *Am J Ophthalmol.* 2005;140(1):45–51.

Tomkins-Netzer O, Taylor SR, Lightman S. Long-term clinical and anatomic outcome of birdshot chorioretinopathy. *JAMA Ophthalmol.* 2014;132(1):57–62.

Acute posterior multifocal placoid pigment epitheliopathy

Acute posterior multifocal placoid pigment epitheliopathy (APMPPE), an uncommon condition presenting in otherwise healthy young adults, typically occurs with an influenza-like illness (50%) and affects men and women equally. A genetic predisposition may be present, given the association of HLA-B7 and HLA-DR2 with the development of this entity. A number of noninfectious systemic conditions have been reported in connection with APMPPE, including erythema nodosum, GPA, PAN, cerebral vasculitis, scleritis and episcleritis, sarcoidosis, and ulcerative colitis. Infectious conditions including group A streptococcal and adenovirus type 5 infections, tuberculosis, Lyme disease, and mumps have also been associated with APMPPE, as has hepatitis B vaccination. These diverse disease associations reinforce the concept that APMPPE is an immune-driven vascular alteration. Of greatest concern is the rare but potentially life-threatening association of APMPPE with cerebral vasculitis. Patients presenting with symptoms suggestive of CNS disease should undergo urgent neurologic evaluation.

Patients typically present with a sudden onset of vision loss associated with central and paracentral scotomata; the fellow eye becomes involved within days to weeks. Photopsias may precede loss of vision. There is minimal or no anterior segment inflammation; vitritis may be present but is usually mild. Funduscopic findings include multiple large, flat, yellow-white placoid lesions at the level of the RPE that vary in size from 1 to 2 disc areas and are located throughout the posterior pole to the equator (Fig 6-27). New peripheral lesions may appear in a linear or radial array over the next 3 weeks. Papillitis may be observed, but CME is uncommon. Atypical findings include retinal vasculitis, retinal vascular occlusive disease, retinal neovascularization, and exudative retinal detachment. The lesions resolve over a period of 2–6 weeks, leaving a permanent, well-defined alteration in the RPE consisting of alternating areas of depigmentation and pigment clumping. Rapid evolution of the pigmentary changes, often over days, is a typical feature of the disease.

The diagnosis of APMPPE is based on the characteristic clinical presentation and FA findings during the acute phase of the disease: early hypofluorescent lesions corresponding to but typically more numerous than those apparent on funduscopy and late hyperfluorescent staining (Fig 6-28). Subacute lesions may show increased central hyperfluorescence with late staining; with resolution, transmission defects are typically

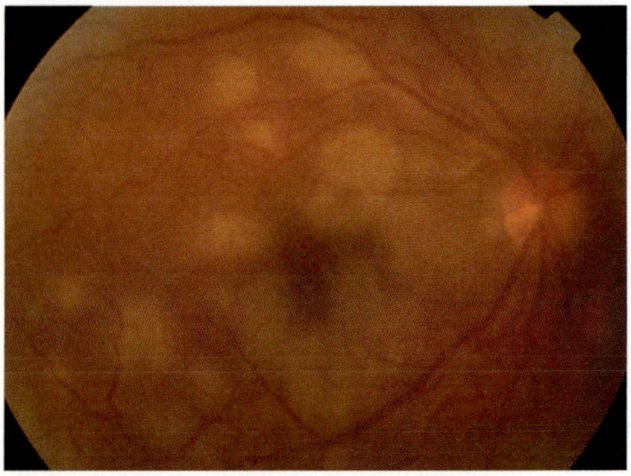

Figure 6-27 Acute posterior multifocal placoid pigment epitheliopathy (APMPPE): fundus photograph showing multifocal, placoid lesions in the macula. *(Courtesy of Albert T. Vitale, MD.)*

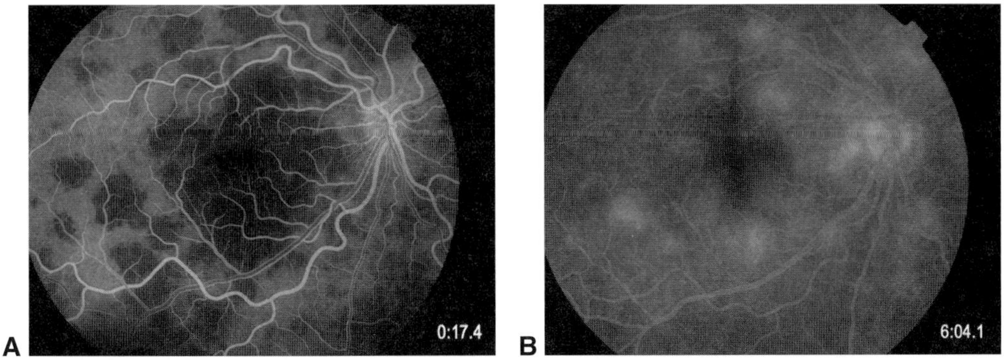

Figure 6-28 Fluorescein angiography image from a patient with APMPPE. **A,** Early blockage of choroidal circulation. **B,** Late-phase staining. *(Courtesy of Albert T. Vitale, MD.)*

observed. ICG angiography reveals choroidal hypofluorescence with hypervisualization of the underlying choroidal vessels in both the acute and inactive stages of the disease; these lesions become smaller in the inactive stages (Fig 6-29). Choroidal perfusion abnormalities revealed early on FA and ICG angiography are more numerous than the overlying placoid lesions. Abnormalities noted on FAF imaging lag the appearance of these lesions, are fewer in number, and lack the perfusion changes observed during angiography; RPE alterations observed during recovery appear well after the choroid is affected. Whether the lesions of APMPPE are due primarily to involvement of the RPE or represent choroidal/choriocapillary perfusion abnormalities with secondary involvement of the RPE and photoreceptors remains controversial; however, taken together, the FA, ICG, and FAF imaging findings suggest a primary choroidal process. OCT of acute lesions demonstrates hyperreflectivity of the outer retinal layers; subretinal or intraretinal fluid may also be present (Fig 6-30). As the lesions resolve, outer retinal and photoreceptor loss can be observed.

An important differential diagnostic consideration—in addition to choroidal metastasis, viral retinitis, sarcoidosis, VKH syndrome, and pneumocystis choroiditis—is serpiginous choroiditis. APMPPE is an acute, usually nonrecurring disease, whereas serpiginous choroiditis is insidious and progressive.

In the majority of patients with APMPPE, visual acuity returns to 20/40 or better within 6 months, although 20% are left with residual visual dysfunction. Risk factors for loss of vision include foveal involvement at presentation, older age at presentation,

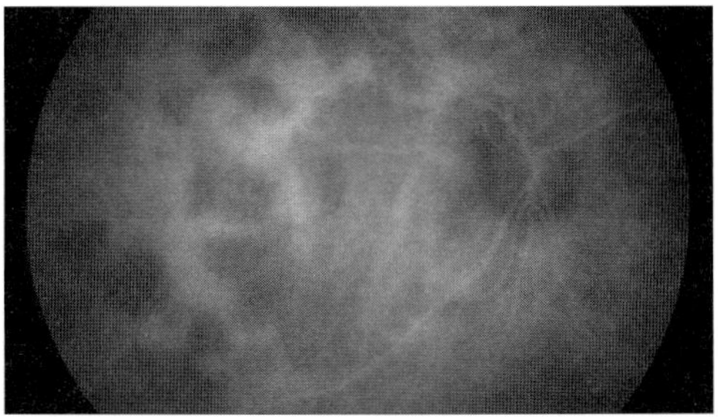

Figure 6-29 Indocyanine green angiography image from a patient with APMPPE showing multiple midphase hypofluorescent spots. *(Courtesy of Albert T. Vitale, MD.)*

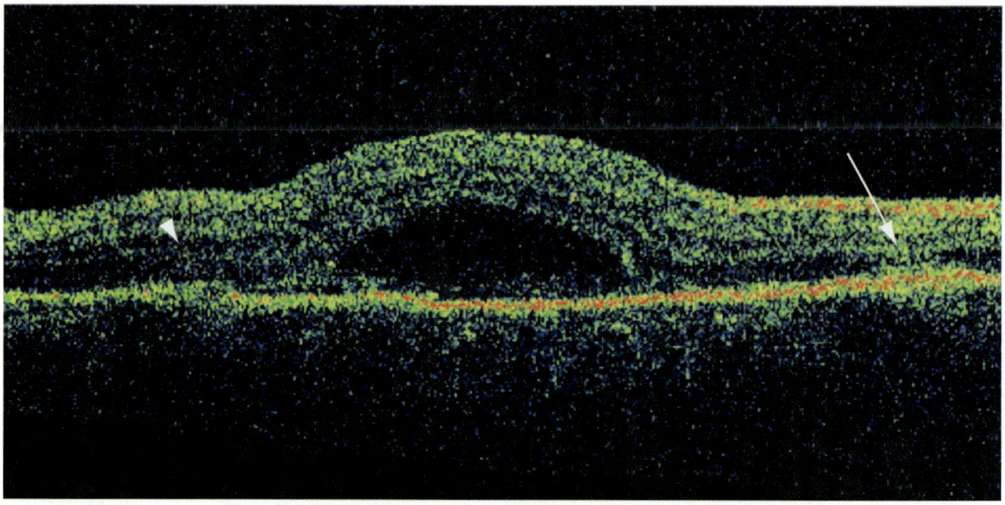

Figure 6-30 OCT scan of APMPPE showing multiple findings, including disruption of the outer retina and RPE *(arrowhead),* a collection of sub- and outer-retinal fluid centrally, and hyperreflectivity of the outer retina and RPE *(arrow). (Courtesy of Debra A. Goldstein, MD.)*

unilateral disease, a longer interval between initial and fellow eye involvement, and recurrence. No convincing data suggest that treatment with systemic corticosteroids is beneficial in altering the visual outcome, although some authorities advocate such treatment in patients presenting with extensive macular involvement in an effort to limit subsequent RPE derangement of the foveal center, and in individuals with an associated CNS vasculitis.

An uncommon variant termed *relentless placoid chorioretinitis* or *ampiginous choroiditis* has features of both serpiginous choroiditis and APMPPE. Men or women between the second and sixth decades of life present with floaters, photopsia, paracentral scotomata, and decreased vision, as well as variable degrees of anterior segment inflammation and vitritis. The acute retinal lesions are similar to those of APMPPE or serpiginous choroiditis, both clinically and angiographically, but the clinical course is atypical for both entities. Patients have numerous posterior and peripheral lesions predating or occurring simultaneously with macular involvement. Acute lesions heal over a period of weeks, with resultant chorioretinal atrophy. Older pigmented areas are observed together with new, active, white placoid lesions that are not necessarily extensions of previous areas of activity. Prolonged periods of disease activity occur, with the appearance of numerous (>50) multifocal lesions scattered throughout the fundus. Relapses are common, and new lesions and the growth of subacute lesions may occur for up to 2 years after the initial presentation. FA demonstrates early hypofluorescence and late staining of these lesions. Although macular involvement can result in vision loss, metamorphopsia, or scotomata, visual acuity is preserved in most patients upon healing of the lesions (Fig 6-31). The precise roles for systemic steroids, antiviral drugs, and IMT in the treatment of relentless placoid chorioretinitis are incompletely understood. Systemic steroids are commonly employed, but the disease may recur despite their use. It is important to rule out the presence of tuberculosis-associated serpiginous-like choroiditis (see discussion in the next

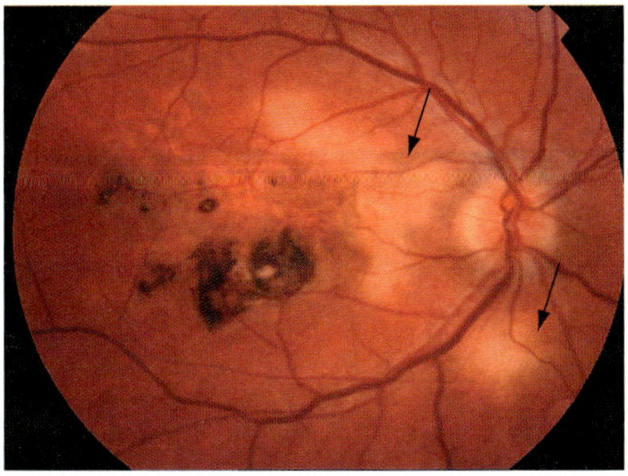

Figure 6-31 Relentless placoid chorioretinitis: fundus photograph showing retinal pigment epithelial hyperpigmentation and atrophy in the central macula in areas of previous inflammation, with new, yellow-white foci of active disease temporal and inferior to the optic nerve *(arrows)*. *(Courtesy of Albert T. Vitale, MD.)*

section). For more information about APMPPE and variants, see the American Academy of Ophthalmology lecture by Kaplan included in the following reference list.

Fiore T, Iaccheri B, Androudi S, et al. Acute posterior multifocal placoid pigment epitheliopathy: outcome and visual prognosis. *Retina.* 2009;29(7):994–1001.

Jones BE, Jampol LM, Yannuzzi LA, et al. Relentless placoid chorioretinitis: a new entity or an unusual variant of serpiginous chorioretinitis? *Arch Ophthalmol.* 2000;118(7):931–938.

Kaplan HJ. APMPPE and "ampiginous choroiditis": how should these be treated? [American Academy of Ophthalmology Annual Meeting Video Program]. San Francisco: American Academy of Ophthalmology; 2012. Available at http://one.aao.org/annual-meeting-video/apmppe-ampiginous-choroiditis-how-should-these-be. Accessed October 27, 2014.

Pagliarini S, Piguet B, Ffytche TJ, Bird AC. Foveal involvement and lack of visual recovery in APMPPE associated with uncommon features. *Eye (Lond).* 1995;9(pt 1):42–47.

Steiner S, Goldstein DA. Imaging in the diagnosis and management of APMPPE. *Int Ophthalmol Clin.* 2012;52(4):211–219.

Serpiginous choroiditis

Serpiginous choroiditis, also known as *geographic* or *helicoid choroidopathy,* is an uncommon, chronic, progressive inflammatory condition affecting adult men and women equally in the second to seventh decades of life. Its etiology is unknown, but it is thought to represent an immune-mediated occlusive vasculitis. Microorganisms may be a potential trigger, but attempts to identify an infectious cause remain inconclusive. Thus, the intraocular inflammation is treated with immunosuppression without the use of antimicrobial drugs. Serpiginous choroiditis has been reported to occur in patients with Crohn disease, sarcoidosis, and PAN, but no consistent systemic disease associations have been identified.

Patients present with painless, unilateral, paracentral scotomata and decreased vision, with minimal vitreous involvement and a quiet anterior chamber. Although patients may present with unilateral symptoms, funduscopy usually reveals asymmetric bilateral scarring. Active areas appear as gray-white lesions at the level of the RPE that project in a pseudopodial or geographic manner from the optic nerve in the posterior fundus (Fig 6-32). Far less commonly, macular or peripheral lesions may present without peripapillary involvement. Disease activity is typically confined to the leading edge of the

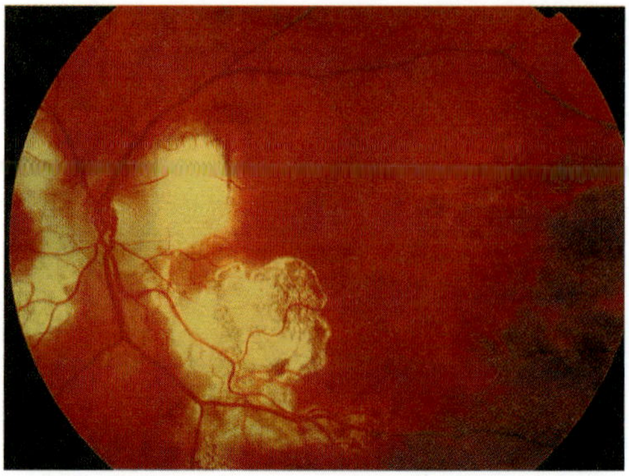

Figure 6-32 Serpiginous choroiditis: fundus photograph. *(Courtesy of Albert T. Vitale, MD.)*

advancing lesion and may be associated with shallow subretinal fluid. Occasionally, vascular sheathing has been reported along with RPE detachment and neovascularization of the disc. Late findings include atrophy of the choriocapillaris, RPE, and retina, with extensive RPE hyperpigmentation and subretinal fibrosis, as well as CNV occurring at the border of an old scar in up to 25% of patients.

The disease course is marked by progressive centrifugal extension, with marked asymmetry between the 2 eyes. New lesions and recurrent attacks are typical; up to 38% of patients reach a final visual acuity of between 20/200 and counting fingers in the affected eye. FA shows blockage of the choroidal flush in the early phase of the study and staining of the active edge of the lesion in the later stage of the angiogram (Fig 6-33). In contrast, early hyperfluorescence with late leakage is indicative of the presence of CNV. ICG angiography reveals hypofluorescence throughout all phases of the study for both acute and old lesions. It may reveal more extensive involvement than FA or clinical examination and may be useful in distinguishing active new serpiginous lesions, which are hypofluorescent, from CNV, which may appear as localized areas of hyperfluorescence during the middle to late phases of the study. FAF imaging may be an exquisitely sensitive modality for detecting damage to the RPE and monitoring the clinical course of serpiginous choroiditis; characteristic hypoautofluorescence corresponds closely to areas of regressed

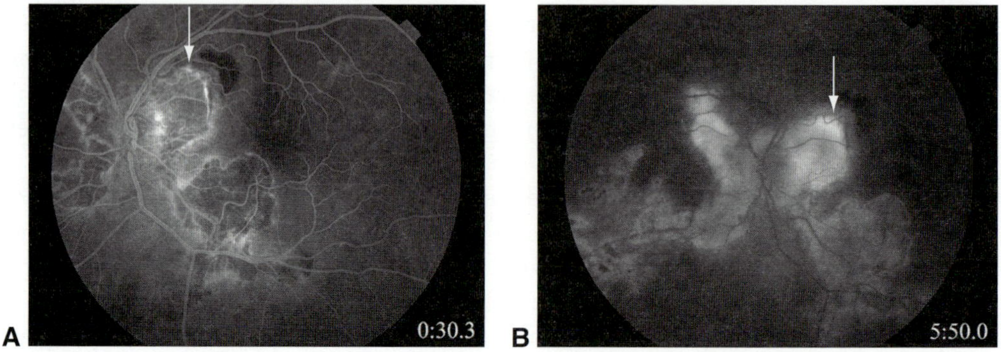

Figure 6-33 Serpiginous choroiditis: fluorescein angiograms. **A,** Early blocked fluorescence *(arrow).* **B,** Late staining and leakage at the active margin of the lesion *(arrow). (Courtesy of Albert T. Vitale, MD.)*

disease activity, and hyperfluorescence highlights areas of active disease (Fig 6-34). OCT imaging can show increased outer retinal reflectivity and disruption in active disease, and atrophic changes in the retina and RPE in quiescent areas.

Given the small number of patients with serpiginous choroiditis, no consensus has evolved regarding the optimal treatment regimen or its efficacy. Systemic, periocular, and even intravitreal corticosteroids may be used in the treatment of active lesions, particularly lesions threatening the fovea. The addition of systemic IMT at the outset has been suggested, as corticosteroids alone are ineffective and patients require prolonged anti-inflammatory therapy. Cyclosporine monotherapy has been effectively used in small numbers of patients, as has triple therapy with prednisone, cyclosporine, and azathioprine. Although this approach may induce rapid remission of acute disease, prolonged therapy is required and disease recurrence is frequently observed as these drugs are tapered. Cytotoxic therapy with cyclophosphamide or chlorambucil has been shown to induce long, drug-free remissions. The intravitreal fluocinolone acetonide implant may be used in patients intolerant of systemic therapy. Intravitreal anti-VEGF drugs, focal laser photocoagulation, and photodynamic therapy are important therapeutic modalities for the treatment of associated CNV.

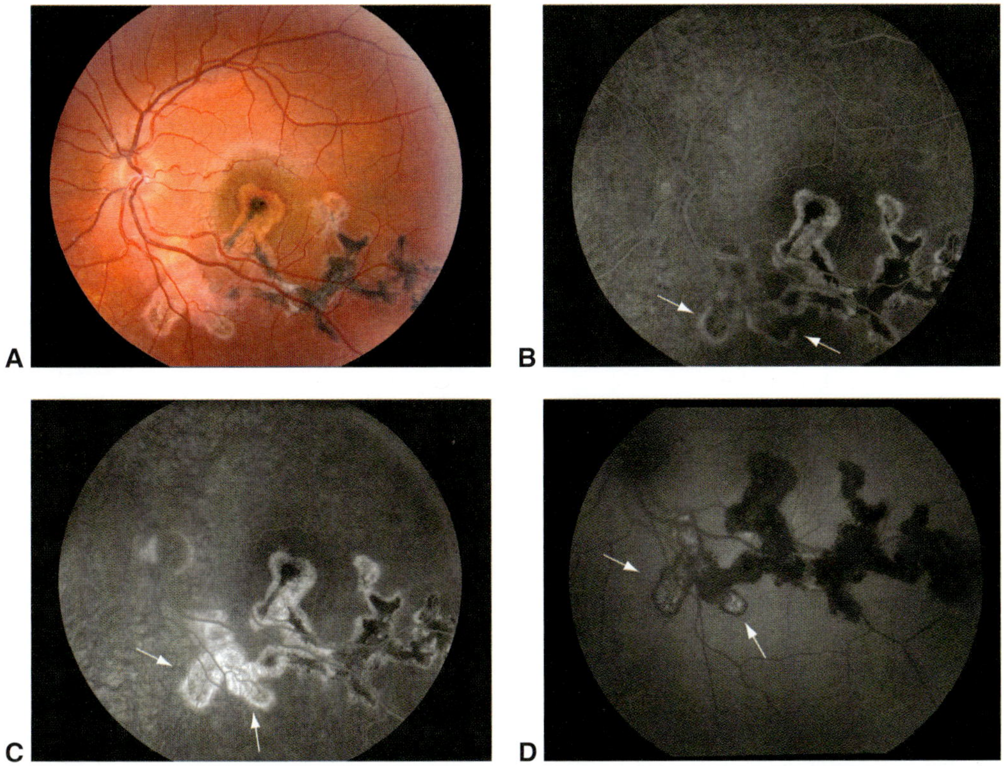

Figure 6-34 Serpiginous choroiditis. **A,** Color photograph showing an area of active inflammation, nasal to the darker areas of previous inflammation and scarring. **B, C,** Fluorescein angiogram images showing early hypofluorescence of the active area followed by late staining *(arrows)*. **D,** Fundus autofluorescence image demonstrating marked autofluorescence in the areas of disease activity *(arrows)*. *(Courtesy of H. Nida Sen, MD.)*

Recent studies highlight the importance of distinguishing presumed immune-mediated serpiginous choroiditis from infectious entities that can simulate the disease. Herpetic and syphilitic choroiditis can occasionally mimic serpiginous choroiditis, but there is increasing recognition that *Mycobacterium tuberculosis* can cause inflammation that also simulates typical serpiginous choroiditis. Tuberculosis (TB)-associated disease has been called *multifocal serpiginoid choroiditis* or *serpiginous-like choroiditis* (see Chapter 7, Fig 7-54).

Patients with serpiginous-like choroiditis tend to be from countries where TB is endemic, have emigrated from such countries, or have been exposed to active pulmonary TB. Results of tuberculin skin testing and the interferon-gamma release assay are usually positive for TB, although the chest X-ray often appears normal. The ocular involvement in TB-related serpiginous-like choroiditis is mostly unilateral, with serpiginoid lesions involving the posterior pole, mid-periphery, and periphery but usually sparing the juxtapapillary area until late in the disease. The lesions tend to appear and progress in multiple areas rather than to spread out centrifugally as they do in serpiginous choroiditis. Patients with serpiginous-like choroiditis exhibit a more prominent inflammatory cellular reaction in the vitreous than do patients with serpiginous choroiditis. The disease usually responds to anti-TB treatment, although complete control may take months and corticosteroids may also be needed to control inflammation. (See Chapter 7 for a full discussion of TB-associated uveitis.) For more information about serpiginous choroiditis and serpiginous-like choroiditis, see the American Academy of Ophthalmology lecture by Rao included in the following reference list.

Akpek EK, Jabs DA, Tessler HH, Joondeph BC, Foster CS. Successful treatment of serpiginous choroiditis with alkylating agents. *Ophthalmology.* 2002;109(8):1506–1513.

Bansal R, Gupta A, Gupta V. Imaging in the diagnosis and management of serpiginous choroiditis. *Int Ophthalmol Clin.* 2012;52(4):229–236.

Christmas NJ, Oh KT, Oh DM, Folk JC. Long-term follow-up of patients with serpiginous choroiditis. *Retina.* 2002;22(5):550–556.

Gupta V, Gupta A, Arora S, Bambery P, Dogra MR, Agarwal A. Presumed tubercular serpiginouslike choroiditis: clinical presentations and management. *Ophthalmology.* 2003;110(9):1744–1749.

Hooper PL, Kaplan HJ. Triple agent immunosuppression in serpiginous choroiditis. *Ophthalmology.* 1991;98(6):944–951.

Nazari Khanamiri H, Rao NA. Serpiginous choroiditis and infectious multifocal serpiginoid choroiditis. *Surv Ophthalmol.* 2013;58(3):203–232.

Rao NA. Serpiginous choroiditis: autoimmune, herpes, or tuberculosis. [American Academy of Ophthalmology Annual Meeting Video Program]. San Francisco: American Academy of Ophthalmology; 2012. Available at http://one.aao.org/annual-meeting-video/serpiginous-choroiditis-autoimmune-herpes-tubercl. Accessed October 27, 2014.

Multifocal choroiditis and panuveitis

Multifocal choroiditis and panuveitis (MCP), PIC, and the subretinal fibrosis and uveitis syndrome represent a subset of the white dot syndromes; some authorities regard them as discrete entities, whereas others view them as a single disease with a variable severity continuum. When the disorders are considered a continuum, the term *multifocal choroiditis* (MFC) may be used to describe all the entities, and the presence of fibrosis or panuveitis is then described separately. For this discussion, the traditional nomenclature is used to discuss the 3 related diseases as discrete entities.

MCP is an idiopathic inflammatory disorder of unknown etiology affecting the choroid, retina, and vitreous; it presents asymmetrically, most often in young women with myopia. Symptoms include floaters, photopsias, enlargement of the physiologic blind spot, and decreased vision. The ophthalmoscopic hallmarks include the presence of multiple old, atrophic lesions that appear as punched-out, white-yellow dots (50–200 µm) in a peripapillary, midperipheral, and anterior equatorial distribution (Fig 6-35). Acute lesions have a creamier, opaque appearance that becomes punched out over time. Varying degrees of anterior segment inflammation and an associated vitritis are uniformly present, effectively excluding a diagnosis of OHS or PIC. The lesions are smaller than those present in birdshot uveitis or APMPPE and evolve into atrophic scars with varying degrees of hyperpigmentation. They are larger and more pigmented than the lesions found in patients with PIC. New lesions may appear, and peripheral chorioretinal streaks and peripapillary pigment changes similar to those present in OHS have been observed. Subretinal fibrosis with RPE clumping is much more common in MCP than in OHS. Structural complications noted at presentation can include cataract, CME, ERM, and CNV. These problems, as well as complications that develop over the chronic course of this disease, are frequent causes of visual impairment.

Fluorescein angiography shows early hypofluorescence with late staining of acute active lesions, whereas atrophic lesions behave as transmission defects (early hyperfluorescence that fades in the late phases of the angiogram). Early hyperfluorescence and late leakage are observed in the presence of macular edema and CNV (Fig 6-36). As in

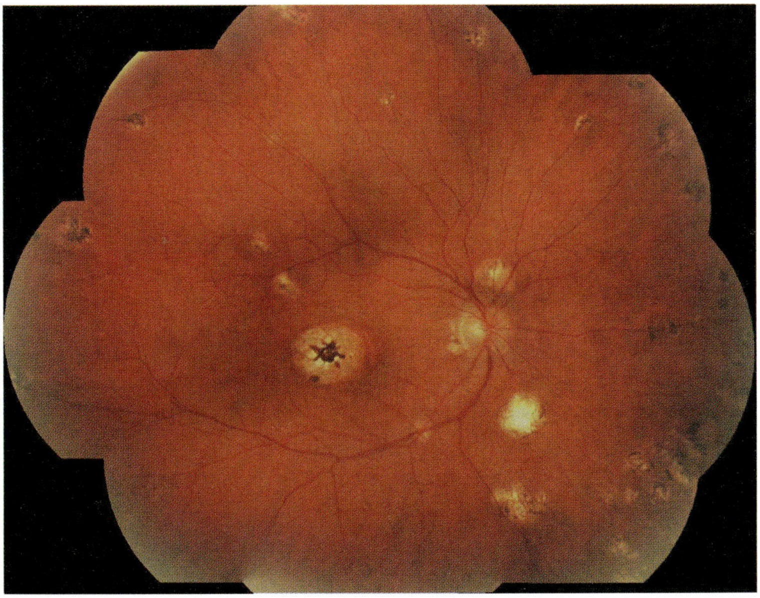

Figure 6-35 Multifocal choroiditis and panuveitis (MCP): fundus photograph. *(Courtesy of Ramana S. Moorthy, MD.)*

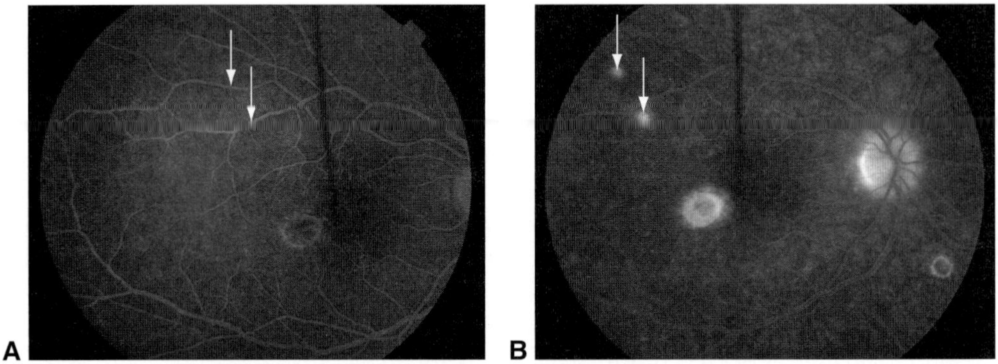

Figure 6-36 Multifocal choroiditis and panuveitis: fluorescein angiogram. **A,** Early blocked fluorescence *(arrows).* **B,** Late staining of lesions *(arrows). (Courtesy of Ramana S. Moorthy, MD.)*

birdshot uveitis, ICG angiography reveals multiple midphase hypofluorescent lesions compatible with active choroiditis that are more numerous than those apparent on clinical examination or FA; they are frequently clustered around the optic nerve. This finding may correlate with an enlarged blind spot revealed by visual field testing. The hypofluorescent spots may fade with treatment and resolution of the intraocular inflammation. The most common finding on FAF imaging is punctate hypoautofluorescent spots (≥125 µm) corresponding to multiple areas of chorioretinal atrophy; however, smaller (<125 µm) spots numbering in the hundreds may be seen in the macular and peripapillary regions that are not visible on fundus photography, some of which will later develop into clinically evident chorioretinal scars (Fig 6-37). Active MCP lesions display hyperautofluorescence that disappears with minimal RPE disruption following anti-inflammatory treatment. FAF imaging in MCP suggests that patients have more widespread involvement of the RPE than indicated by other imaging modalities and therefore that the modality may be useful in monitoring response to treatment. OCT imaging may show drusenlike material beneath the RPE at the site of visible spots that can be associated with more widespread disruption of the overlying outer retina. There is also choroidal hyperreflectivity beneath the deposits.

A viral etiology involving herpes simplex and Epstein-Barr virus has been postulated, but neither has been conclusively demonstrated. Pathologic specimens obtained from eyes with MCP have shown variable findings, ranging from large numbers of B lymphocytes in the choroid to a predominance of T lymphocytes, suggesting that different immune mechanisms may produce a similar clinical picture and that an initial viral infection may trigger an autoimmune process.

The diagnosis is one of exclusion, as many other conditions such as sarcoidosis, syphilis, and TB may produce lesions similar in appearance to those of MCP. The visual prognosis is guarded, with permanent vision loss in at least 1 eye occurring in up to 75% of patients as a result of the complications associated with chronic, recurrent inflammation. In one study, the incidence of vision loss to 20/200 or worse was 12% per eye-year in the affected eye.

Systemic and periocular corticosteroids may be effective for the treatment of macular edema and have been shown to induce regression of CNV in some patients. Corticosteroid-sparing strategies with IMT are frequently required because of the chronic, recurrent nature of the inflammation; these treatments have been successful in achieving not only

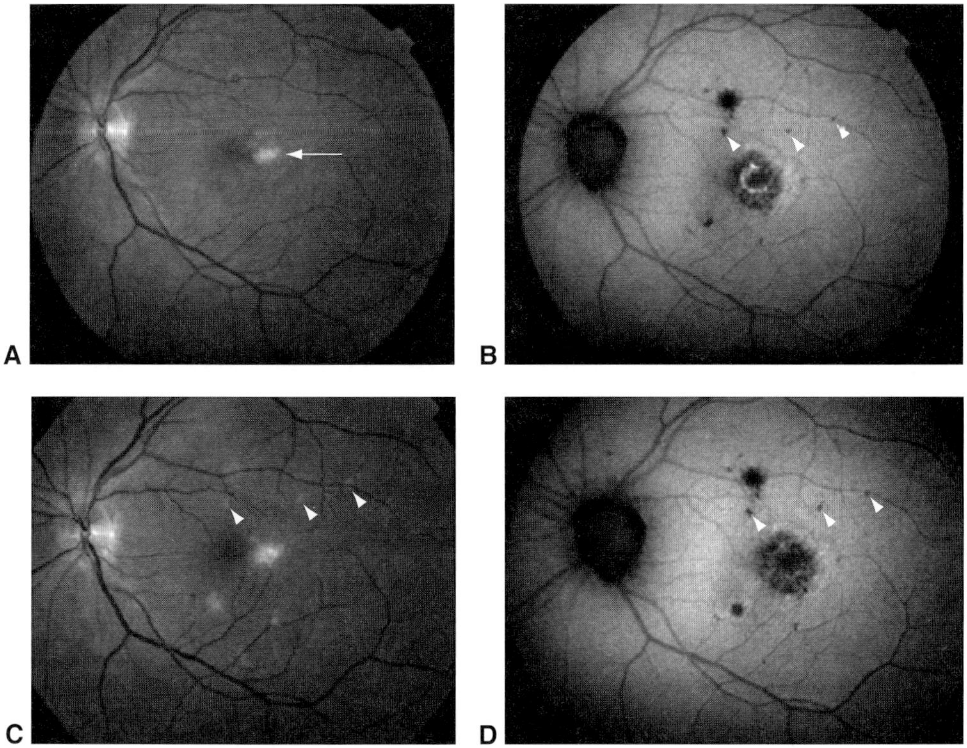

Figure 6-37 Images from a 36-year-old woman with MCP. **A,** Fundus photograph showing an area of choroidal neovascularization (CNV) *(arrow)* treated with photodynamic therapy 3 years earlier. **B,** Fundus autofluorescence (FAF) photograph shows multiple hypoautofluorescent spots *(arrowheads)* that did not correspond to ophthalmoscopically visible lesions. **C,** Three years later, fundus photograph shows multiple visible spots *(arrowheads)* corresponding to previously visualized hypoautofluorescent spots. **D,** FAF photograph taken at the same time as **C** shows corresponding hypoautofluorescent spots *(arrowheads),* which are slightly enlarged from the previous study. *(Reprinted with permission from Haen SP, Spaide RF. Fundus autofluorescence in multifocal choroiditis and panuveitis.* Am J Ophthalmol. *2008;145(5):850.)*

inflammatory quiescence, but also an 83% reduction in the risk of posterior pole complications (CME, ERM, and CNV) and a 92% reduction in the risk of vision loss to 20/200 or worse in affected eyes. The intravitreal fluocinolone acetonide implant is also a potential treatment option. Intravitreal anti-VEGF drugs and laser modalities (thermal photocoagulation and photodynamic therapy) are important adjuncts for the treatment of CNV. However, active inflammation can stimulate neovascularization and blunt the effects of these treatments, so it is important that any inflammatory component be well controlled. (The same concept applies to any uveitic entity complicated by CNV.)

Dreyer RF, Gass DJ. Multifocal choroiditis and panuveitis. A syndrome that mimics ocular histoplasmosis. *Arch Ophthalmol.* 1984;102(12):1776–1784.

Essex RW, Wong J, Jampol LM, Dowler J, Bird AC. Idiopathic multifocal choroiditis: a comment on present and past nomenclature. *Retina.* 2013;33(1):1–4.

Haen SP, Spaide RF. Fundus autofluorescence in multifocal choroiditis and panuveitis. *Am J Ophthalmol.* 2008;145(5):847–853.

Michel SS, Ekong A, Baltatzis S, Foster CS. Multifocal choroiditis and panuveitis: immunomodulatory therapy. *Ophthalmology.* 2002;109(2):378–383.

Spaide RF, Goldberg N, Freund KB. Redefining multifocal choroiditis and panuveitis and punctate inner choroidopathy through multimodal imaging. *Retina.* 2013;33(7):1315–1324.

Thorne JE, Wittenberg S, Jabs DA, et al. Multifocal choroiditis with panuveitis: incidence of ocular complications and loss of visual acuity. *Ophthalmology.* 2006;113(12):2310–2316.

Yeh S, Forooghian F, Wong WT, et al. Fundus autofluorescence imaging of the white dot syndromes. *Arch Ophthalmol.* 2010;128(1):46–56.

Punctate inner choroiditis

PIC is an idiopathic inflammatory disorder that, like MCP, occurs in otherwise healthy myopic white women, but it presents at a younger median age (29 vs 45 years, respectively). Patients with PIC can present with metamorphopsia, paracentral scotomata, photopsias, and asymmetric loss of central acuity. In contrast to the lesions of MCP, those of PIC (100–200 µm) rarely extend to the midperiphery and are never associated with vitritis (Fig 6-38). They progress to atrophic scars, typically leaving a halo of pigmentation, and are deeper and more punched out than those of MCP. New lesions and CME are rarely observed, whereas serous retinal detachment may be found over confluent PIC lesions. With the exception of CNV, patients with PIC have few structural complications (cataract, CME, or ERM) at presentation, unlike patients with MCP, a difference undoubtedly related to the presence of chronic intraocular inflammation in MCP. CNV, a common vision-threatening complication in both entities, may be more frequent at presentation in patients with PIC (79%) than with MCP (28%), but patients with MCP are more likely to have bilateral visual impairment of visual acuity 20/50 or worse (Fig 6-39).

Fluorescein angiography studies in patients with PIC show early hypofluorescence of the inflammatory lesions with late staining, although early hyperfluorescence can also occur, especially if a CNV is present (Figs 6-40, 6-41). ICG angiography displays midphase hypofluorescence throughout the posterior pole in a peripapillary distribution that corresponds to the lesions apparent on FA and clinical examination; such imaging studies may be useful in delineating disease extent and monitoring its activity (Fig 6-42). OCT can show findings similar to those of MCP, as well as CNV if present.

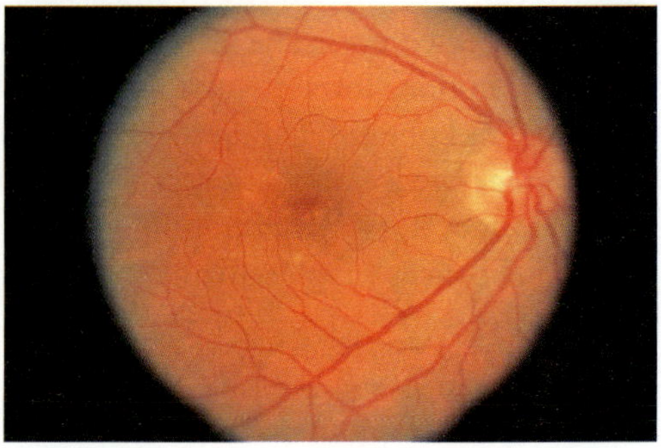

Figure 6-38 Punctate inner choroiditis (PIC): fundus photograph. *(Courtesy of E. Mitchel Opremcak, MD.)*

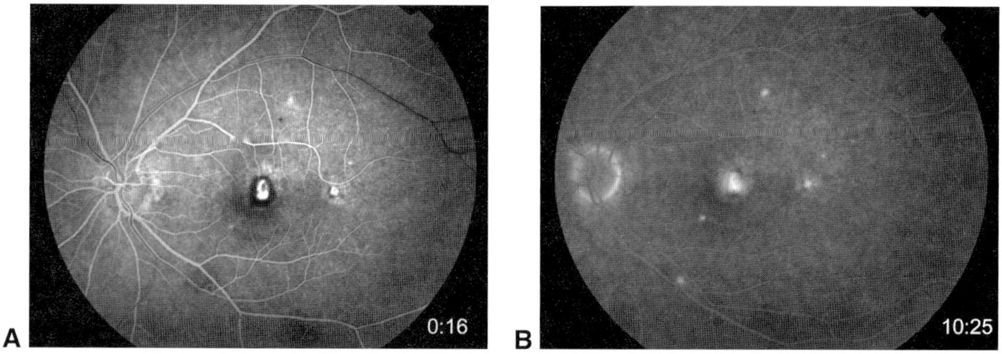

Figure 6-39 PIC with associated CNV. **A,** Fluorescein angiogram showing early hyperfluorescence of the PIC lesions, with lacy hyperfluorescence of CNV. **B,** Late hyperfluorescence and staining of PIC lesions and leakage due to CNV. *(Courtesy of Albert T. Vitale, MD.)*

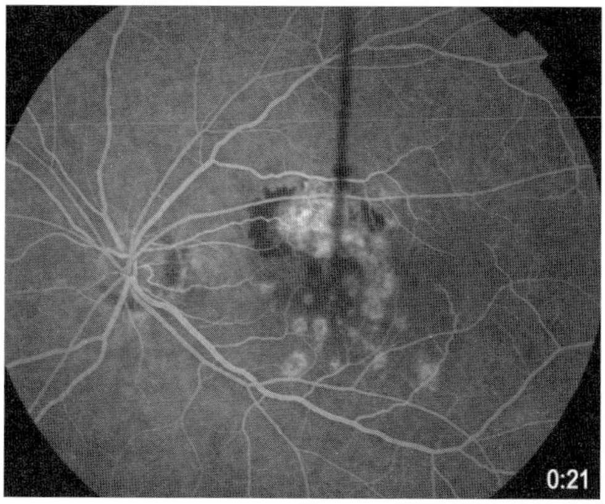

Figure 6-40 Fluorescein angiogram showing early hyperfluorescence of PIC lesions and CNV. *(Courtesy of Albert T. Vitale, MD.)*

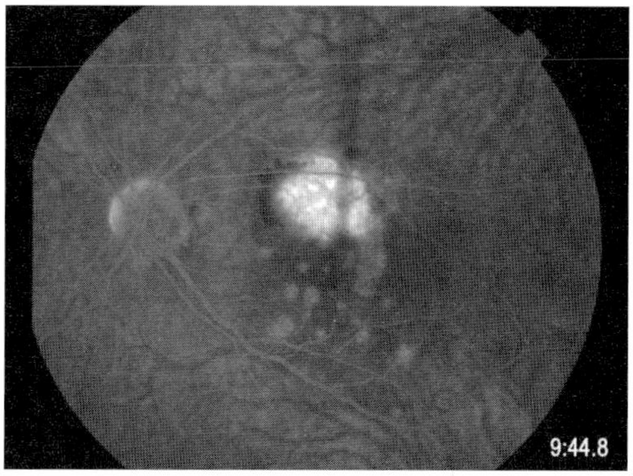

Figure 6-41 Fluorescein angiogram showing late staining of PIC lesions with leakage from CNV. *(Courtesy of Albert T. Vitale, MD.)*

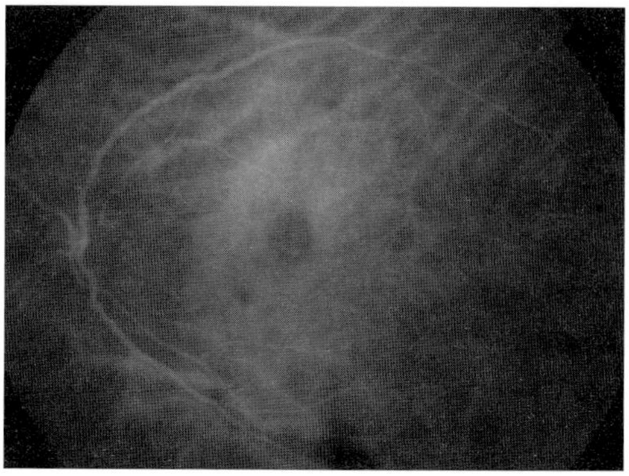

Figure 6-42 PIC: indocyanine green angiogram showing multiple midphase hypofluorescent spots. *(Courtesy of Albert T. Vitale, MD.)*

The visual prognosis is favorable in eyes without CNV involving the foveal center. Treatment options include observation or periocular and/or systemic corticosteroids for eyes presenting with poor initial visual acuity or multiple acute PIC lesions proximate to the fovea. Intravitreal anti-VEGF drugs, laser photocoagulation, photodynamic therapy with or without intravitreal corticosteroids, and submacular surgery may be considered in eyes with CNV, as previously described.

Kedhar SR, Thorne JE, Wittenberg S, Dunn JP, Jabs DA. Multifocal choroiditis with panuveitis and punctate inner choroidopathy: comparison of clinical characteristics at presentation. *Retina.* 2007;27(9):1174–1179.

Leung TG, Moradi A, Liu D, et al. Clinical features and incidence rate of ocular complications in punctate inner choroidopathy. *Retina.* 2014;34(8):1666–1674.

Subretinal fibrosis and uveitis syndrome

Subretinal fibrosis and uveitis syndrome is an extremely uncommon panuveitis of unknown etiology affecting otherwise healthy myopic females between the ages of 14 and 34 years. Significant anterior segment inflammation and mild to moderate vitritis are typically present bilaterally, with white-yellow lesions (50–500 μm) located in the posterior pole to midperiphery at the level of the RPE. These lesions may fade without RPE alterations, become atrophic, or enlarge and coalesce into large, white, stellate zones of subretinal fibrosis (Figs 6-43, 6-44). Serous neurosensory retinal detachment, CME, and CNV may also be observed.

Immune mechanisms have been implicated in the pathogenesis of subretinal fibrosis and uveitis syndrome, as suggested by the presence of local antibodies directed against the RPE, granulomatous infiltration of the choroid, enhanced expression of the Fas-Fas ligand in the retina, choroidal scars, and choroidal granulomas. A predominance of B lymphocytes, plasma cells, and subretinal fibrotic tissue with islands of RPE and Müller cells is observed histologically. The disease course is marked by chronic recurrent inflammation, and the visual prognosis is guarded. Treatment with systemic corticosteroids and

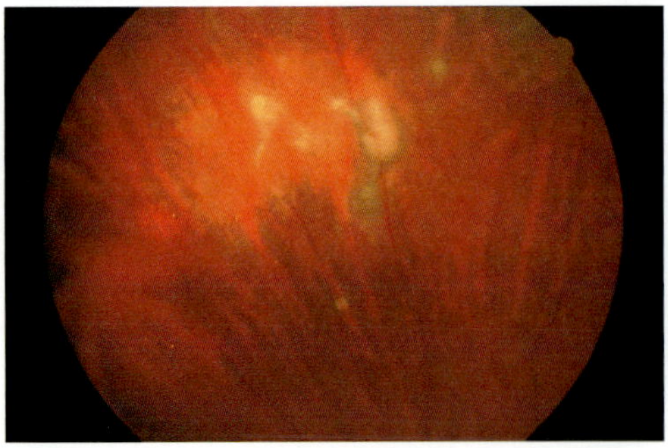

Figure 6-43 Subretinal fibrosis and uveitis syndrome: fundus photograph showing multifocal white subretinal lesions. *(Courtesy of E. Mitchel Opremcak, MD.)*

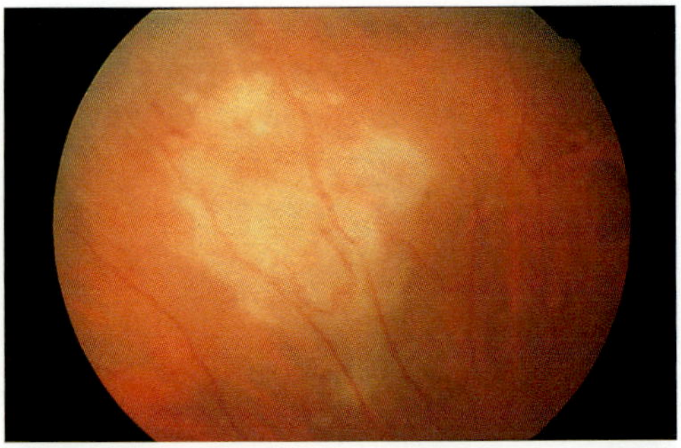

Figure 6-44 Subretinal fibrosis and uveitis syndrome: fundus photograph from the same patient as in Figure 6-43, showing progressive subretinal fibrosis. *(Courtesy of E. Mitchel Opremcak, MD.)*

IMT is of equivocal efficacy, although a recent report suggests rituximab may have some utility.

Fluorescein angiography shows multiple areas of blocked choroidal fluorescence and hyperfluorescence in the early stages of the study; in the late phase, staining of the lesions without leakage is observed. OCT shows variable retinal edema, subretinal fluid, and subretinal fibrosis. Again, the differential diagnosis includes ocular inflammatory conditions producing panuveitis and disorders in the differential diagnosis of the white dot syndromes, including sarcoidosis, OHS, APMPPE, syphilis, TB, birdshot uveitis, pathologic myopia, sympathetic ophthalmia, and toxoplasmosis.

Brown J Jr, Folk JC. Current controversies in the white dot syndromes. Multifocal choroiditis, punctate inner choroidopathy, and the diffuse subretinal fibrosis syndrome. *Ocul Immunol Inflamm.* 1998;6(2):125–127.

Kim MK, Chan CC, Belfort R Jr, et al. Histopathologic and immunohistopathologic features of subretinal fibrosis and uveitis syndrome. *Am J Ophthalmol.* 1987;104(1):15–23.

Spiteri Cornish K, Kuffova L, Forrester JV. Treatment of diffuse subretinal fibrosis uveitis with rituximab [epub ahead of print May 30, 2014]. *Br J Ophthalmol.* doi:10.1136/bjophthalmol-2013-304686.

Multiple evanescent white dot syndrome

MEWDS is an uncommon idiopathic inflammatory condition of the retina that typically affects otherwise healthy, young, moderately myopic females in the second to fourth decades of life. Patients present with acute unilateral (80%) blurred or decreased vision, photopsias, and central or paracentral scotomata corresponding to an enlarged physiologic blind spot. An antecedent viral prodrome occurs in approximately one-third of cases. Funduscopy during the acute phase of the disease reveals multiple, discrete, white-to-orange spots (100–200 µm) at the level of the RPE or deep retina, typically in a perifoveal location (Fig 6-45). These spots are transitory and frequently missed; they leave instead a granular macular pigmentary change—a pathognomonic finding that can be very useful in making the diagnosis when patients present with symptoms after the white dots have faded. Bilateral cases have been reported, and a small minority of patients with chronic MEWDS may develop choroidal scarring. There may be variable degrees of vitreous inflammation, mild blurring of the optic disc, and, in rare instances, isolated vascular sheathing.

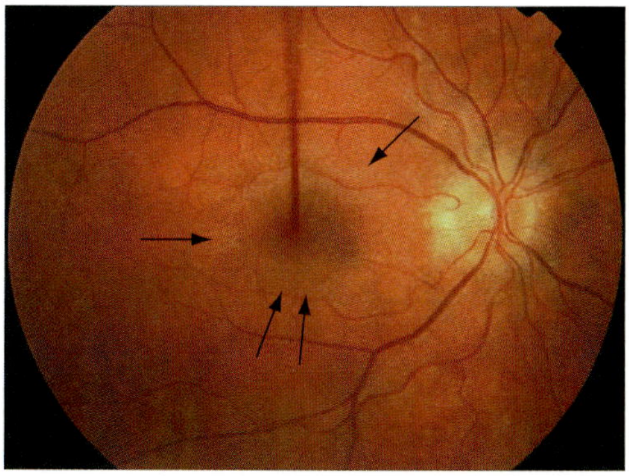

Figure 6-45 Multiple evanescent white dot syndrome (MEWDS). Multiple discrete, punctate yellowish perifoveal dots *(arrows)*. *(Courtesy of Albert T. Vitale, MD.)*

Fluorescein angiography reveals late-staining, characteristic punctate hyperfluorescent lesions in a wreathlike configuration surrounding the fovea (Fig 6-46). ICG angiography shows multiple hypofluorescent lesions that are more numerous than those apparent on clinical examination or FA and that typically fade with resolution of the disease (Fig 6-47). FAF imaging shows hyperfluorescent spots corresponding to those found on clinical examination and may also show small, punctate hypoautofluorescent areas localized around the optic disc and posterior pole. Visual field abnormalities are variable and include generalized depression, paracentral or peripheral scotomata, and enlargement of the blind spot. The ERG reveals diminished a-wave and early receptor potential (ERP) amplitudes, both of which are reversible. Results of the multifocal ERG (mfERG) and electro-oculogram (EOG) localize the disease process to the RPE–photoreceptor complex rather than to the choroid. Further support for localization of the disease process to the RPE–photoreceptor complex comes from the demonstration of abnormal photoreceptor inner/outer segment line (ellipsoid zone) reflectivity on spectral-domain optical coherence tomography (SD-OCT) and the correspondence of this finding with hypofluorescent spots visualized on ICG angiography and changes in microperimetry sensitivity. These abnormalities completely resolve during the course of the disease (Fig 6-48).

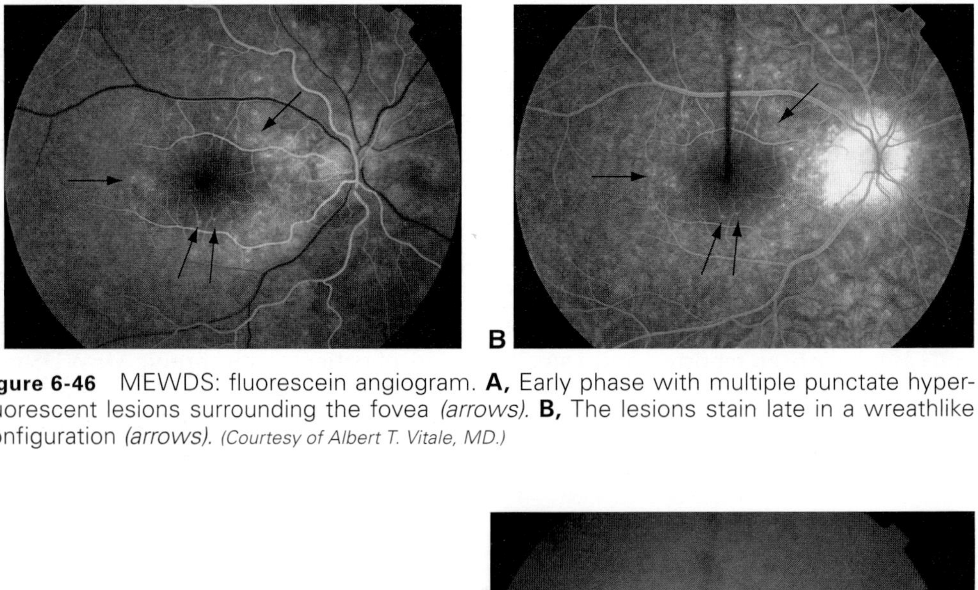

A B

Figure 6-46 MEWDS: fluorescein angiogram. **A,** Early phase with multiple punctate hyperfluorescent lesions surrounding the fovea *(arrows).* **B,** The lesions stain late in a wreathlike configuration *(arrows). (Courtesy of Albert T. Vitale, MD.)*

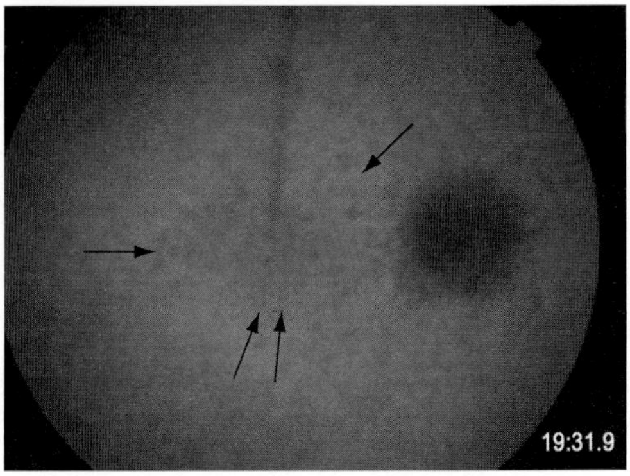

Figure 6-47 MEWDS: indocyanine green angiogram of the same patient as in Figure 6-46, showing multiple midphase, hypofluorescent spots, more numerous than appreciated on fluorescein angiography or clinical examination *(arrows). (Courtesy of Albert T. Vitale, MD.)*

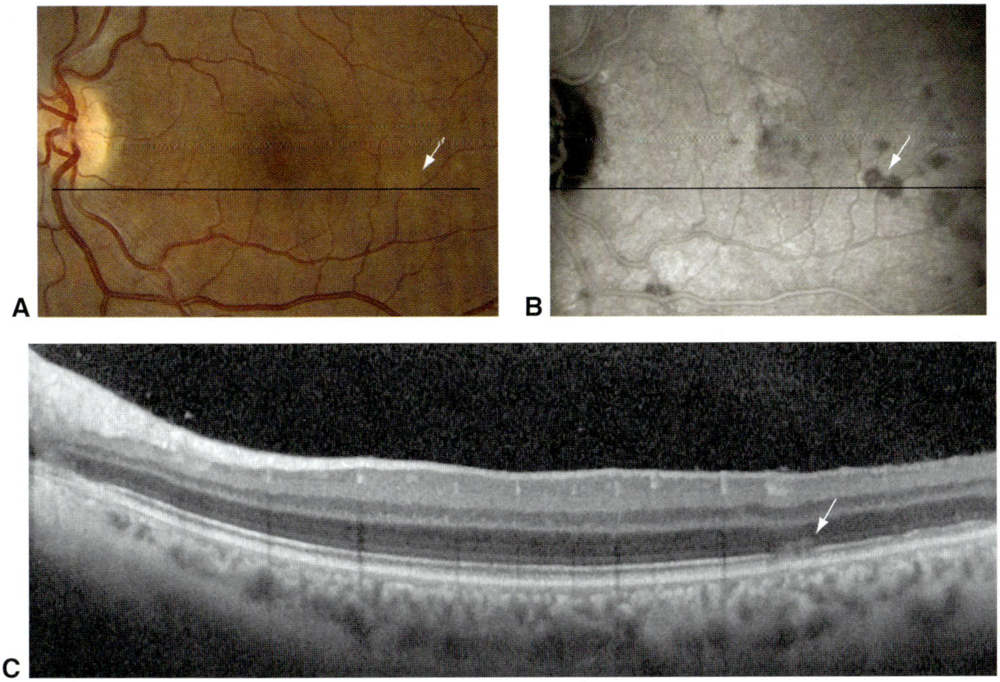

Figure 6-48 MEWDS. **A,** Color fundus photograph shows subtle spots *(arrow)* and foveal granularity. **B,** ICG angiogram shows more spots *(arrow)* than are apparent on the color photograph. **C,** Spectral-domain OCT image of the spots (positioned at *horizontal lines* in **A** and **B**) shows disruption of the inner/outer segment line (ellipsoid zone) *(arrow)*. *(Courtesy of Janet L. Davis, MD, and Charles Wycoff, MD.)*

The prognosis is excellent, with recovery of vision within 2–10 weeks without treatment; however, residual symptoms including photopsias and enlargement of the blind spot may persist for months. Recurrences are uncommon (10%–15% of patients) and have a similarly good prognosis.

MEWDS has been reported in association with MCP, acute zonal occult outer retinopathy, and acute macular neuroretinopathy, suggesting a common genetic susceptibility and/or pathogenetic factor. Acute macular neuroretinopathy (AMN) is a rare condition, occurring among otherwise healthy young women, and is characterized by the acute onset of visual impairment and multifocal scotomata that correspond precisely to reddish, flat, wedge-shaped lesions in the macula. Although most patients with AMN experience a minimal decrease in visual acuity, symptoms frequently persist despite resolution of the fundus lesions. No treatment is required for AMN, given the condition's favorable natural history.

Hangai M, Fujimoto M, Yoshimura N. Features and function of multiple evanescent white dot syndrome. *Arch Ophthalmol.* 2009;127(10):1307–1313.

Jampol LM, Sieving PA, Pugh D, Fishman GA, Gilbert H. Multiple evanescent white dot syndrome. I. Clinical findings. *Arch Ophthalmol.* 1984;102(5):671–674.

Thomas BJ, Albini TA, Flynn HW Jr. Multiple evanescent white dot syndrome: multimodal imaging and correlation with proposed pathophysiology. *Ophthalmic Surg Lasers Imaging Retina.* 2013;44(6):584–587.

Acute retinal pigment epitheliitis

Acute retinal pigment epitheliitis, or Krill disease, is a benign self-limited inflammatory disorder of the RPE of unknown etiology. It typically presents in otherwise healthy young adults between the ages of 16 and 40 years with acute unilateral vision loss, central metamorphopsia, and scotomata. Ophthalmoscopic findings include clusters of small, discrete, hyperpigmented lesions, typically with a yellow halo in the posterior pole unassociated with vitritis or other abnormalities noted on funduscopy (Fig 6-49). FA shows early hyperfluorescence of the pinpoint dots with a surrounding halo of hyperfluorescence and late staining. Visual field testing shows central scotomata. Normal results on ERG with abnormal results on EOG serve to localize the disease process to the RPE. OCT shows transient disruption of the inner/outer segment line (ellipsoid zone), along with wider disruption of the RPE inner band. No treatment is required, as the lesions resolve without sequelae with excellent visual acuity over 6–12 weeks.

Baillif S, Wolff B, Paoli V, Gastaud P, Mauget-Faÿsse M. Retinal fluorescein and indocyanine green angiography and spectral-domain optical coherence tomography findings in acute retinal pigment epitheliitis. *Retina.* 2011;31(6):1156–1163.

Cho HJ, Han SY, Cho SW, et al. Acute retinal pigment epitheliitis: spectral-domain optical coherence tomography findings in 18 cases. *Invest Ophthalmol Vis Sci.* 2014;55(5): 3314–3319.

Deutman AF. Acute retinal pigment epitheliitis. *Am J Ophthalmol.* 1974;78(4):571–578.

Acute zonal occult outer retinopathy

Acute zonal occult outer retinopathy (AZOOR) is typified by acute loss of one or more zones of outer retinal function associated with photopsia, minimal funduscopic changes, and abnormal ERG findings; unilateral disease is more common at first, but 1 or both eyes may be affected. Patients are typically young, myopic women who present with acute unilateral visual disturbances not infrequently associated with a mild vitritis (50%), apparently normal results on funduscopic examination, and visual acuity in the 20/40 range. Electrophysiological studies may demonstrate a consistent pattern of dysfunction, not only at the photoreceptor–RPE complex but also at the inner retinal level. Essentially, this dysfunction consists of a delayed 30-Hz–flicker ERG and a reduction in the EOG

A 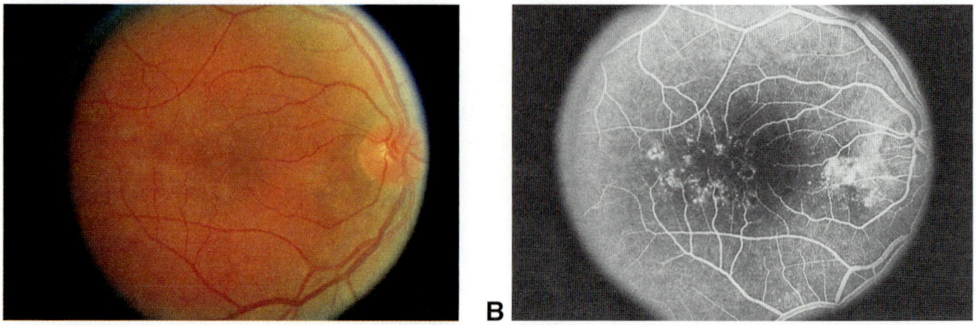 B

Figure 6-49 Acute retinal pigment epitheliitis. **A,** Fundus photograph. **B,** Fluorescein angiogram showing honeycomb lesions at the level of the RPE. *(Courtesy of E. Mitchel Opremcak, MD.)*

light rise, which when present with classic symptomatology may be helpful diagnostically, obviating extensive neurologic evaluation. Visual field defects include enlargement of the blind spot and paracentral inferior, superior, and temporal defects with no corresponding retinal defect. Results of mfERG show decreased response from the blind spots and other visual field defects with corresponding loss or irregularity of the inner/outer segment line (ellipsoid zone) shown on OCT, suggesting that photoreceptor outer segment dysfunction and/or degeneration are the primary lesions in AZOOR. During the early disease stages, FA findings may be normal, showing only a prolonged retinal circulation time. With disease progression, however, diffuse areas of hyperfluorescence and hypofluorescence and window defects corresponding to zones of RPE derangement become common. FAF imaging may be particularly useful in monitoring patients with AZOOR, as it reveals conspicuous areas of central hypoautofluorescence corresponding to RPE and choriocapillary atrophy; peripheral hyperautofluorescence is found at the border of the expanding lesion due to the presence of lipofuscin-laden cells that presage RPE cell death (Fig 6-50). There may also be diffuse zones of speckled hyperautofluorescence in areas of subacute disease activity. These evolve into areas of speckled hypoautofluorescence as atrophic changes ensue.

With extended follow-up, the majority of patients are found to develop bilateral disease, with recurrences in approximately one-third. Similarly, the funduscopic appearance varies with the stage of the disease, ranging from initial, subtle RPE changes with depigmentation in areas of vision loss to vessel attenuation, late pigment migration, and focal perivenous sheathing. Occasionally a demarcation line can be seen at the edge of active disease expansion. Visual field abnormalities typically stabilize in approximately 75% of

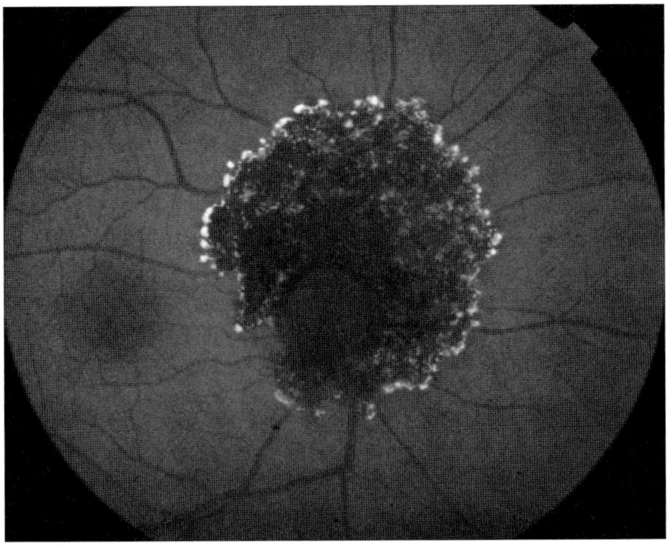

Figure 6-50 Acute zonal occult outer retinopathy: FAF photograph showing peripapillary hypoautofluorescence corresponding to atrophy of the RPE–choriocapillaris. Intense hyperautofluorescence at the outer border of the lesion corresponds to the yellowish drusenlike material thought to represent the accumulation of large amounts of lipofuscin. *(Reprinted with permission from Spaide RF. Collateral damage in acute zonal occult outer retinopathy.* Am J Ophthalmol. *2004;138(5):889.)*

patients and partially improve in about 25%. Visual acuity remains in the 20/40 range in 68% of patients; however, legal blindness has been reported in as many as 18% with long-term follow-up.

Cancer-associated retinopathy and retinitis pigmentosa should be considered in the differential diagnosis of AZOOR. It is unclear whether treatment with systemic corticosteroids or IMT alters the disease course or vision outcome.

The considerable similarities between AZOOR and other white dot syndromes—namely, MEWDS, MCP, OHS, PIC, acute macular neuroretinopathy, and acute idiopathic blind spot enlargement syndrome—have led some investigators to group these entities together in the so-called *AZOOR complex* of diseases. Although an infectious etiology has been postulated, systemic autoimmune disease has been observed in 28% of patients, supporting the notion that these diseases are of an inflammatory etiology and arise in patients with a common non–disease-specific genetic background, possibly triggered by some exogenous agent.

Francis PJ, Marinescu A, Fitzke FW, Bird AC, Holder GE. Acute zonal occult outer retinopathy: towards a set of diagnostic criteria. *Br J Ophthalmol.* 2005;89(1):70–73.

Monson DM, Smith JR. Acute zonal occult outer retinopathy. *Surv Ophthalmol.* 2011; 56(1):23–35.

Mrejen S, Khan S, Gallego-Pinazo R, Jampol LM, Yannuzzi LA. Acute zonal occult outer retinopathy: a classification based on multimodal imaging [epub ahead of print June 19, 2014]. *JAMA Ophthalmol.* doi:10.1001/jamaophthalmol.2014.1683.

Panuveitis

By definition, *panuveitis* (or *diffuse uveitis*) requires involvement of all anatomical compartments of the eye—namely, the anterior chamber, vitreous, and retina or choroid—with no single predominant site of inflammation. As with posterior uveitis, structural complications such as macular edema, retinal or choroidal neovascularization, and peripheral vasculitis, although not infrequent accompaniments, are not considered essential in the anatomical classification of panuveitis. Generally, panuveitis is bilateral, although 1 eye may be affected first and the severity is not necessarily symmetric. The discussion of panuveitis in this chapter is limited to the noninfectious entities.

Sarcoidosis

Sarcoidosis is a multisystem granulomatous disorder of unknown etiology with protean systemic and ocular manifestations. Although intrathoracic manifestations are most common (90%), other sites frequently involved include the lymph nodes, skin, eyes, CNS, bones and joints, liver, and heart. Ocular involvement may be present in up to 50% of patients with systemic disease, and uveitis is the most frequent manifestation. In most large series, sarcoidosis accounts for up to 10% of all cases of uveitis. The basic lesion of sarcoidosis is a noncaseating granuloma without histologic evidence of infection or foreign body (Fig 6-51). See BCSC Section 4, *Ophthalmic Pathology and Intraocular Tumors,* for a more detailed description of the pathology of sarcoidosis.

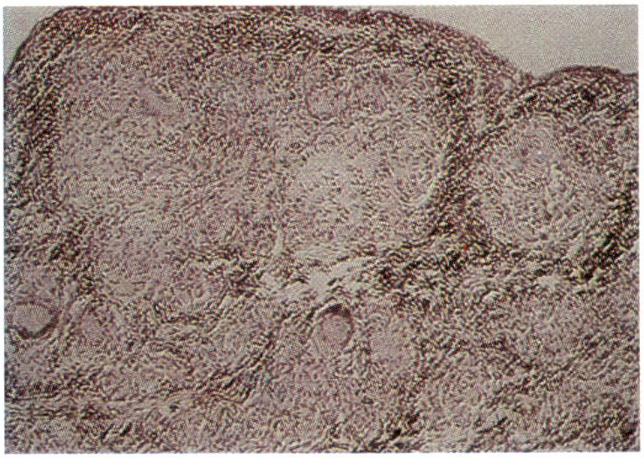

Figure 6-51 Sarcoidosis: histologic view of conjunctival biopsy. Note the giant cells and granulomatous inflammation.

Sarcoidosis has a worldwide distribution and affects all ethnic groups; the highest prevalence is in the northern European countries (40 cases per 100,000 people). In the United States, the disease is up to 20 times more prevalent among African Americans than whites. Both sexes are affected, albeit with a slight female predominance. Although onset usually occurs between the ages of 20 and 50 years, sarcoidosis is also an important diagnostic consideration in older patients. In a recent review, sarcoidosis was a common cause of newly diagnosed uveitis among patients ages 60 years and older. Patients with late-onset sarcoidosis may be more likely to have uveitis and less likely to have asymptomatic chest radiograph abnormalities than younger patients with the disease.

Pediatric involvement is uncommon, and the clinical course is atypical. Children with early-onset sarcoidosis (younger than 5 years) are less likely than adults to manifest pulmonary disease and far more likely to have cutaneous and articular involvement; the disease course in older children (8–15 years) approximates that in adults.

Although numerous environmental, infectious, and genetic factors have been implicated in causing the disease, no single etiologic agent or genetic locus has been clearly identified in the pathogenesis of sarcoidosis. For instance, the ACCESS (A Case Control Etiologic Study of Sarcoidosis) project suggests that exposure to microbe-rich environments may modestly increase the risk of developing sarcoidosis; however, no dominant factor could be determined. Molecular studies of tissue specimens provide evidence suggesting that mycobacterial and, less convincingly, propionibacterial organisms may be important etiologic factors. A genetic predisposition for the disease is suggested by familial clustering; siblings of patients have a fivefold increased risk of developing the disease.

Systemic sarcoidosis may present acutely, frequently with associated anterior uveitis in young patients, and spontaneously remit within 2 years of onset. One form of acute sarcoidosis, called *Löfgren syndrome,* consists of erythema nodosum, febrile arthropathy, bilateral hilar adenopathy, and acute iritis and is quite responsive to systemic corticosteroids; it has a good long-term prognosis. Another, termed *Heerfordt syndrome* (uveoparotid fever), is characterized by uveitis, parotitis, fever, and facial nerve palsy. Chronic sarcoidosis presents insidiously and is characterized by persistent disease of more than 2 years' duration, frequently with interpulmonary involvement and chronic uveitis. Extended corticosteroid therapy may be required. Pulmonary disease is the major cause of morbidity; overall mortality from sarcoidosis approaches 5% but may be as high as 10% with neurosarcoidosis.

Sarcoidosis can affect any ocular tissue, including the orbit and adnexa. Cutaneous involvement is frequent, and orbital and eyelid granulomas are common (Fig 6-52). Palpebral and bulbar conjunctival nodules may also be observed and provide a readily accessible site for tissue biopsy (Fig 6-53). Lacrimal gland infiltration may cause keratoconjunctivitis sicca.

Anterior uveitis, presenting either acutely or as a chronic granulomatous uveitis, is the most common ocular lesion, occurring in approximately two-thirds of patients with ocular sarcoidosis. Symptoms of uveal involvement are variable and frequently include mild to moderate blurring of vision and aching around the eyes. Typical biomicroscopic findings include

- mutton-fat KPs (Fig 6-54), including those involving the anterior chamber angle
- Koeppe and Busacca iris nodules (Fig 6-55)
- white clumps of cells ("snowballs") in the inferior anterior vitreous

Although the cornea is infrequently involved, nummular corneal infiltrates and inferior corneal endothelial opacification may be present; band keratopathy may develop

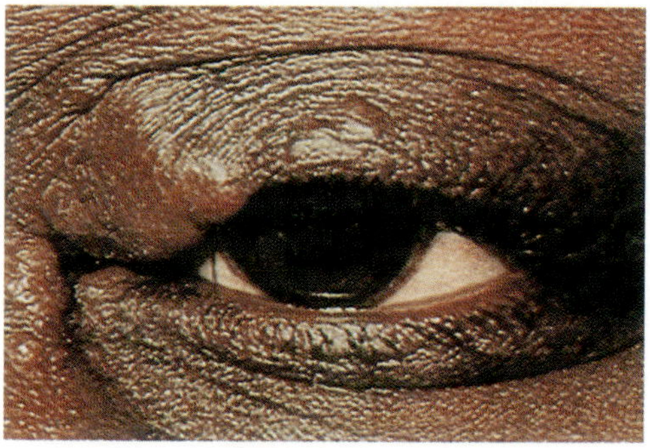

Figure 6-52 Sarcoidosis: skin lesions.

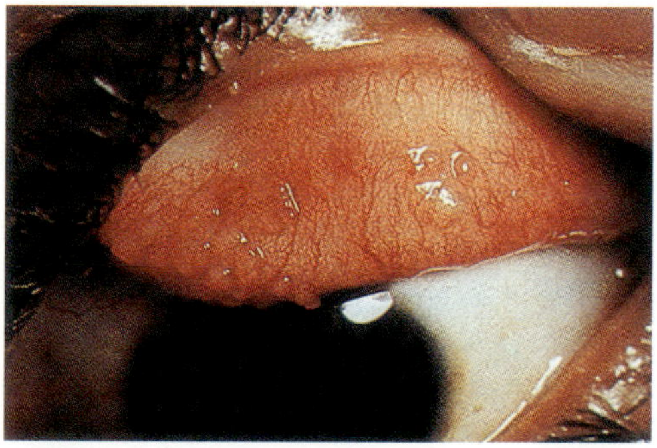

Figure 6-53 Sarcoidosis: conjunctival nodules.

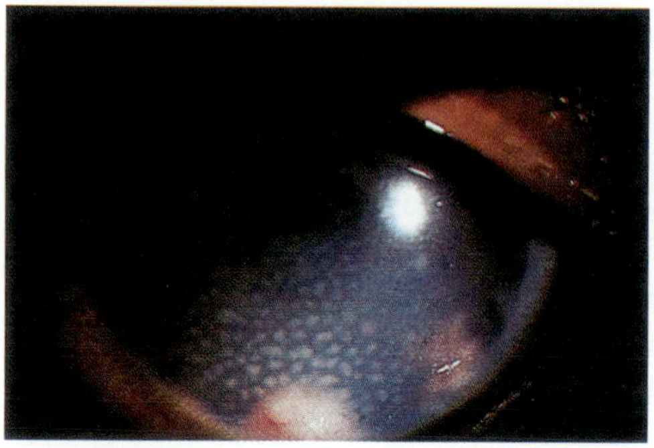

Figure 6-54 Sarcoidosis with keratic precipitates and anterior uveitis.

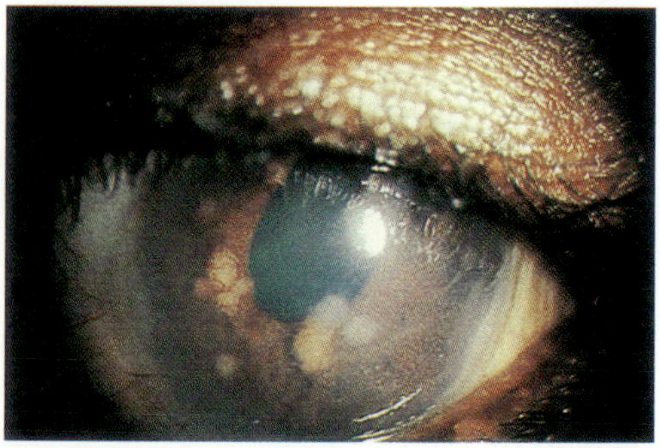

Figure 6-55 Sarcoidosis: iris nodules. Busacca nodules are in the iris stroma, and Koeppe nodules are found at the pupil margin.

as a result of either chronic uveitis or hypercalcemia. Large iris granulomas may also be noted. Extensive posterior synechiae may lead to iris bombé and angle-closure glaucoma. Peripheral anterior synechiae may also be extensive, encompassing the entire angle for 360° in advanced cases. Secondary glaucoma, together with sarcoid uveitis, may be severe and portends a poor prognosis with associated severe vision loss.

Posterior segment lesions occur in up to 20% of patients with ocular sarcoidosis. Vitreous involvement is common and often presents as clumps of snowballs with or without diffuse cellular infiltration. Vitreous cells may also form linear strands known as "string of pearls." Nodular granulomas measuring ¼–1 disc diameter may be present on the optic nerve, in both the retina and the choroid, either posteriorly or peripherally (Fig 6-56). Perivascular sheathing is also common, appearing most often as either a linear or segmental periphlebitis (Fig 6-57). Irregular nodular granulomas along venules have been termed *candle-wax drippings,* or *taches de bougie.* Occlusive retinal vascular disease, especially branch retinal vein occlusion and, less commonly, central retinal vein occlusion, together

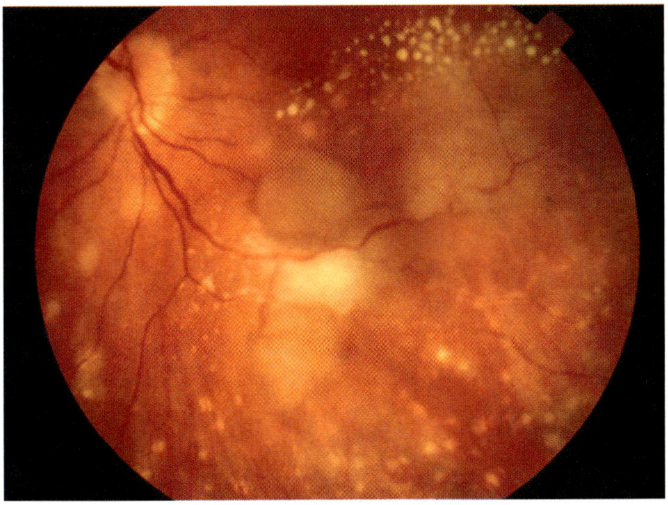

Figure 6-56 Fundus photograph showing numerous retinal and choroidal nodular granulomas, perivasculitis, and vitritis in a patient with sarcoidosis-associated posterior segment involvement. *(Courtesy of Albert T. Vitale, MD.)*

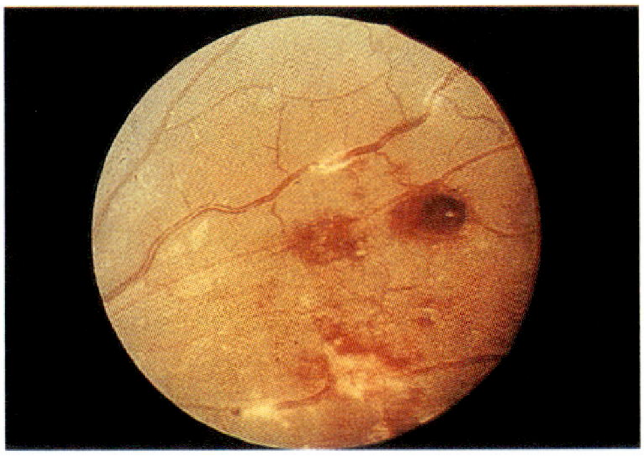

Figure 6-57 Sarcoidosis: fundus photograph showing retinal vascular sheathing.

with peripheral retinal capillary nonperfusion, may lead to retinal neovascularization and vitreous hemorrhage. CME is frequently present, and optic disc edema without granulomatous invasion of the optic nerve may be observed in patients with papilledema and neurosarcoidosis.

Diagnosis and treatment

Given its heterogeneous presentation, sarcoidosis should be considered in the differential diagnosis of any patient presenting with intraocular inflammation. Early-onset sarcoidosis in children (5 years of age or younger) must be differentiated from JIA-associated anterior uveitis and from familial juvenile systemic granulomatosis (Blau syndrome), given the overlap of ocular and articular involvement. Familial juvenile systemic granulomatosis, an autosomal dominantly inherited syndrome with 100% phenotypic correspondence to mutations in the *NOD2* gene (also known as *CARD15*), may produce ocular disease that is virtually identical to sarcoidosis and should be suspected in patients with a family history of granulomatous disease.

Chest radiograph abnormalities are present at some point in up to 90% of sarcoid patients, but these abnormalities do not persist throughout the disease course and thus may be absent at the time of workup. High-resolution computed tomography (CT) is a more sensitive imaging modality and may be particularly valuable in patients with a normal appearance on chest radiograph but for whom a high clinical index of suspicion remains; the risk of increased radiation must be weighed against the clinical utility of the information gained in such cases. Although the serum ACE and lysozyme levels may be abnormally elevated, neither result is diagnostic nor specific; rather, they are reflective of total-body granuloma content and, as such, may be useful in tracking active disease. (Note that the ACE levels may be artificially low in patients taking ACE-inhibitor medications.) Other laboratory evaluations that have been suggested include those for serum and urinary calcium levels and liver function. These assessments are not specific for sarcoidosis, but they may suggest more widespread involvement in patients likely to have the disease.

Gallium scanning has been used to check for occult disease activity, but it has limited sensitivity. Fluorine-18-fluorodeoxyglucose positron emission tomography is considered more accurate in pulmonary and extrapulmonary sarcoidosis, but its utility in ophthalmic sarcoidosis is not well defined. The finding of mononuclear alveolitis with increased $CD4^+$ lymphocytes, as revealed by bronchoalveolar lavage, can also help support the diagnosis.

The traditional approach for suspected ophthalmic involvement with sarcoidosis is to obtain a chest radiograph, possibly along with ACE and lysozyme levels. Some experts recommend repeating the tests annually in patients with negative results but for whom a strong suspicion for the disease exists. The additional tests mentioned above can then supplement the workup, depending on the degree of suspicion and/or preference of the managing physician.

Ultimately, the diagnosis of sarcoidosis is made histologically from tissue obtained from the lungs, mediastinal lymph nodes, skin, peripheral lymph nodes, liver, conjunctiva, minor salivary glands, or lacrimal glands. Readily accessible and clinically evident lesions (such as those on the skin, palpable lymph nodes, and nodules on the conjunctiva) should be sought for biopsy, because they are associated with a high yield and low morbidity and may obviate the need for more invasive transbronchial biopsy. Diagnostic criteria for ocular sarcoidosis were proposed in an international workshop of ophthalmologists but have yet to be validated. These criteria consist of diagnostic grades ranging from "definitive" (based on tissue biopsy), to "presumed" (based on typical ocular findings with bilateral hilar adenopathy), to "probable" or "possible" disease (with supporting ancillary evidence).

Topical, periocular, and systemic corticosteroids are the mainstays of therapy for ocular sarcoidosis. Cycloplegia is useful for comfort and prevention of synechiae. Vision-threatening posterior segment lesions generally require, and are responsive to, systemic corticosteroids (prednisone, 40–80 mg/day). Intravitreal corticosteroids, including the fluocinolone acetonide implant, are potential treatment options for patients intolerant of systemic therapy, but they leave the systemic disease untreated. Systemic IMT with methotrexate, azathioprine, mycophenolate mofetil, or cyclosporine can provide good control of the disease while minimizing the risks of long-term corticosteroid therapy. Recently, the TNF-α inhibitors infliximab and adalimumab have been shown to be effective in the treatment of sarcoidosis-associated uveitis. (Paradoxically, the TNF-α inhibitor etanercept has been reported to cause a sarcoidlike syndrome in some patients.) The likelihood of significant visual improvement is substantially increased with systemic therapy; patients with chronic vision-threatening sarcoidosis seem to respond better to IMT than to management that simply treats flare-ups with intermittent local or systemic corticosteroids.

Prognostic factors associated with vision loss in patients with ocular sarcoidosis include the presence of chronic posterior uveitis, glaucoma, a delay in presentation to a uveitis specialist of more than 1 year, and the presence of intermediate or posterior uveitis. Poor patient adherence also leads to vision loss, so patients should be educated about the importance of careful monitoring, even if they are asymptomatic.

Baughman RP, Lower EE, Ingledue R, Kaufman AH. Management of ocular sarcoidosis. *Sarcoidosis Vasc Diffuse Lung Dis.* 2012;29(1):26–33.

Chen ES, Moller DR. Etiology of sarcoidosis. *Clin Chest Med.* 2008;29(3):365–377.

Dana MR, Merayo-Lloves J, Schaumberg DA, Foster CS. Prognosticators for visual outcome in sarcoid uveitis. *Ophthalmology.* 1996;103(11):1846–1853.

Herbort CP, Rao NA, Mochizuki M; members of Scientific Committee of First International Workshop on Ocular Sarcoidosis. International criteria for the diagnosis of ocular sarcoidosis: results of the first International Workshop on Ocular Sarcoidosis (IWOS). *Ocul Immunol Inflamm.* 2009;17(3):160–169.

Sympathetic Ophthalmia

Sympathetic ophthalmia (SO) is a rare, bilateral, diffuse, granulomatous, nonnecrotizing panuveitis that may develop after either surgical or accidental trauma to 1 eye (called the *exciting eye*), followed by a latent period and the appearance of uveitis in the uninjured fellow eye (the *sympathizing eye*). Although the precise incidence of SO is difficult to ascertain because of its rarity, significant improvements in the management of ocular trauma, together with the more widespread use of IMT, have led to an overall decrease. Earlier estimates of the incidence of SO ranged from up to 0.5% in eyes with nonsurgical trauma and 10/100,000 cases after intraocular surgery. Although the most recent minimum incidence estimate is low (0.03/100,000), SO remains a disease with a persistent and potentially devastating presence.

Until recently, accidental penetrating ocular trauma was the most common precipitating event for SO. Ocular surgery—particularly vitreoretinal surgery—has now emerged as the main risk for the development of SO. In the early 1980s, the prevalence of SO in patients who had undergone pars plana vitrectomy was reported to be 0.01%, increasing to 0.06% when the procedure was performed in the context of other penetrating ocular injuries. More recent studies suggest that the risk of developing SO following pars plana vitrectomy is more than twice this figure and may be significantly higher than the risk of infectious endophthalmitis after vitrectomy. Improved access to emergency surgical care following penetrating ocular trauma and improved microsurgical technique have undoubtedly influenced this etiologic shift from penetrating injury to surgical trauma. Similarly, the demographic of SO has changed from earlier reports, in which there was higher prevalence among men, children, and older patients (due to their presumed increased risk of accidental trauma), to more recent studies, which show no sex predominance and a lower risk in children (resulting in part from a reduced incidence of pediatric ocular injuries) as well as an increased risk in older patients (likely stemming from an increased frequency of ocular surgery and retinal detachment in this population). In addition, although SO has traditionally been reported to develop in 80% of patients within 3 months of injury and in 90% within 1 year, these time intervals may actually be longer than previously thought. In a recent series, only one-third of patients developed SO within 3 months and less than one-half did so within 1 year of injury.

Patients with SO typically present with asymmetric bilateral panuveitis, in which the exciting eye exhibits more severe inflammation than the sympathizing eye, at least initially. Signs and symptoms in the sympathizing eye vary in their severity and onset; they range from minimal problems in near vision, mild photophobia, and slight redness to severe granulomatous anterior uveitis. Both eyes may show mutton-fat KPs, thickening of the iris from lymphocytic infiltration, posterior synechiae formation, and elevated IOP due to trabeculitis or hypotony as a result of ciliary body shutdown (Fig 6-58).

Posterior segment findings include moderate to severe vitritis with characteristic yellowish white, midequatorial choroidal lesions (so-called *Dalen-Fuchs nodules*) that may become confluent. Peripapillary choroidal lesions and exudative retinal detachment may also develop (Fig 6-59). Structural complications of SO include cataract, chronic CME,

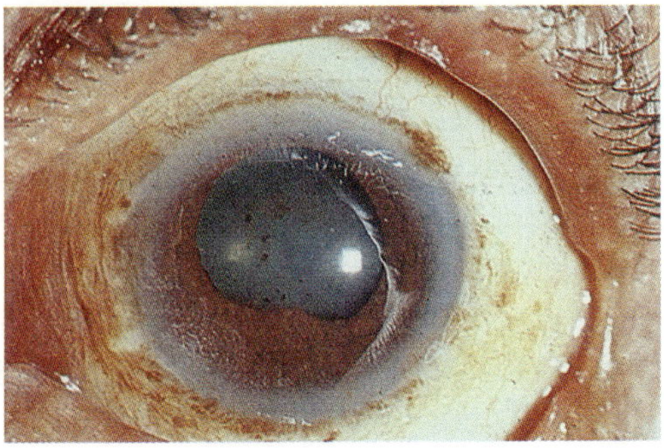

Figure 6-58 Sympathetic ophthalmia: photograph shows sympathizing eye with synechiae.

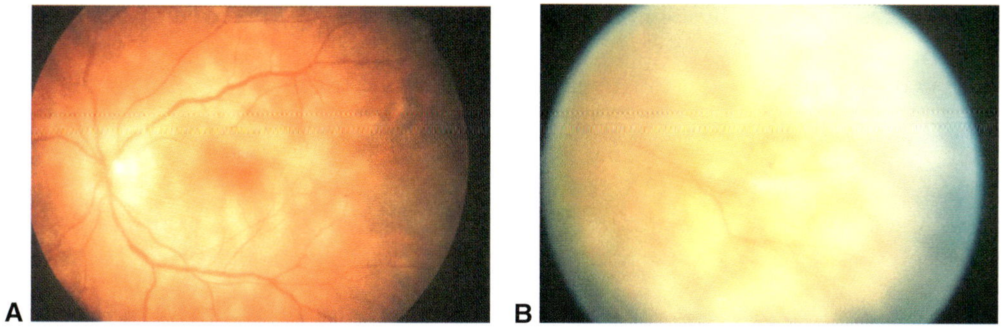

Figure 6-59 Sympathetic ophthalmia. **A,** Fundus photograph showing peripapillary and multifocal choroiditis (yellowish subretinal inflammatory infiltrates) with exudative retinal detachment in the macula. **B,** Fundus photograph showing peripheral multifocal choroiditis and hazy view due to vitritis. *(Courtesy of Ramana S. Moorthy, MD.)*

peripapillary and macular CNV, and optic atrophy. In a recent study, complications in the sympathizing eye at presentation were frequent (up to 47%); cataract and optic nerve abnormalities were most often associated with decreased vision and the further development of new complications, which occurred at a rate of 40% per person-year. Furthermore, traumatic etiology, the presence of active intraocular inflammation, and exudative retinal detachment correlated with poorer vision in the sympathizing eye. Extraocular findings similar to those observed with VKH syndrome, including cerebral spinal fluid pleocytosis, sensory neural hearing disturbance, alopecia, poliosis, and vitiligo, may be noted, although they are uncommon.

During the acute stage of the disease, FA reveals multiple hyperfluorescent sites of leakage at the level of the RPE during the venous phase, which persists into the late stage of the study (Fig 6-60). Pooling of dye is observed beneath areas of exudative neurosensory retinal detachment. Less-common fluorescein angiographic patterns are determined by the status of the overlying RPE. Multiple chorioretinal lesions may be present and may appear hypofluorescent early in the study, simulating the pattern seen in APMPPE, or

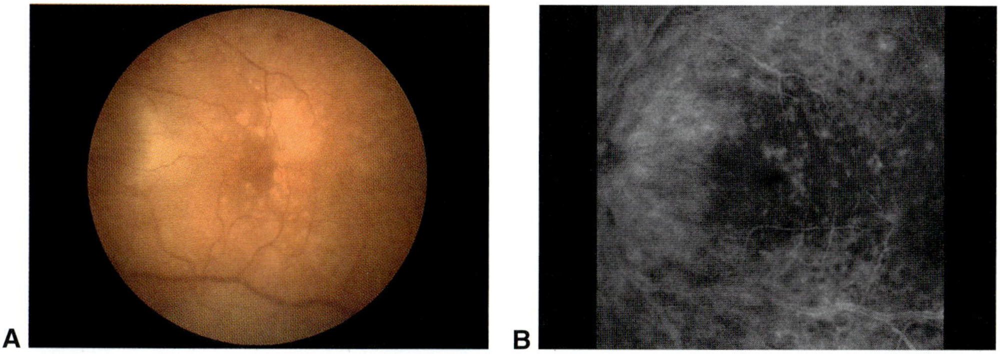

Figure 6-60 Sympathetic ophthalmia. **A,** Fundus photograph showing a multifocal choroiditis. **B,** Corresponding fluorescein angiogram disclosing multiple areas of alternating hyperfluorescence and blocked fluorescence at the level of the RPE. *(Courtesy of Albert T. Vitale, MD.)*

hyperfluorescent with late staining. These lesions are commonly referred to clinically as "Dalen-Fuchs nodules," even though that term refers to the histopathologic finding of clusters of epithelioid cells located between the RPE and the Bruch membrane. ICG angiography reveals numerous hypofluorescent foci, which are best visualized during the intermediate phase of the angiogram; some of these foci may become isofluorescent in the late stage of the study (Fig 6-61). OCT imaging may demonstrate a shallow, serous retinal detachment and/or intraretinal edema, and monitoring these findings can help determine the efficacy of treatment. B-scan ultrasonography frequently reveals choroidal thickening.

The histologic features of SO are similar for both the exciting and sympathizing eyes. Findings include diffuse, granulomatous, nonnecrotizing infiltration of the choroid that classically spares the choriocapillaris in the early stage. Dalen-Fuchs nodules are present in about one-third of patients. The nodules are not specific to SO and can also be found in VKH syndrome and sarcoidosis (see BCSC Section 4, *Ophthalmic Pathology and Intraocular Tumors*).

The precise etiology of SO is unknown; however, in the overwhelming majority of patients, there is a history of surgery or penetrating ocular injury complicated by incarceration of uveal tissue. The disorder may result from altered T-lymphocyte responses to previously sequestered ocular self-antigens and antigens derived from the RPE or choroid. The penetrating wound itself may facilitate exposure of uveoretinal antigens to conjunctival lymphatic channels and thereby initiate this immunopathologic response. Furthermore, there may be a genetic predisposition to the development of the disease, as patients with SO are more likely to express HLA-DR4, -DRw53, and -DQw3 haplotypes. It should be noted that the immunogenetics of SO and VKH syndrome are virtually identical, as the same associations have been found in both diseases.

The diagnosis of SO is clinical, and the disorder should be suspected in the presence of bilateral uveitis following any ocular trauma or surgery. Differential diagnostic considerations include other causes of panuveitis, including TB, sarcoidosis, syphilis, and fungal infections, as well as traumatic or postoperative endophthalmitis. Lens-associated uveitis has been reported with SO in up to 25% of cases and may present with a similar clinical picture. The clinical presentations of SO and VKH syndrome may be strikingly similar; however, a history of prior ocular injury is by definition absent in patients with VKH syndrome.

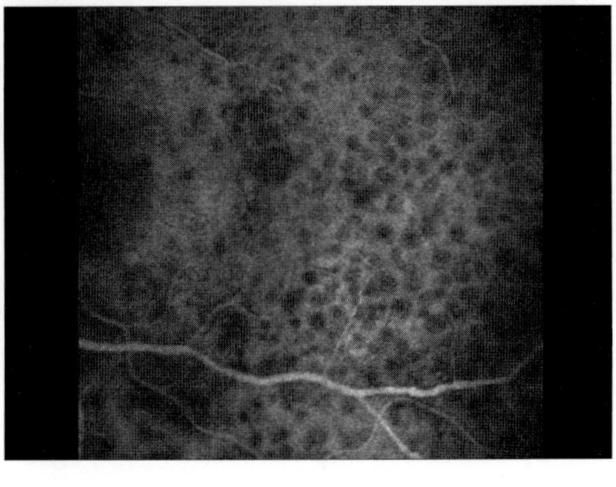

Figure 6-61 Sympathetic ophthalmia: indocyanine green angiogram of the same patient as in Figure 6-60. Multiple midphase hypofluorescent foci corresponding to, and more numerous than, the choroidal lesions found on clinical examination or fluorescein angiography.

The course of SO is chronic, with frequent exacerbations; left untreated, SO leads to loss of vision and phthisis bulbi. Every attempt should be made to salvage eyes with a reasonable prognosis for useful vision through meticulous and prompt closure of penetrating injuries; however, enucleation within 2 weeks of injury to prevent the development of SO should be considered in patients with grossly disorganized globes with no discernible visual function. Although controversial, enucleation may still be preferred to evisceration as the operation of choice for the removal of ocular contents in severely injured eyes because it eliminates the possibility of residual uveal tissue, which may predispose to the development of sympathetic disease. BCSC Section 7, *Orbit, Eyelids, and Lacrimal System,* discusses the advantages and disadvantages of enucleation and evisceration in greater detail. Regardless of visual potential, once SO has become established, enucleation of the exciting eye has not been shown to be beneficial in altering the disease course of the sympathizing eye. In fact, the exciting eye may eventually become the better-seeing eye.

The initial treatment of SO involves systemic corticosteroids, with the frequent addition of corticosteroid-sparing drugs such as azathioprine, methotrexate, mycophenolate mofetil, cyclosporine, chlorambucil, and cyclophosphamide, as extended therapy is anticipated in most patients. Topical corticosteroids, together with cycloplegic and mydriatic agents, are essential in the treatment of the acute anterior uveitis associated with SO. Periocular corticosteroids are used to manage inflammatory recurrences and CME. Intravitreal corticosteroids, including the intravitreal fluocinolone acetonide implant, represent an option for patients intolerant of systemic corticosteroid therapy. With prompt and aggressive systemic therapy, the visual prognosis of SO is good; 60% of patients achieve a final visual acuity of 20/40, although up to 25% may decline to 20/200 or worse in the sympathizing eye.

Castiblanco C, Adelman RA. Imaging for sympathetic ophthalmia: impact on the diagnosis and management. *Int Ophthalmol Clin.* 2012;52(4):173–181.

Chu XK, Chan CC. Sympathetic ophthalmia: to the twenty-first century and beyond. *J Ophthalmic Inflamm Infect.* 2013;3(1):49.

Galor A, Davis JL, Flynn HW Jr, et al. Sympathetic ophthalmia: incidence of ocular complications and vision loss in the sympathizing eye. *Am J Ophthalmol.* 2009;148(5): 704–710.

Lubin JR, Albert DM, Weinstein M. Sixty-five years of sympathetic ophthalmia. A clinicopathologic review of 105 cases (1913–1978). *Ophthalmology.* 1980;87(2):109–121.

Vogt-Koyanagi-Harada Syndrome

VKH syndrome is an uncommon multisystem disease of presumed autoimmune etiology that is characterized by chronic, bilateral, diffuse, granulomatous panuveitis with accompanying integumentary, neurologic, and auditory involvement. Although the disease most commonly affects certain ethnic groups (people with Asian, Asian Indian, Hispanic, Native American, and Middle Eastern ancestry) and is uncommon among whites, VKH syndrome is also rare among sub-Saharan Africans, suggesting that other factors, in addition to skin pigmentation, are important in its pathogenesis. The incidence of VKH syndrome varies geographically, accounting for up to 4% of all uveitis referrals in the United States and 8% in Japan. In Brazil and Saudi Arabia, it is the most commonly encountered cause of noninfectious uveitis.

The precise etiology and pathogenesis of VKH syndrome are unknown, but current clinical and experimental evidence suggests a cell-mediated autoimmune process driven by T lymphocytes directed against self-antigens associated with melanocytes of all organ systems in genetically susceptible individuals. A genetic predisposition for the development of the disease and an immune dysregulatory pathogenesis are further supported by the strong association with HLA-DR4 among Japanese patients and with HLA-DR1 or HLA-DR4 among Hispanic patients from southern California.

There are 4 stages of VKH syndrome: prodromal, acute uveitic, convalescent, and chronic recurrent. Histologic findings vary depending on the stage. During the acute uveitic stage, there is a diffuse, nonnecrotizing, granulomatous inflammation virtually identical to that seen in SO, consisting of lymphocytes and macrophages admixed with epithelioid and multinucleate giant cells, with preservation of the choriocapillaris. Proteinaceous fluid exudates are observed in the subretinal space between the detached neurosensory retina and the RPE. Although the peripapillary choroid is the predominant site of the granulomatous inflammatory infiltration, the ciliary body and iris may also be affected. The convalescent stage is characterized by nongranulomatous inflammation, with uveal infiltration of lymphocytes, few plasma cells, and the absence of epithelioid histiocytes. The number of choroidal melanocytes decreases with loss of melanin pigment, which corresponds with the characteristic clinical feature known as *sunset-glow fundus.* In addition, the appearance of numerous nummular chorioretinal scars in the peripheral retina histologically corresponds to the focal loss of RPE cells with chorioretinal adhesions. The chronic recurrent stage is characterized by granulomatous choroiditis with damage to the choriocapillaris. The numerous clinical, pathologic, and genetic similarities between SO and VKH syndrome suggest that they share a similar immunopathogenesis, albeit with different triggering events and modes of sensitization.

The clinical features of VKH syndrome also vary depending on the stage of the disease. The prodromal stage is marked by flulike symptoms. Several days preceding the onset of ocular symptoms, patients may present with headache, nausea, meningismus, dysacusia, tinnitus, fever, orbital pain, photophobia, and hypersensitivity of the skin and hair to touch. Focal neurologic signs, although rare, may develop and include cranial neuropathies, hemiparesis, aphasia, transverse myelitis, and ganglionitis. Cerebrospinal fluid analysis reveals lymphocytic pleocytosis with normal levels of glucose in more than 80% of patients; this finding may persist for up to 8 weeks. Auditory problems are observed in 75% of patients, frequently coincident with the onset of ocular disease. Central dysacusia, usually involving higher frequencies or tinnitus, occurs in approximately 30% of patients early in the disease course, typically improving within 2–3 months; however, persistent deficits may remain.

The acute uveitic stage is heralded by the onset of sequential blurring of vision in both eyes, 1–2 days after the onset of CNS signs, and is marked by bilateral granulomatous anterior uveitis, a variable degree of vitritis, thickening of the posterior choroid with elevation of the peripapillary retinal choroidal layer, hyperemia and edema of the optic nerve, and multiple serous retinal detachments (Fig 6-62). The focal serous retinal detachments are often shallow, exhibiting a cloverleaf pattern around the posterior pole, but they may coalesce and evolve into large, bullous, exudative detachments (Fig 6-63). Profound vision loss may occur during this phase. Less commonly, mutton-fat KPs and iris nodules at the pupillary margin may be observed. IOP may be elevated; also, the anterior chamber may be shallow because of forward displacement of the lens–iris diaphragm as the result of ciliary body edema or annular choroidal detachment, or it may be low, secondary to ciliary body shutdown.

The convalescent stage occurs several weeks later and is marked by resolution of the exudative retinal detachments and gradual depigmentation of the choroid, resulting in the classic orange-red discoloration, or sunset-glow fundus (Fig 6-64). In addition, small, round, discrete depigmented lesions develop in the inferior peripheral fundus (Fig 6-65). Juxtapapillary depigmentation may also be seen (see Fig 6-64). In Hispanic patients, the

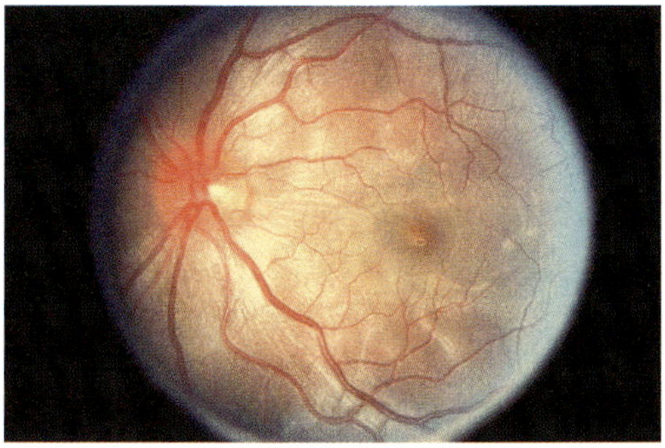

Figure 6-62 Vogt-Koyanagi-Harada (VKH) syndrome: fundus photograph showing disc hyperemia and multiple serous retinal detachments in the posterior pole of the left eye of a Hispanic patient in the acute uveitic stage. *(Reprinted with permission from Moorthy RS, Inomata H, Rao NA. Vogt-Koyanagi-Harada syndrome.* Surv Ophthalmol. *1995;39(4):271.)*

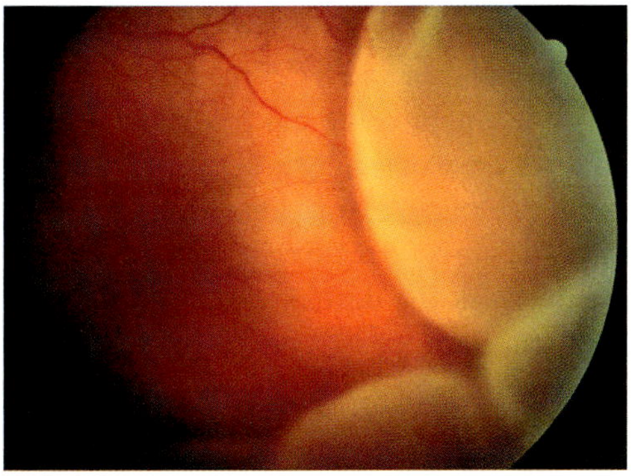

Figure 6-63 VKH syndrome: fundus photograph showing bullous exudative retinal detachment in the acute uveitic stage. *(Courtesy of Albert T. Vitale, MD.)*

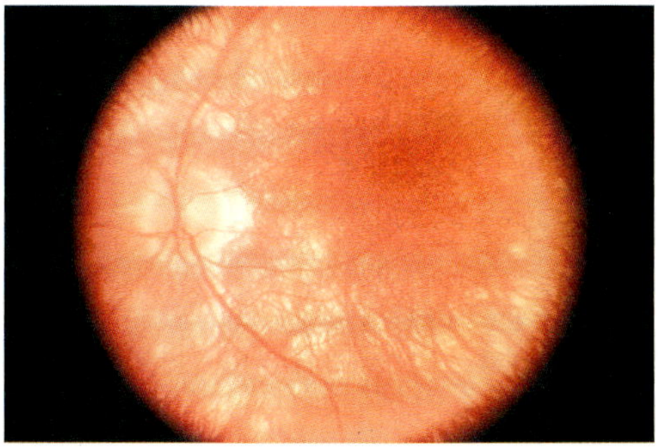

Figure 6-64 VKH syndrome: fundus photograph showing sunset-glow fundus appearance with juxtapapillary detachment in a Hispanic patient in the convalescent stage. *(Reprinted with permission from Moorthy RS, Inomata H, Rao NA. Vogt-Koyanagi-Harada syndrome.* Surv Ophthalmol. *1995;39(4):272.)*

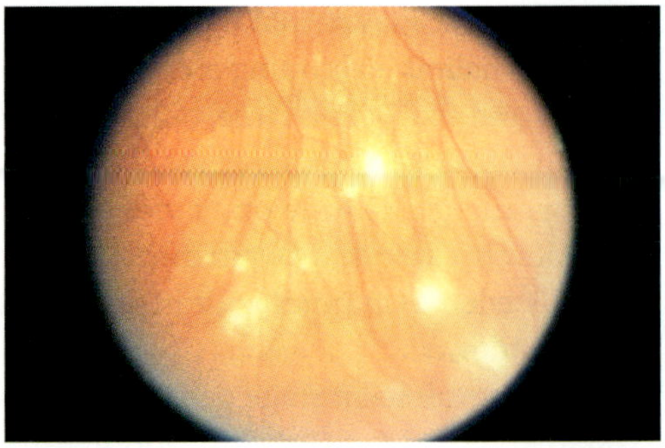

Figure 6-65 VKH syndrome: fundus photograph showing multiple inferior, peripheral, punched-out chorioretinal lesions in a patient in the convalescent stage. *(Courtesy of Ramana S. Moorthy, MD.)*

sunset-glow fundus may show focal areas of retinal hyperpigmentation or hypopigmentation. Perilimbal vitiligo (Sugiura sign) may be present in up to 85% of Japanese patients but is rarely observed among white patients (Fig 6-66). Integumentary changes, including vitiligo, alopecia, and poliosis, typically appear during the convalescent stage in about 30% of patients and correspond with the development of fundus depigmentation (Fig 6-67). In general, skin and hair changes occur weeks to months after the onset of ocular inflammation, but in some cases they may appear simultaneously. Between 10% and 63% of patients develop vitiligo, depending on ethnic background; among Hispanic patients, the incidence of cutaneous and other extraocular manifestations is relatively low.

The chronic recurrent stage is marked by repeated bouts of granulomatous anterior uveitis, with the development of KPs, posterior synechiae, iris nodules, iris depigmentation, and stromal atrophy. Posterior segment recurrences (vitritis, papillitis, multifocal choroiditis, and exudative retinal detachment) have been reported but are uncommon during this stage. Anterior segment recurrence, however, may occur concomitantly with subclinical choroidal inflammation, requiring systemic therapy. Visually debilitating sequelae of chronic inflammation develop during this stage and include posterior subcapsular cataract, glaucoma, CNV, and subretinal fibrosis.

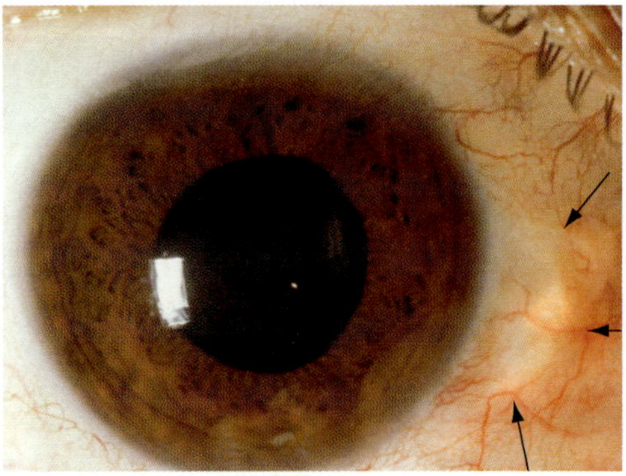

Figure 6-66 Perilimbal vitiligo (Sugiura sign) *(arrows)*. *(Courtesy of Albert T. Vitale, MD.)*

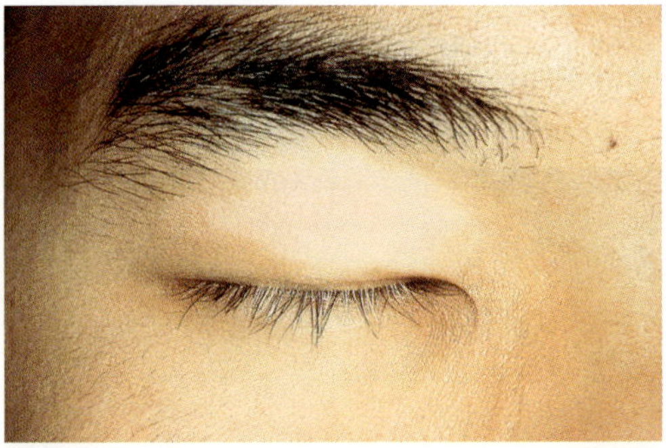

Figure 6-67 VKH syndrome: vitiligo of the upper eyelid and marked poliosis in the convalescent stage. *(Courtesy of Ramana S. Moorthy, MD.)*

Based on these clinical features and their distinctive appearance within the overall disease course, comprehensive diagnostic criteria for the complete, incomplete, and probable forms of VKH syndrome were revised in 2001 (Table 6-3). Regardless of the form of the disease, essential features for the diagnosis of VKH syndrome include bilateral involvement, no history of penetrating ocular trauma, and no evidence of other ocular or systemic disease.

The diagnosis of VKH syndrome is essentially clinical; exudative retinal detachment during the acute disease and sunset-glow fundus during the chronic phase are highly

Table 6-3 Revised Diagnostic Criteria for Vogt-Koyanagi-Harada Syndrome

Complete Vogt-Koyanagi-Harada syndrome

I. No history of penetrating ocular trauma or surgery
II. No clinical or laboratory evidence of other ocular or systemic disease
III. Bilateral ocular disease (either A or B below must be met):
   A. Early manifestations
      1. Diffuse choroiditis as manifested by either:
         a. Focal areas of subretinal fluid, or
         b. Bullous serous subretinal detachments
      2. With equivocal fundus findings, then both:
         a. Fluorescein angiography showing focal delayed choroidal perfusion, pinpoint leakage, large placoid areas of hyperfluorescence, pooling of dye within subretinal fluid, and optic nerve staining
         b. Ultrasonography showing diffuse choroidal thickening without evidence of posterior scleritis
   B. Late manifestations
      1. History suggestive of findings from IIIA, and either both 2 and 3 below, or multiple signs from 3
      2. Ocular depigmentation
         a. Sunset-glow fundus, or
         b. Sugiura sign
      3. Other ocular signs
         a. Nummular chorioretinal depigmentation scars, or
         b. RPE clumping and/or migration, or
         c. Recurrent or chronic anterior uveitis
IV. Neurologic/auditory findings (may have resolved by time of examination):
   A. Meningismus
   B. Tinnitus
   C. Cerebrospinal fluid pleocytosis
V. Integumentary findings (not preceding central nervous system or ocular disease)
   A. Alopecia
   B. Poliosis
   C. Vitiligo

Incomplete Vogt-Koyanagi-Harada syndrome

Criteria I to III and either IV or V from above

Probable Vogt-Koyanagi-Harada syndrome

Criteria I to III from above must be present
Isolated ocular disease

Adapted from Read RW, Holland GN, Rao NA, et al. Revised diagnostic criteria for Vogt-Koyanagi-Harada disease: report of an international committee on nomenclature. *Am J Ophthalmol.* 2001;131(5):647–652.

specific to this entity. In patients presenting without extraocular changes, FA, ICG angiography, OCT, FAF imaging, lumbar puncture, and ultrasonography may be useful confirmatory tests. During the acute uveitic stage, FA typically reveals numerous punctate hyperfluorescent foci at the level of the RPE in the early stage of the study, followed by pooling of dye in the subretinal space in areas of neurosensory detachment (Fig 6-68). The vast majority of patients show disc leakage, but CME and retinal vascular leakage are uncommon. In the convalescent and chronic recurrent stages, focal RPE loss and atrophy produce multiple hyperfluorescent window defects without progressive staining.

ICG angiography highlights the choroidal pathology, disclosing a delay in choriocapillaris and choroidal vessel perfusion, early choroidal stromal vessel hyperfluorescence and leakage, disc hyperfluorescence, multiple hypofluorescent spots throughout the fundus thought to correspond to foci of lymphocytic infiltration, and hyperfluorescent pinpoint changes within areas of exudative retinal detachment. The hypofluorescent spots may be present even when the funduscopic and FA findings are unremarkable; thus, they serve as sensitive markers for the detection and monitoring of subclinical choroidal inflammation.

Ultrasonography may be helpful in establishing the diagnosis, especially in the presence of media opacity. Findings include diffuse, low to medium reflective thickening of the posterior choroid that is most prominent in the peripapillary area, with extension to the equatorial region; exudative retinal detachment; vitreous opacification; and posterior thickening of the sclera.

OCT may be useful in the diagnosis and monitoring of serous macular detachments, CME, and choroidal neovascular membranes. Patients may have characteristic fibrin bands extending from the retina to the RPE in the acute phase, and choroidal thickening is commonly seen (Fig 6-69). SD-OCT using enhanced depth imaging demonstrates choroidal thickening in the acute phase that decreases with treatment. The combined use of SD-OCT and FAF imaging, which shows granular hyperautofluorescence in areas of inflammation, offers a noninvasive assessment of RPE and outer retinal inflammation that may not be apparent on clinical examination in patients with chronic VKH syndrome.

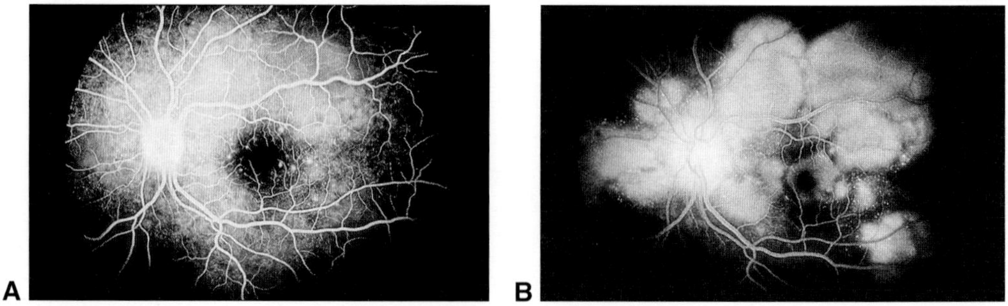

Figure 6-68 VKH syndrome. **A,** Early arteriovenous phase fluorescein angiogram showing multiple pinpoint foci of hyperfluorescence in the posterior pole of the left eye of a patient in the acute uveitic stage. **B,** Late arteriovenous phase fluorescein angiogram showing fluorescein pooling in multiple serous retinal detachments in the posterior pole in the same eye. *(Courtesy of Ramana S. Moorthy, MD.)*

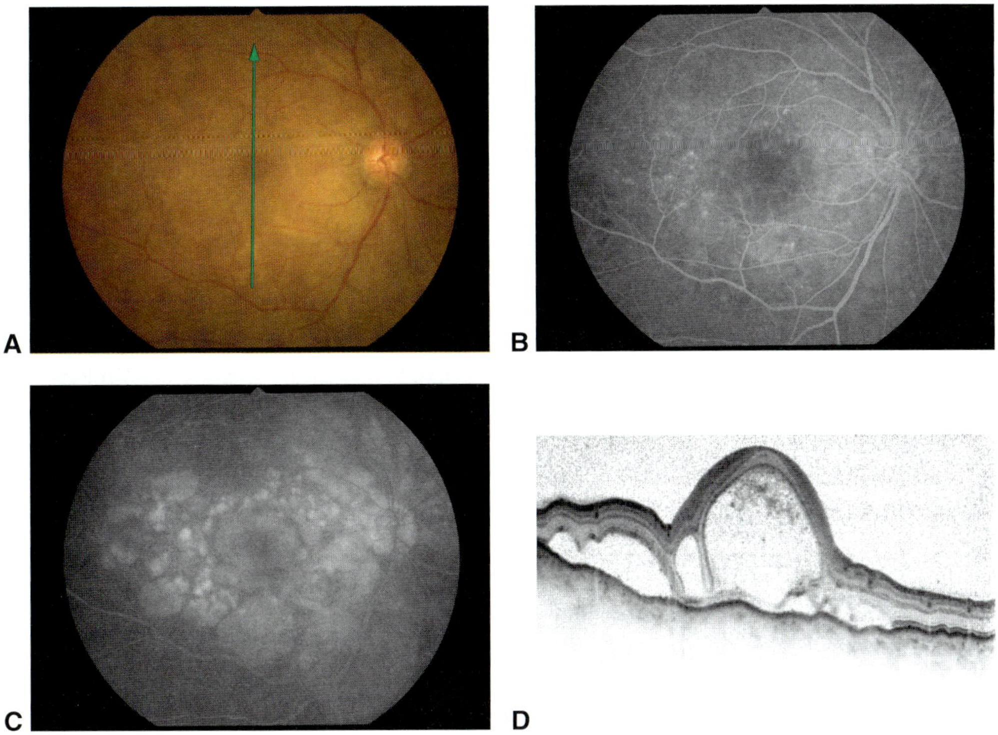

Figure 6-69 VKH syndrome. **A,** Color photograph showing multiple serous retinal detachments. **B, C,** Fluorescein angiograms showing early punctate hyperfluorescence **(B)** followed by late filling of the subretinal spaces with dye **(C)**. **D,** OCT scan showing characteristic loculated spaces of subretinal fluid, with bands extending from the retina to the RPE. The location of the OCT scan is indicated by the *green arrow* in **A.** *(Courtesy of Annabelle Okada, MD.)*

In highly atypical cases—particularly patients presenting early in the course of the disease with prominent neurologic signs and a paucity of ocular findings—a lumbar puncture, revealing lymphocytic pleocytosis, may be useful diagnostically. However, in the vast majority of cases, the history and clinical examination, together with results of FA and/or ultrasonography, are sufficient to establish the diagnosis.

The differential diagnosis of VKH syndrome includes SO, uveal effusion syndrome, posterior scleritis, primary intraocular lymphoma, uveal lymphoid infiltration, APMPPE, and sarcoidosis. These entities may be differentiated from VKH syndrome by a thorough history, review of systems, and physical examination, together with a directed laboratory evaluation.

The acute stage of VKH syndrome is responsive to early and aggressive treatment with corticosteroids. Initial dosages typically are 1–1.5 mg/kg/day of oral prednisone or up to 1 g of intravenous methylprednisolone daily for 3 days followed by high-dose oral corticosteroids. Oral versus intravenous routes of administration show no demonstrable differences in visual acuity outcome or the development of visually significant complications. For patients intolerant of systemic therapy, use of intravitreal corticosteroids, including the intravitreal fluocinolone acetonide implant, is an option. Systemic corticosteroids are tapered slowly according to the clinical response, on average over a 6–12 month period, in an effort to prevent progression of the disease to the chronic recurrent stage and to minimize the incidence and severity of extraocular manifestations. Tapering corticosteroids too soon can result in early recurrence.

Despite adequate initial treatment with systemic corticosteroids, many patients experience recurrent episodes of inflammation. This risk has led many experts to initiate IMT (including cyclosporine, azathioprine, mycophenolate mofetil, chlorambucil, cyclophosphamide, and infliximab) earlier to achieve more prompt inflammatory control and to facilitate more rapid tapering of corticosteroids. The overall visual prognosis for patients treated in this fashion is fair, with up to 70% of patients retaining visual acuity of 20/40 or better. Structural complications associated with ocular morbidity include cataract formation (50%); glaucoma (33%); CNV (up to 15%); and subretinal fibrosis, the development of which is associated with increased disease duration, more frequent recurrences, and an older age at disease onset. Recently, the use of either oral corticosteroids or IMT with extended follow-up was shown to reduce the risk of vision loss and the development of some structural complications. Specifically, oral corticosteroids reduced the risk of CNV and subretinal fibrosis by 82% and the risk of visual acuity decline to 20/200 or worse in better-seeing eyes by 67%. IMT was associated with risk reductions of 67% for vision loss to 20/50 or worse and 92% for vision loss to 20/200 or worse in better-seeing eyes.

Bykhovskaya I, Thorne JE, Kempen JH, Dunn JP, Jabs DA. Vogt-Koyanagi-Harada disease: clinical outcomes. *Am J Ophthalmol.* 2005;140(4):674–678.

Fang W, Yang P. Vogt-Koyanagi-Harada syndrome. *Curr Eye Res.* 2008;33(7):517–523.

Greco A, Fusconi M, Gallo A, et al. Vogt-Koyanagi-Harada syndrome. *Autoimmun Rev.* 2013; 12(11):1033–1038.

Jap A, Chee SP. Imaging in the diagnosis and management of Vogt-Koyanagi-Harada disease. *Int Ophthalmol Clin.* 2012;52(4):163–172.

Rao NA. Pathology of Vogt-Koyanagi-Harada disease. *Int Ophthalmol.* 2007;27(2–3):81–85.

Rao NA, Gupta A, Dustin L, et al. Frequency of distinguishing clinical features in Vogt-Koyanagi-Harada disease. *Ophthalmology.* 2010;117(3):591–599.

Read RW, Holland GN, Rao NA, et al. Revised diagnostic criteria for Vogt-Koyanagi-Harada disease: report of an international committee on nomenclature. *Am J Ophthalmol.* 2001; 131(5):647–652.

Read RW, Rechodouni A, Butani N, et al. Complications and prognostic factors in Vogt-Koyanagi-Harada disease. *Am J Ophthalmol.* 2001;131(5):599–606.

Vasconcelos-Santos DV, Sohn EH, Sadda S, Rao NA. Retinal pigment epithelial changes in chronic Vogt-Koyanagi-Harada disease: fundus autofluorescence and spectral domain-optical coherence tomography findings. *Retina.* 2010;30(1):33–41.

Behçet Disease

Behçet disease (BD) is a chronic, relapsing, occlusive systemic vasculitis (Fig 6-70) of unknown etiology that is characterized, in part, by a uveitis that can affect both the anterior and the posterior segments of the eye, often simultaneously. The symptoms of this disease were described as early as 2500 years ago, but it was only in the early 20th century that its clinical features were more completely characterized by Adamantiades and Behçet. BD occurs in many ethnic populations all over the world. It is most common in the Northern

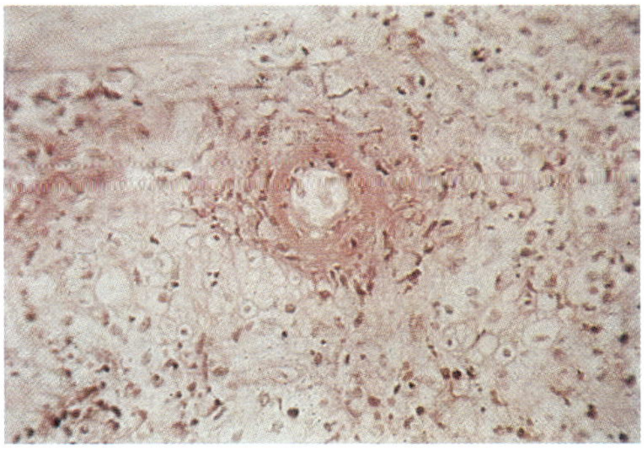

Figure 6-70 Behçet disease: histologic view of perivascular inflammation.

Hemisphere in the countries of the eastern Mediterranean and on the eastern rim of Asia, particularly along the Old Silk Route. The prevalence of BD varies from as high as 80–300 cases per 100,000 inhabitants in Turkey to 8–10 per 100,000 in Japan and 0.4 per 100,000 in the United States. The "complete" type of BD (fulfilling 4 major diagnostic criteria; Table 6-4) is more common in men, and the "incomplete" type (fulfilling 3 major criteria or ocular involvement with 1 other major criterion; see Table 6-4) is equally frequent in men and women. Throughout the world, the typical age of onset is between 25 and 35 years, but BD can also develop as early as age 10–15 years. Although there have been some familial cases of BD, most are sporadic.

The diagnosis of BD is clinical and is based on the presence of multiple systemic findings. The diagnostic system for BD given in Table 6-4 was suggested by researchers in Japan, and another diagnostic system was suggested by the International Study Group for Behçet's Disease (Table 6-5). Although BD is a multisystem disease, it can have its predominant effect on a single system; thus, special clinical types of BD occur—namely, neuro-BD, ocular BD, intestinal BD, and vascular BD.

Table 6-4 Diagnostic System for Behçet Disease (Japan)

Major criteria
Recurrent oral aphthous ulcers
Skin lesions (erythema nodosum, acneiform pustules, folliculitis)
Recurrent genital ulcers
Ocular inflammatory disease
Minor criteria
Arthritis
Gastrointestinal ulceration
Epididymitis
Systemic vasculitis or associated complications
Neuropsychiatric symptoms
Types of Behçet disease
Complete (4 major criteria)
Incomplete (3 major criteria or ocular involvement with 1 other major criterion)
Suspect (2 major criteria with no ocular involvement)
Possible (1 major criterion)

Information from Behçet's Disease Research Committee of Japan. Behçet's disease: guide to diagnosis of Behçet's disease. *Jpn J Ophthalmol.* 1974;18:291–294.

Table 6-5 Diagnostic System for Behçet Disease (International Study Group for Behçet's Disease)

Recurrent oral aphthous ulcers (at least 3 or more times per year) plus 2 of the following criteria:

1. Recurrent genital ulcers
2. Ocular inflammation
3. Skin lesions
4. Positive cutaneous pathergy test

Adapted from International Study Group for Behçet's Disease. Criteria for diagnosis of Behçet's disease. *Lancet.* 1990;335(8697):1078–1080.

Nonocular systemic manifestations

Oral aphthae are the most frequent finding in BD (Fig 6-71). These lesions are recurrent mucosal ulcers that produce significant discomfort and pain. They can occur on the lips, gums, palate, tongue, uvula, and posterior pharynx. They are discrete, round or oval, white ulcerations with red rims that vary in size from 2 to 15 mm. They recur every 5–10 days or every month, last 7–10 days, and heal with little scarring unless large.

Skin lesions can include painful or recurrent erythema nodosum, often over extensor surfaces such as the tibia, but also on the face, neck, and buttocks. They disappear with minimal, if any, scarring. Acne vulgaris or folliculitis-like skin lesions may frequently appear on the upper thorax and face. Nearly 40% of patients with BD exhibit cutaneous pathergy, which is characterized by the development of a sterile pustule at the site of a venipuncture or an injection but is not pathognomonic of BD.

Genital ulcers appear grossly similar to oral aphthous ulcers. In male patients, they can occur on the scrotum or penis. In female patients, they can appear on the vulva and the vaginal mucosa. These lesions are associated with variable amounts of pain. Genital lesions can be deep and leave scars that may be apparent on examination even if patients have no acute symptoms.

Systemic vasculitis may also occur in up to 25% of patients with BD, and any size artery or vein in the body may be affected. Four different vascular complications can develop from the systemic vasculitis of BD: arterial occlusion, aneurysm, venous occlusion, and varices. Cardiac involvement from BD can include granulomatous endocarditis, myocarditis, endomyocardial fibrosis, coronary arteritis, and pericarditis; cardiac effects can

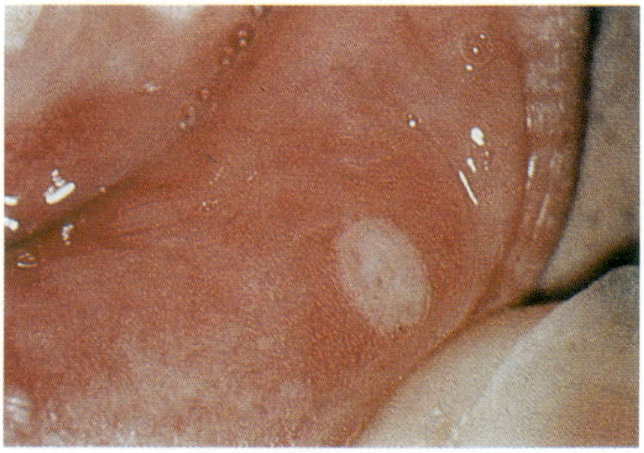

Figure 6-71 Behçet disease: mucous membrane ulcers (oral aphthae).

occur in up to 17% of patients. Gastrointestinal lesions can include multiple ulcers involving the esophagus, stomach, and intestines. Pulmonary involvement is mainly pulmonary arteritis with aneurysmal dilatation of the pulmonary artery. Fifty percent of patients with BD develop arthritis; in 50% of these, the knee is most affected.

Neurologic involvement is the most serious of all manifestations of BD and may occur in up to 10% of patients. Ten percent of patients with neuro-BD can have ocular disease, and 30% of patients with ocular BD may have neurologic involvement. CNS involvement affects mainly areas of motor control. Widespread vasculitis in the CNS can result in headaches. CNS symptoms such as strokes, palsies, and a confusional state may develop in 25% of patients. Mortality has previously been reported to be as high as 10% in patients with neuro-BD, but it may be lower currently, especially with the use of IMT. More men than women appear to develop neuro-BD. Neuro-ophthalmic involvement can include cranial nerve palsies, central scotomata caused by papillitis, visual field defects, and papilledema resulting from thrombosis of the superior sagittal sinus or other venous sinuses.

Ocular manifestations

Ocular manifestations affect up to 70% of patients with BD. They carry serious implications because they are often recurrent and relapsing, resulting in permanent, often irreversible, ocular damage. Severe vision loss can occur in up to 25% of patients with BD. Ocular disease appears to be more severe in men, and more men are affected; up to 80% of cases are bilateral. Ocular involvement as an initial presenting problem is relatively uncommon, occurring in about 10% of patients. The intraocular inflammation is characterized by a nongranulomatous, necrotizing, obliterative vasculitis that can affect any or all portions of the uveal tract.

Anterior uveitis may be the only ocular manifestation of BD; it presents with a transient hypopyon in up to 25% of cases (Fig 6-72). The inflammation is nongranulomatous, and redness, pain, photophobia, and blurred vision are common findings. On clinical examination, the hypopyon can shift with the patient's head position or disperse with head shaking, and it may not be visible unless viewed by gonioscopy. Although anterior uveitis may be very severe, it can spontaneously resolve even without treatment; however, the nature of ocular BD is one of explosive onset over the course of just a few hours. With relapses, posterior synechiae, iris bombé, and angle-closure glaucoma may all develop.

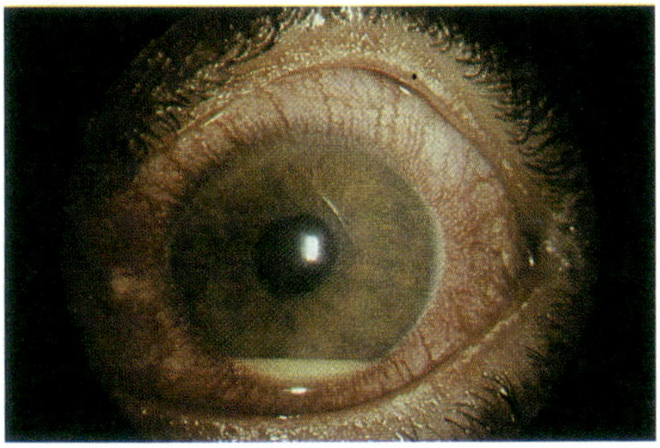

Figure 6-72 Behçet disease: hypopyon.

Other less-common anterior segment findings of BD include cataract, episcleritis, scleritis, conjunctival ulcers, and corneal immune ring opacities.

The posterior segment manifestations of ocular BD are often profoundly sight threatening. The essential retinal finding is that of an obliterative, necrotizing retinal vasculitis that affects both the arteries and the veins in the fundus (Fig 6-73). This form is the most common type of uveitis found in children and adults with BD. Posterior manifestations can include branch retinal vein occlusion, isolated branch artery occlusions, combined branch retinal vein and branch retinal artery occlusions, and vascular sheathing with variable amounts of vitritis, plus associated CME. Retinal ischemia can lead to the development of retinal neovascularization and even of neovascularization of the iris and neovascular glaucoma. After repeated episodes of retinal vasculitis and vascular occlusions, retinal vessels may become white and sclerotic. Active areas of retinal vasculitis may be accompanied by multifocal areas of chalky white retinitis. The ischemic nature of the vasculitis and accompanying retinitis may produce a funduscopic appearance that may be confused with acute retinal necrosis syndrome or other necrotizing herpetic entities (Fig 6-74; see also Chapter 7). The optic nerve is affected in 25% of patients with BD. Optic papillitis can occur, but progressive optic atrophy may occur as a result of the vasculitis affecting the arterioles that supply blood to the optic nerve.

Pathogenesis

The immunopathogenesis of BD remains unknown. Many environmental factors have been suggested as potential causes, but none has been proved. No infectious agent or microorganism has been reproducibly isolated from the lesions of patients with BD. The disorder is clinically and experimentally unlike other autoimmune diseases.

Specific HLA associations have been found in certain systemic forms of BD: HLA-B12 with mucocutaneous lesions and HLA-B51 with ocular lesions. These associations are not reproducible in all populations and are of little diagnostic value. Histologically, the lesions

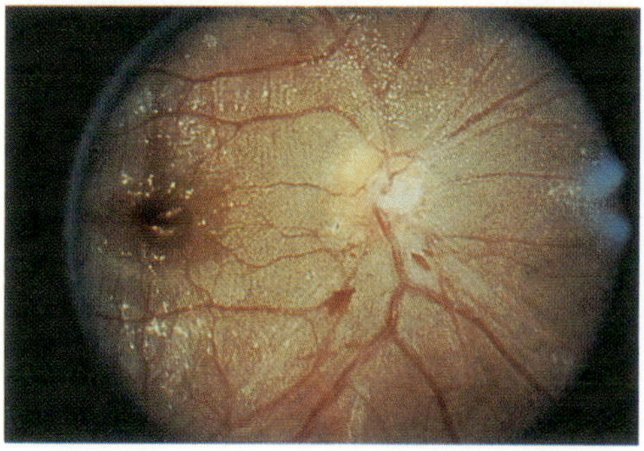

Figure 6-73 Behçet disease: fundus photograph of retinal vasculitis.

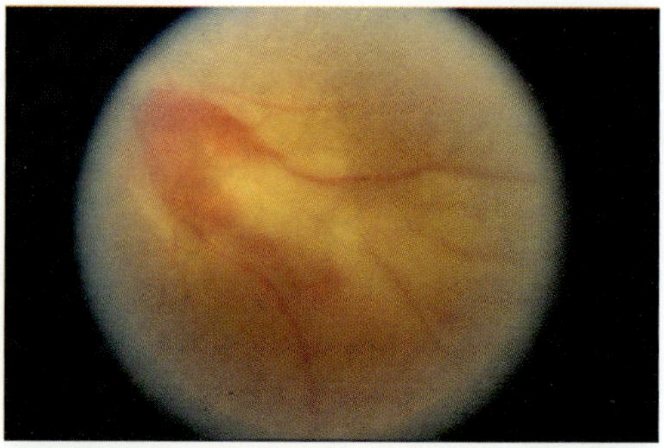

Figure 6-74 Behçet disease: fundus photograph of retinitis and vasculitis with retinal hemorrhage. The retinitis shown here appears similar to necrotizing herpetic retinitis with retinal whitening and occlusive retinal vasculitis. *(Courtesy of Ramana S. Moorthy, MD.)*

of BD resemble those of delayed-type hypersensitivity reactions early on; late lesions resemble those of immune-complex–type reactions.

Diagnosis

Diagnosis of BD is based on clinical findings and the diagnostic criteria given in Tables 6-4 and 6-5. Laboratory tests—for example, HLA typing, cutaneous pathergy testing, and testing for nonspecific serologic markers of inflammation such as ESR and levels of C-reactive protein—are of little value in confirming the diagnosis. Fluorescein angiography demonstrates marked dilatation and occlusion of retinal capillaries with perivascular staining, evidence of retinal ischemia, leakage of fluorescein into the macula with the development of CME, and retinal neovascularization that may leak (Fig 6-75). Subtle vascular leakage may be present on FA before there is clinical evidence of disease activity, and adjusting therapy in response to this leakage may prevent the development of inflammatory damage. OCT imaging can show structural alterations caused by the vasculitis in the form of

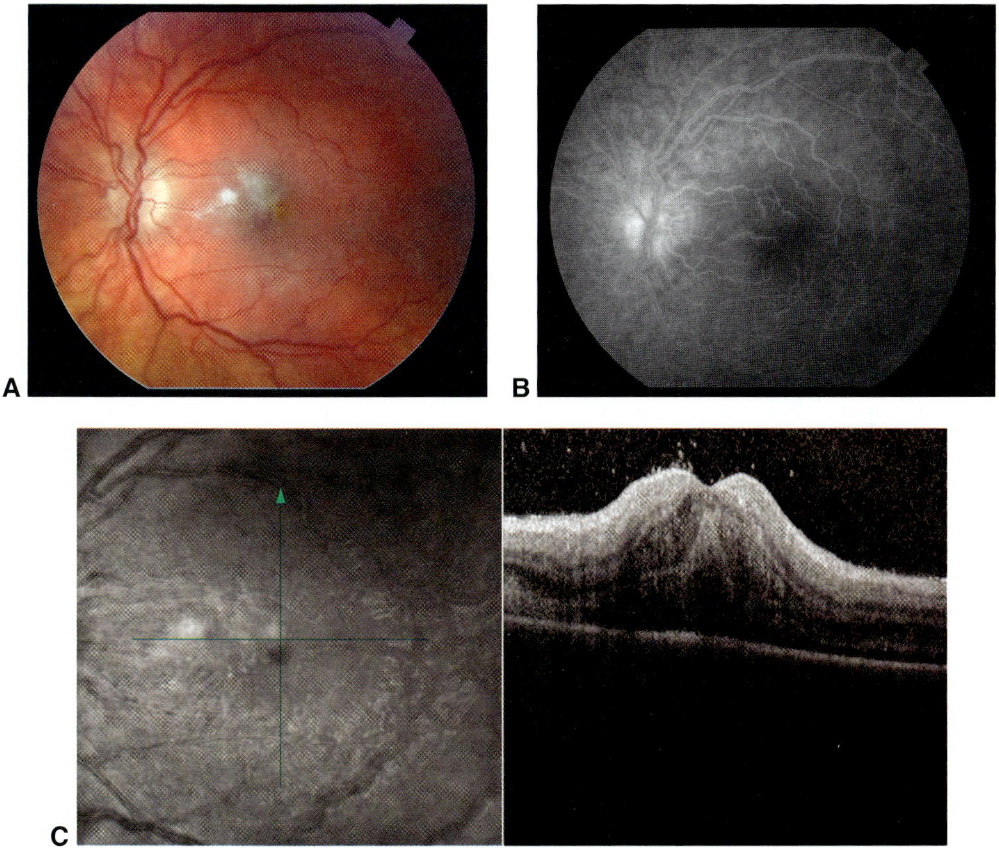

Figure 6-75 Behçet disease. **A,** Color fundus photograph indicating vasculitis and localized retinitis. **B,** Fluorescein angiogram showing disc staining and perivascular leakage. **C,** OCT scan revealing macular edema and inflammatory disruption of the retinal microarchitecture. *(Courtesy of David J. Browning, MD, PhD.)*

macular edema and disruption of the retinal architecture (see Fig 6-75). Radiologic imaging, including chest x-ray, chest CT, and brain MRI with contrast enhancement, may be helpful, as indicated by clinical presentation.

Differential diagnosis

The differential diagnosis for BD includes HLA-B27–associated anterior uveitis, reactive arthritis syndrome, sarcoidosis, and systemic vasculitides including systemic lupus erythematosus, PAN, and GPA. Necrotizing herpetic retinitis can also mimic occlusive BD retinal vasculitis.

Treatment

The goal of treatment is not only to treat the explosive onset of acute disease with systemic corticosteroids but also to control chronic inflammation and prevent or decrease the number of relapses of ocular inflammation with IMT.

Corticosteroids These drugs may be used to treat explosive-onset anterior segment and posterior segment inflammation, although most patients eventually become resistant to corticosteroid therapy. Nevertheless, systemic corticosteroids (eg, 1.5 mg/kg/day of prednisone with a gradual taper) are extremely useful in controlling acute inflammation. Periocular and intravitreal steroids may also be useful in selected patients.

Immunomodulatory medications Patients who present with sight-threatening posterior segment ocular BD require prompt initiation of systemic corticosteroids together with IMT, which may include azathioprine, infliximab, cyclosporine, tacrolimus, mycophenolate mofetil, chlorambucil, or cyclophosphamide. Colchicine is used for treatment of mucocutaneous disease; it is ineffective for treating ocular BD. In prospective clinical trials, azathioprine has been found to be useful in preserving visual acuity in patients with established ocular BD. It can also be effective in controlling oral and genital ulcers and arthritis. Open-label clinical trials have confirmed the efficacy of infliximab in controlling inflammation, and many uveitis specialists consider infliximab the treatment of choice for Behçet retinal vasculitis. Infliximab can result in rapid remission of disease activity and provide long-term disease control. However, there is concern that infliximab, particularly at doses of 10 mg/kg or more, carries a greater risk of long-term therapeutic complications such as disseminated TB or possibly malignancy.

A European League Against Rheumatism panel has recommended using azathioprine (with corticosteroids) as first-line IMT for ocular BD and cyclosporine or infliximab as second-line treatment. A recent American expert panel recommended anti-TNF therapy with infliximab (good-quality evidence) or adalimumab (moderate-quality evidence) as first- or second-line corticosteroid-sparing therapy. Infliximab was recommended as first- or second-line treatment for acute exacerbations of preexisting Behçet disease. Cyclosporine has been used with limited success in the management of ocular BD, but it is not as effective as other cytotoxic drugs and may carry risks of nephrotoxicity. There may also be an increased risk of neuro-BD in patients treated with cyclosporine. Tacrolimus is less toxic and may be used as a substitute for cyclosporine; it has been used successfully in Japan to treat BD. Mycophenolate mofetil has also been successful in treating ocular BD in small case series. Recent reports in the European literature emphasize that interferon alfa-2a is efficacious and well tolerated; it is highly effective in Behçet uveitis and somewhat less effective in non–Behçet uveitis.

Chlorambucil has been found to be effective in the treatment of BD, even at relatively low doses. Some experts believe that chlorambucil may be the most effective of the immunomodulatory drugs in achieving durable remission. Cyclophosphamide is an alternative to chlorambucil and can be used orally or as pulsed intravenous therapy. Both chlorambucil and cyclophosphamide have been shown to be more effective than cyclosporine in the management of posterior segment ocular BD but carry a greater risk of systemic complications. Effective therapeutic reduction of white blood cell counts and proper hematologic monitoring are essential and can be quite complex with these alkylating agents. The availability of biologic drugs has led some experts to reserve the use of alkylating agents for patients with refractory disease.

Prognosis

Prognosis for vision is guarded in patients with BD. Nearly 25% of patients worldwide with chronic ocular BD have visual acuity less than 20/200, most commonly caused by macular edema, occlusive retinal vasculitis, optic atrophy, and glaucoma. Adult men tend to have poorer vision outcomes. Compared with the results achieved in the 1980s, however, current patients appear to have a better visual prognosis because of earlier and more aggressive use of IMT. Complications such as macular edema, complex cataract, glaucoma, secondary and neovascular glaucoma, retinal and optic disc neovascularization, retinal detachment, and vitreous hemorrhage may require complex medical and surgical intervention (see Chapter 10), and all have profound impacts on final visual outcomes. The presence of posterior synechiae, persistent inflammation, elevated IOP, and hypotony are all statistically significant predictive factors for vision loss. The chronic relapsing nature of this disease, with frequent exacerbations after long periods of remission, makes it difficult to predict visual outcomes.

Hatemi G, Silman A, Bang D, et al; EULAR Expert Committee. EULAR recommendations for the management of Behçet disease. *Ann Rheum Dis.* 2008;67(12):1656–1662.

Kaçmaz RO, Kempen JH, Newcomb C, et al; Systemic Immunosuppressive Therapy for Eye Diseases Cohort Study Group. Ocular inflammation in Behçet disease: incidence of ocular complications and of loss of visual acuity. *Am J Ophthalmol.* 2008;146(6):828–836.

Kitaichi N, Miyazaki A, Iwata D, Ohno S, Stanford MR, Chams H. Ocular features of Behçet's disease: an international collaborative study. *Br J Ophthalmol.* 2007;91(12):1579–1582.

Levy-Clarke G, Jabs DA, Read RW, Rosenbaum JT, Vitale A, Van Gelder RN. Expert panel recommendations for the use of anti–tumor necrosis factor biologic agents in patients with ocular inflammatory disorders. *Ophthalmology.* 2014;121(3):785–796.

Tugal-Tutkun I, Gupta V, Cunningham ET. Differential diagnosis of Behçet uveitis. *Ocul Immunol Inflamm.* 2013;21(5):337–350.

Tugal-Tutkun I, Onal S, Altan-Yaycioglu R, Huseyin Altunbas H, Urgancioglu M. Uveitis in Behçet disease: an analysis of 880 patients. *Am J Ophthalmol.* 2004;138(3):373–380.

Zierhut M, Abu El-Asrar AM, Bodaghi B, Tugal-Tutkun I. Therapy of ocular Behçet disease. *Ocul Immunol Inflamm.* 2014;22(1):64–76.

CHAPTER 7

Infectious Ocular Inflammatory Diseases

This chapter includes a related video, which can be accessed by scanning the QR code provided in the text or going to www.aao.org/bcscvideo_section09.

Viruses, fungi, protozoa, helminths, and bacteria can all cause infectious uveitis. Because infection with these organisms may produce inflammation in different parts of the uveal tract, this chapter has been organized according to the causative organism and, if appropriate, subcategorized by the anatomical location of the intraocular inflammation. The most common primary site of inflammation has been identified for each entity. Some diseases, such as herpes simplex virus infection, may cause anterior and/or posterior uveitis. Other illnesses, such as syphilis, Lyme borreliosis, and onchocerciasis, may also cause panuveitis.

Viral Uveitis

Herpesviridae Family

Herpes simplex virus and varicella-zoster virus

Anterior uveitis Acute anterior uveitis can be associated with herpetic viral disease. BCSC Section 8, *External Disease and Cornea,* extensively discusses herpes simplex virus (HSV) and varicella-zoster virus (VZV) infections (Figs 7-1, 7-2). Anterior uveitis in herpetic viral infections may be associated with corneal involvement (keratouveitis) but also occurs without noticeable keratitis. In many cases, the inflammation becomes chronic. VZV infection may be considered in the differential diagnosis of chronic unilateral anterior uveitis, even if the cutaneous component of the condition occurred in the past or was minimal when present. Some patients may develop anterior uveitis without ever having had a cutaneous component (varicella-zoster sine herpete).

Chickenpox (varicella), which is caused by the same virus that is responsible for secondary VZV reactivation, may be associated with an acute, mild, nongranulomatous, self-limiting, and bilateral anterior uveitis. Cutaneous vesicles at the tip of the nose (Hutchinson sign) indicate nasociliary nerve involvement and a greater likelihood that the eye will be affected (see Fig 7-1). Most patients are asymptomatic but, monitored prospectively, up to 40% of patients with primary VZV infection may develop anterior uveitis.

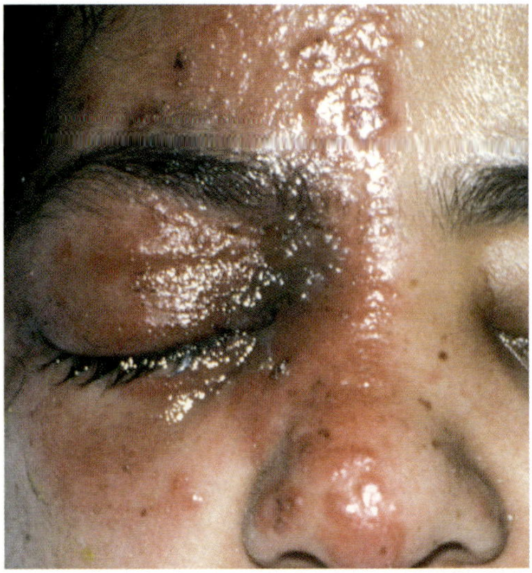

Figure 7-1 Varicella-zoster virus infection: skin lesions. *(Courtesy of Debra A. Goldstein, MD.)*

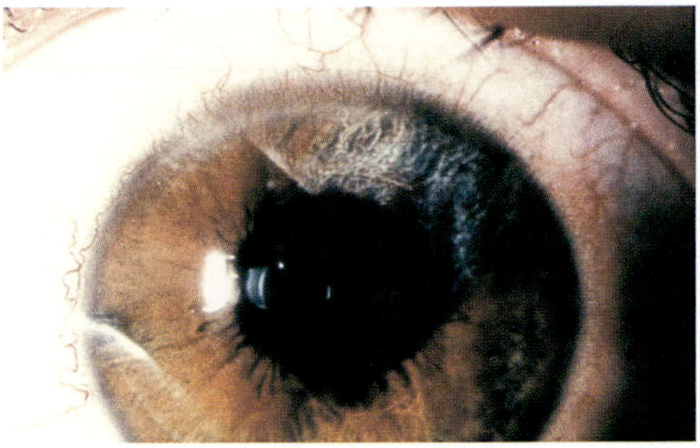

Figure 7-2 Iris stromal atrophy in a patient with varicella-zoster anterior uveitis. *(Courtesy of David Forster, MD.)*

Patients with intraocular viral infections, particularly with herpes group viruses, may occasionally exhibit stellate keratic precipitates (KPs). This morphology is also present in Fuchs heterochromic uveitis. These stellate KPs usually assume a diffuse distribution, as opposed to a regional distribution in the inferior third of the cornea within the *Arlt triangle.* In addition, the KPs are fine and fibrillar and often exhibit a distinctly stellate pattern on high-magnification biomicroscopy. Although the identification of diffuse or stellate KPs may be useful in the differential diagnosis of anterior segment inflammation, it is not diagnostic of any particular condition. In patients with herpetic disease and concomitant keratopathy, mild anterior segment inflammation may also be associated with diffuse or localized decreased corneal sensation and neurotrophic keratitis.

Ocular hypertension is a frequent complication of herpetic uveitis and is thus a helpful diagnostic hallmark. Most other inflammatory syndromes are associated with decreased intraocular pressure (IOP) as a result of ciliary body hyposecretion. However, just as the herpesvirus can localize to corneal, cutaneous, or conjunctival tissues, herpetic reactivation may directly cause trabeculitis and thus increase IOP, often to as high as 50–60 mm Hg. In addition, inflammatory cells may contribute to trabecular obstruction and congestion. Other findings include hyphema, hypopyon, posterior synechia, KP, and corneal edema.

Iris atrophy is characteristic of herpetic inflammation and can be present with HSV-, VZV-, or cytomegalovirus (CMV)-associated anterior uveitis. The atrophy may be patchy or sectoral (see Fig 7-2) and is best demonstrated with retroillumination at the slit lamp.

Viral retinitis (discussed in the following section) may occur with these entities, particularly in immunocompromised hosts. Vasculitis may occur with herpes-zoster ophthalmicus, and it may lead to anterior segment ischemia, retinal artery occlusion, and scleritis. Vasculitis in the orbit gives rise to cranial nerve palsies.

Treatment for viral anterior uveitis includes topical corticosteroids and cycloplegic agents. Topical antiviral drugs are usually ineffective for herpetic uveitis but may be indicated in patients with herpes simplex keratouveitis to prevent dendritic keratitis as a complication of topical corticosteroid therapy. Systemic antiviral drugs such as acyclovir (400–800 mg, 5 times/day), famciclovir (250–500 mg, 3 times/day), or valacyclovir (500 mg to 1 g, 3 times/day) are often beneficial in intraocular inflammation associated with HSV or VZV uveitis, with the higher doses used for VZV uveitis. Initiation of oral antiviral therapy at the onset of VZV uveitis is recommended. Patients with herpetic uveitis may require prolonged corticosteroid therapy with very gradual tapering. In fact, some patients with VZV infection require very long-term, albeit extremely low, doses of topical corticosteroids (as infrequent as 1 drop per week) for the condition to remain quiescent. Systemic corticosteroids are sometimes necessary. Long-term, suppressive, low-dose antiviral therapy may be indicated in patients with herpetic uveitis, but controlled studies are lacking. The oral prophylactic dosages for patients with herpes simplex are acyclovir, 400 mg 2 times/day, or valacyclovir, 500 mg/day. For VZV disease, dosages are acyclovir, 800 mg 2 times/day, or valacyclovir, 1 g/day.

Barron BA, Gee L, Hauck WW, et al. Herpetic Eye Disease Study: a controlled trial of oral acyclovir for herpes simplex stromal keratitis. *Ophthalmology.* 1994;101(12):1871–1882.

Siverio Júnior CD, Imai Y, Cunningham ET Jr. Diagnosis and management of herpetic anterior uveitis. *Int Ophthalmol Clin.* 2002;42(1):43–48.

van der Lelij A, Ooijman FM, Kijlstra A, Rothova A. Anterior uveitis with sectoral iris atrophy in the absence of keratitis: a distinct clinical entity among herpetic eye diseases. *Ophthalmology.* 2000;107(6):1164–1170.

Wilhelmus KR, Gee L, Hauck WW, et al. Herpetic Eye Disease Study. A controlled trial of topical corticosteroids for herpes simplex stromal keratitis. *Ophthalmology.* 1994;101(12):1883–1895.

Acute retinal necrosis, progressive outer retinal necrosis, and nonnecrotizing herpetic retinitis Acute retinal necrosis (ARN) is part of a spectrum of necrotizing herpetic retinopathies, the clinical expression of which appear to be influenced by host and viral factors. Originally described in 1971 among otherwise healthy adults, ARN has also been reported in children and among immunocompromised patients, including those with HIV infection. Acute, fulminant disease may arise without a systemic prodrome years after primary infection or following cutaneous or systemic herpetic infection such as dermatomal zoster, chickenpox, or herpetic encephalitis. The prevalence is nearly equal between the sexes, with the majority of cases clustering in patients between the fifth and seventh decades of life. The American Uveitis Society has established criteria for the diagnosis of ARN solely on the basis of clinical findings and disease progression, independent of viral etiology or host immune status (Table 7-1). Retinal lesions of presumed herpetic etiology that are not characteristic of well recognized syndromes such as ARN, CMV retinitis, or progressive outer retinal necrosis are grouped under the umbrella designation *necrotizing herpetic retinopathy.*

Patients with ARN usually present with acute unilateral loss of vision, photophobia, floaters, and pain. Fellow eye involvement occurs in approximately 36% of cases, usually within 6 weeks of disease onset, but involvement may be delayed for extended periods (up to 26 years has been reported) after initial presentation. Panuveitis is observed, beginning with significant anterior segment inflammation, KPs, posterior synechiae, and elevated IOP, together with heavy vitreous cellular infiltration. Within 2 weeks, the classic triad of occlusive retinal arteriolitis, vitritis, and a multifocal yellow-white peripheral retinitis has evolved. Early on, the peripheral retinal lesions are discontinuous and have scalloped edges that appear to arise in the outer retina. Within days the lesions coalesce to form a confluent 360° creamy retinitis that progresses in a posterior direction, leaving full-thickness retinal necrosis, arteriolitis, phlebitis, and occasional retinal hemorrhage in its wake (Figs 7-3, 7-4). Widespread necrosis of the midperipheral retina, multiple posterior retinal breaks, and proliferative vitreoretinopathy predispose eyes to combined tractional–rhegmatogenous retinal detachments in 75% of patients (Fig 7-5). The posterior pole tends to be spared, but an exudative retinal detachment may arise with severe inflammation. The optic nerve is frequently involved, as evidenced by disc swelling and a relative afferent pupillary defect.

Table 7-1 American Uveitis Society Criteria for Diagnosis of Acute Retinal Necrosis

One or more foci of retinal necrosis with discrete borders, located in the peripheral retina*
Rapid progression in the absence of antiviral therapy
Circumferential spread
Occlusive vasculopathy with arteriolar involvement
Prominent vitritis, anterior chamber inflammation
Optic neuropathy/atrophy, scleritis, pain supportive but not required

*Macular lesions do not exclude diagnosis in the presence of peripheral retinitis.

Data from Holland GN and the Executive Committee of the American Uveitis Society. Standard diagnostic criteria for the acute retinal necrosis syndrome. *Am J Ophthalmol.* 1994;117(5):663–667.

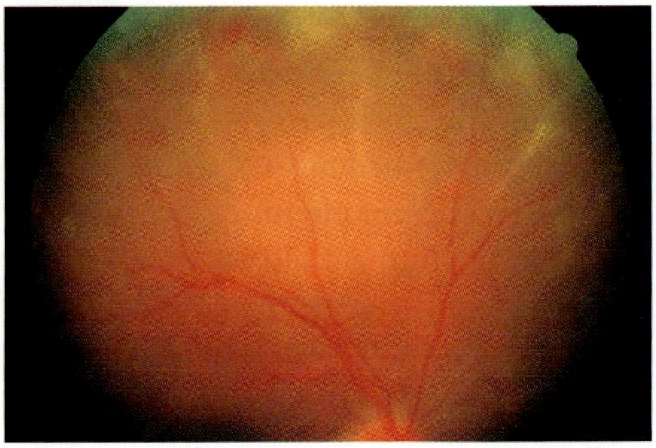

Figure 7-3 Fundus photograph demonstrating acute retinal necrosis, vitritis, arteriolitis, and multiple peripheral "thumbprint" areas of retinitis. *(Courtesy of E. Mitchel Opremcak, MD.)*

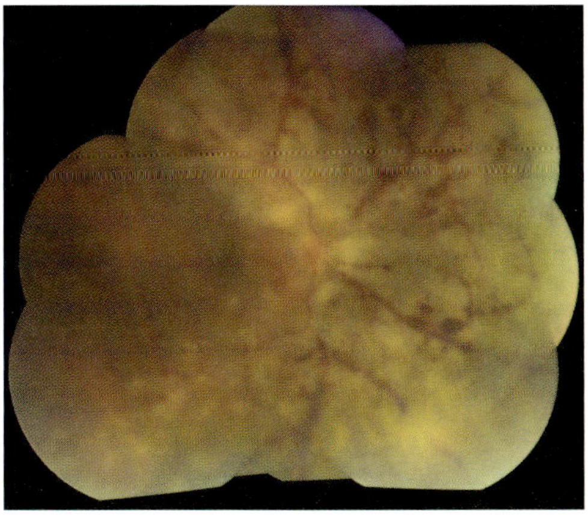

Figure 7-4 Fundus photograph of acute retinal necrosis showing confluent peripheral retinitis. *(Courtesy of H. Nida Sen, MD.)*

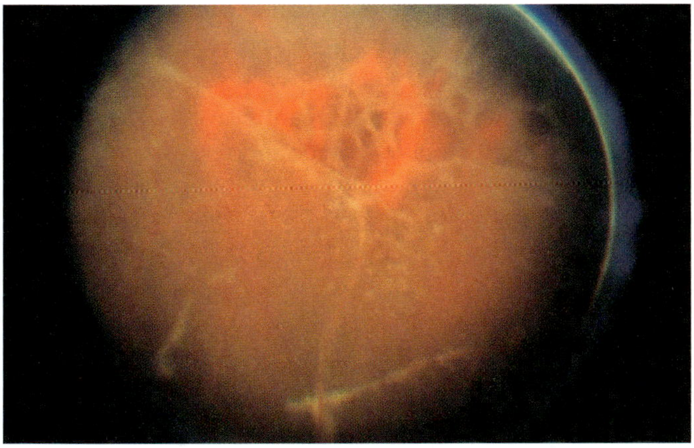

Figure 7-5 Acute retinal necrosis: retinal detachment with multiple, posterior retinal breaks. *(Courtesy of E. Mitchel Opremcak, MD.)*

In most instances, the diagnosis is made clinically; important differential diagnostic considerations include CMV retinitis, atypical toxoplasmic retinochoroiditis, syphilis, lymphoma, leukemia, and autoimmune retinal vasculitis such as that of Behçet disease. ARN may also be present in association with concurrent or antecedent herpetic encephalitis (HSV-1 or -2). When the diagnosis is uncertain, polymerase chain reaction (PCR) testing of aqueous and/or vitreous samples or retinal choroidal biopsy should be performed.

Intraocular antibody production as a measure of the host response to a specific microbial pathogen can be computed using the Goldmann-Witmer (GW) coefficient. The GW coefficient for a specific pathogen is calculated by dividing the amount of immunoglobulin G (IgG) reactive to a specific pathogen (xIgG) in aqueous by the total amount of IgG in the aqueous, and then dividing that ratio by a ratio created by dividing the amount of the same specific antigen IgG (xIgG) in serum by the total amount of IgG in serum:

$$\text{GW} = \frac{(\text{xIgG in aqueous/total IgG in aqueous})}{(\text{xIgG in serum/total IgG in serum})}$$

For example, in order to calculate the GW for *Toxoplasma gondii,* one would obtain both aqueous and serum samples and determine the amount of IgG reactive to *T gondii* (*Toxoplasma* IgG) in the aqueous and serum as well as the total amounts of IgG in aqueous and serum. Then the GW coefficient would be determined as follows:

$$GW = \frac{(\textit{Toxoplasma}\ \text{IgG in aqueous/total IgG in aqueous})}{(\textit{Toxoplasma}\ \text{IgG in serum/total IgG in serum})}$$

A ratio of greater than 3 is considered diagnostic of local antibody production. Aqueous humor analysis is most frequently performed following anterior chamber paracentesis. It has been used more widely in Europe than in the United States as an adjunct to the diagnosis of toxoplasmosis and uveitis caused by HSV and VZV infection, but it is of little value in the diagnosis of CMV retinitis. Combining the GW coefficient with PCR analysis may increase diagnostic yield, especially in viral infections.

PCR testing is probably the most sensitive, specific, and rapid diagnostic method for detecting infectious posterior uveitis in general and ARN specifically. It has largely supplanted viral culture, intraocular antibody titers, and serology. PCR testing may be performed on either aqueous humor or vitreous biopsy specimens; however, for most cases of ARN, aqueous sampling is usually sufficient. Quantitative PCR may add additional information with respect to viral load, disease activity, and response to therapy. Recent studies using PCR-based assays suggest that the most common cause of ARN is VZV infection, followed by infections with HSV-1, HSV-2, and, in rare instances, CMV. Patients with ARN caused by HSV-1 or VZV infection tend to be older (mean age, 40 years), whereas those with ARN due to HSV-2 infection tend to be younger (below age 25 years). There is a higher risk of encephalitis and meningitis among patients with ARN caused by HSV-1 infection than by VZV infection. In rare instances in which PCR results are negative but the clinical suspicion for herpetic necrotizing retinitis is high, endoretinal biopsy may be diagnostic.

Timely diagnosis and prompt initiation of antiviral therapy are essential given the rapidity of disease progression, the frequency of retinal detachment, and the guarded visual prognosis. Intravenous acyclovir, 10 mg/kg every 8 hours for 10–14 days, is effective against HSV and VZV. Reversible elevations in levels of serum creatinine and liver enzymes may occur; in the presence of frank renal insufficiency, the dosage will need to be reduced. After 24–48 hours of antiviral therapy, systemic corticosteroids (prednisone, 1 mg/kg/day) are introduced to treat active inflammation and are subsequently tapered over several weeks. Aspirin and other anticoagulants have been used to treat an associated hypercoagulable state and prevent vascular occlusions, but the results have been inconclusive. Following intravenous antiviral induction for VZV infection, treatment with acyclovir at 800 mg orally 5 times daily, valacyclovir at 1 g orally 3 times daily, or famciclovir at 500 mg orally 3 times daily should be continued for 3 months. For ARN associated with HSV-1 infection, the follow-on oral dose is one-half of that for VZV. Extended antiviral therapy may reduce the incidence of contralateral disease or bilateral ARN by 80% over 1 year.

Oral valacyclovir at doses of up to 2 g 3 times daily has been used successfully as an alternative to intravenous acyclovir as induction therapy. In addition, intravitreal ganciclovir (0.2–2.0 mg/0.1 mL) and foscarnet (1.2–2.4 mg/0.1 mL) have been used to achieve a rapid induction in combination with both intravenous and oral antivirals as first-line therapy or for disease that fails to respond to systemic acyclovir (see Chapter 11). High-dose systemic oral therapy, alone or in combination with intravitreal antiviral drugs, has not been demonstrated as superior to the classic intravenous approach. Given the short intravitreal half-life of these drugs, injections may need to be repeated twice weekly until the retinitis is controlled. Effective treatment inhibits the development of new lesions and promotes lesion regression over 4 days.

Retinal detachment occurs within the first weeks to months following the onset of retinitis. Given the location and multiplicity of retinal breaks, prophylactic barrier laser photocoagulation, applied to the areas of healthy retina at the posterior border of the necrotic lesions, may prevent retinal detachment and is recommended as soon as the view permits. Early vitrectomy combined with endolaser photocoagulation has been proposed to help eliminate the contribution of vitreous traction on the necrotic retina. Due to the presence of proliferative vitreoretinopathy and multiple posterior retinal tears, internal repair using vitrectomy techniques, air–fluid exchange, endolaser photocoagulation, or long-acting gas or silicone oil tamponade is more successful in achieving a higher rate of anatomical attachment than are standard scleral buckling procedures. Untreated, approximately two-thirds of eyes obtain a final visual acuity of 20/200 or worse because of retinal detachment, concurrent optic atrophy, or macular pathology. With early recognition, aggressive antiviral therapy, and laser photocoagulation, this prognosis may be significantly improved, as shown in one study in which 46% of 13 eyes achieved a visual acuity of 20/40 or better and 92% achieved a visual acuity of better than 20/400.

Progressive outer retinal necrosis (PORN) is a morphologic variant of acute necrotizing herpetic retinitis, occurring in those who are profoundly immunosuppressed, most often in advanced AIDS ($CD4^+$ T lymphocytes ≤50 cells/μL). The most common cause of PORN is VZV infection; HSV has also been isolated. As with ARN, the retinitis begins as patchy areas of outer retinal whitening that coalesce rapidly; however, in contrast to ARN, the posterior pole may be involved early in the course of the disease, vitreous inflammatory cells are typically absent, and the retinal vasculature is minimally involved, at least initially (Fig 7-6). Patients with PORN and human immunodeficiency virus (HIV)

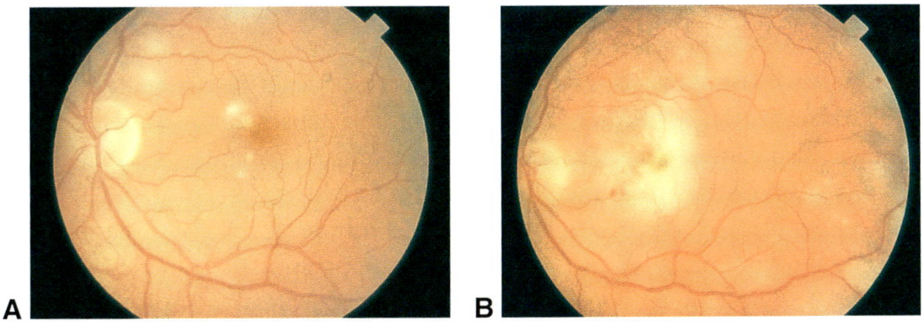

Figure 7-6 **A,** Fundus photograph showing multifocal areas of white retinitis in a patient with progressive outer retinal necrosis (PORN). **B,** Fundus photograph taken 5 days later, showing rapid disease progression and confluence of the areas of the viral retinitis. *(Courtesy of E. Mitchel Opremcak, MD.)*

infection or AIDS frequently have a history of cutaneous zoster (67%) and eventually incur bilateral involvement (71%); they also have a similarly high rate (70%) of retinal detachment as in ARN. The visual prognosis is poor; in the largest series reported to date, 67% of patients had a final visual acuity of no light perception. Although PORN is often resistant to treatment with intravenous acyclovir alone, successful management has been reported with combination systemic and intraocular therapy using foscarnet and ganciclovir. Long-term suppressive antiviral therapy is required in patients with HIV/AIDS who are not able to achieve immune reconstitution through combination antiretroviral treatment. See also BCSC Section 12, *Retina and Vitreous,* for additional discussion of viral retinitis.

Nonnecrotizing herpetic retinitis (nonnecrotizing posterior uveitis) may occur in patients with herpetic infections, including acute retinochoroiditis with diffuse hemorrhages following acute VZV infection in children and chronic choroiditis or retinal vasculitis in adults. In a study using PCR-based assays and local antibody analysis of aqueous fluid samples for herpesviruses, a viral etiology was confirmed in 13% of cases deemed "idiopathic posterior uveitis." Inflammation is typically bilateral, and the disorder may present with cystoid macular edema (CME), as a birdshot uveitis–like retinochoroidopathy, or as an occlusive bilateral retinitis. The disease is initially resistant to conventional therapy with systemic corticosteroids and/or immunomodulatory therapy (IMT), but favorable response is achieved when patients are switched to systemic antiviral medication.

Aizman A, Johnson MW, Elner SG. Treatment of acute retinal necrosis syndrome with oral antiviral medications. *Ophthalmology.* 2007;114(2):307–312.

Chau Tran TH, Cassoux N, Bodaghi B, Lehoang P. Successful treatment with combination of systemic antiviral drugs and intravitreal ganciclovir injections in the management of severe necrotizing herpetic retinitis. *Ocul Immunol Inflamm.* 2003;11(2):141–144.

Engstrom RE Jr, Holland GN, Margolis TP, et al. The progressive outer retinal necrosis syndrome. A variant of necrotizing herpetic retinopathy in patients with AIDS. *Ophthalmology.* 1994;101(9):1488–1502.

Goldstein DA, Pyatetsky D. Necrotizing herpetic retinopathies. *Focal Points: Clinical Modules for Ophthalmologists.* San Francisco, CA: American Academy of Ophthalmology: 2008, module 10.

Cytomegalovirus

Cytomegalovirus is a double-stranded DNA virus in the Herpesviridae family. It is the most common cause of congenital viral infection and causes clinically relevant disease in neonates; it also causes illness in immunocompromised patients with leukemia, lymphoma, or HIV/AIDS; transplant recipients; and those with conditions requiring systemic immunomodulation. CMV retinitis is the most common ophthalmic manifestation of both congenital CMV infection and of CMV as an opportunistic coinfection in patients with HIV/AIDS. The clinical appearance is similar regardless of clinical context, with 3 distinct variants:

- a classic or fulminant retinitis with large areas of retinal hemorrhage against a background of whitened, edematous, or necrotic retina; the retinitis typically appears in

the posterior pole, from the disc to the vascular arcades, in the distribution of the nerve fiber layer, and associated with blood vessels (Fig 7-7)
- a granular or indolent form found more often in the retinal periphery, characterized by little or no retinal edema, hemorrhage, or vascular sheathing, and with active retinitis progressing from the borders of the lesion (Fig 7-8)
- a perivascular form often described as a variant of "frosted-branch" angiitis, an idiopathic retinal perivasculitis initially described in immunocompetent children (Fig 7-9)

Early CMV retinitis may present as a small, white retinal infiltrate masquerading as a cotton-wool spot; it is commonly associated with an HIV-related microvasculopathy, from which it may be distinguished by its inevitable progression without treatment.

The diagnosis of congenital disease is suggested by the clinical appearance of the lesions, coupled with evidence of viral inclusion bodies or positive results of PCR testing in urine, saliva, and subretinal fluid, as well as associated systemic disease findings. The complement-fixation test for cytomegalic inclusion disease is of value 5–24 months after the loss of the maternal antibodies transferred during pregnancy. Likewise, the diagnosis of CMV retinitis in patients with HIV/AIDS or undergoing IMT is essentially clinical,

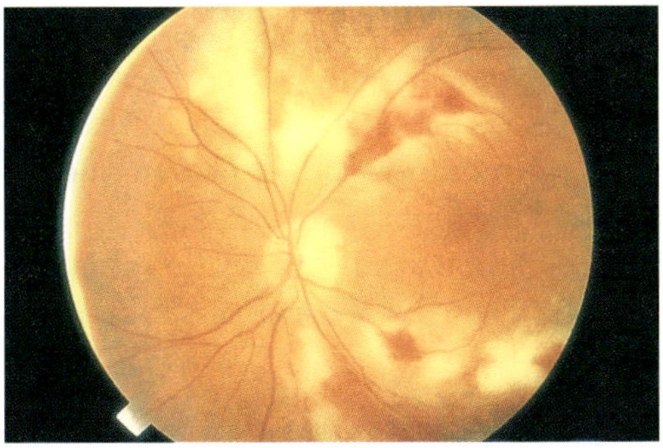

Figure 7-7 Fundus photograph of cytomegalovirus (CMV) retinitis. *(Courtesy of E. Mitchel Opremcak, MD.)*

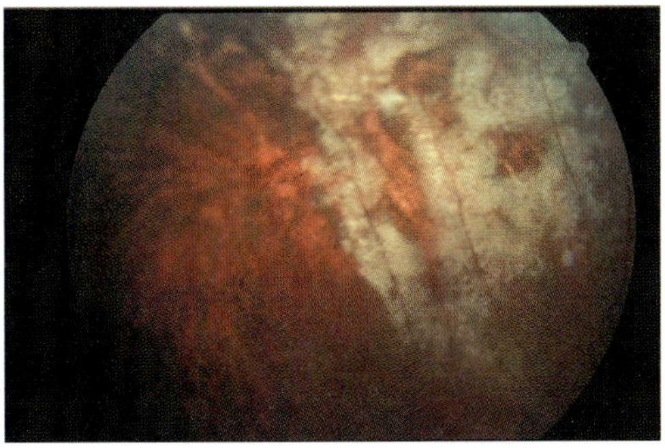

Figure 7-8 Fundus photograph of granular CMV retinitis. *(Courtesy of Careen Lowder, MD.)*

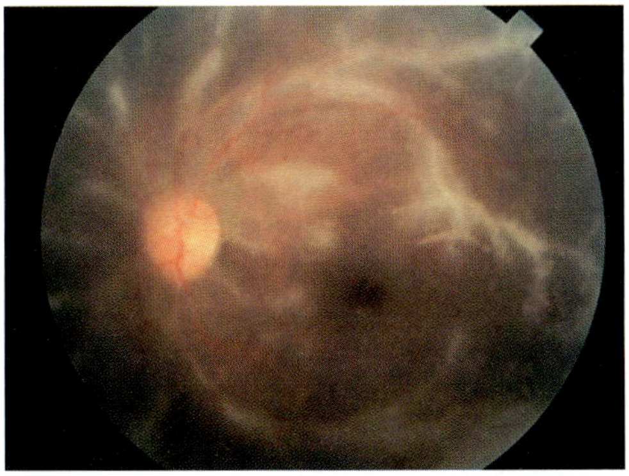

Figure 7-9 Fundus photograph of "frosted branch" CMV perivasculitis. *(Courtesy of Albert T. Vitale, MD.)*

according to the features just described. In immunocompromised patients with atypical lesions or whose disease is not responding to anti-CMV therapy, PCR-based analysis of the aqueous or vitreous samples may provide crucial diagnostic information of high sensitivity and specificity that allows the clinician to differentiate CMV from other herpetic causes of necrotizing retinitis and from toxoplasmic retinochoroiditis.

CMV reaches the eye hematogenously, with passage of the virus across the blood–ocular barrier, infection of retinal vascular endothelial cells, and cell-to-cell transmission of the virus within the retina. The histologic features of both congenital and acquired disease include a primary, full-thickness, coagulative necrotizing retinitis and secondary diffuse choroiditis. Infected retinal cells show pathognomonic cytomegalic changes consisting of large eosinophilic intranuclear inclusions and small, multiple, basophilic cytoplasmic inclusions (Fig 7-10A). Viral inclusions may also be present in the retinal pigment epithelium (RPE) and vascular endothelium. Electron microscopy of infected retinal tissue reveals viral particles with the typical morphology of the herpes family (Fig 7-10B).

Congenital CMV retinitis is usually associated with other systemic manifestations of disseminated infection, including fever, thrombocytopenia, anemia, pneumonitis, and hepatosplenomegaly; the reported prevalence in children with congenital CMV infection is between 11% and 22%. However, CMV retinitis has been reported to occur later in life among children with no discernible lesions ophthalmoscopically and no evidence of systemic disease reactivation. This pattern suggests that even asymptomatic children with evidence of congenital CMV infection should be monitored at regular intervals for potential ocular involvement later into childhood. Resolution of the retinitis leaves both pigmented and atrophic lesions, with retinal detachment occurring in up to one-third of children. Optic atrophy and cataract formation are not uncommon sequelae.

Prior to the introduction of potent combination antiretroviral therapy, an estimated 30% of patients with HIV/AIDS, typically with $CD4^+$ T lymphocyte counts ≤50 cells/μL,

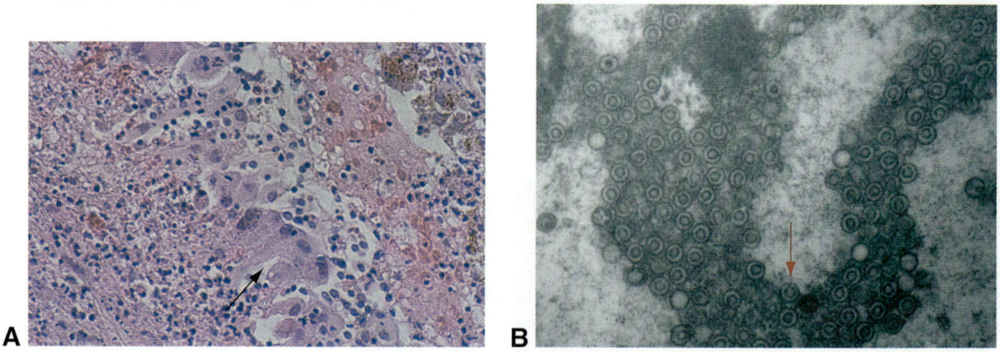

Figure 7-10 **A,** Photomicrograph of a retinal biopsy specimen demonstrating a necrotic retina and giant (megalo) cells with eosinophilic intracytoplasmic inclusions *(arrow)* consistent with CMV retinitis (H&E stain). **B,** Electron photomicrograph of the same specimen showing intranuclear inclusions containing scattered nucleocapsids, relative electron lucency of the central core *(arrow)*, and the typical envelope consistent with CMV. *(Part A courtesy of Careen Lowder, MD. Part B reproduced with permission from Spaide RF, Vitale AT, Toth IR, Oliver JM. Frosted branch angiitis associated with cytomegalovirus retinitis.* Am J Ophthalmol. *1992;113(5):525; courtesy of Albert T. Vitale, MD.)*

incurred CMV retinitis at some point during their disease. Rhegmatogenous retinal detachments with multiple breaks, particularly in areas of peripheral retinal necrosis, occurred at a rate of approximately 33% per eye per year. The availability of combination antiretroviral regimens resulted not only in a significant decline in HIV/AIDS–associated mortality, but also in an 80% decline in new cases per year of CMV retinitis and its associated complications, including retinal detachment, which is itself associated with CMV lesion size. This decrease appears to have stabilized, and new cases of CMV retinitis continue to occur among patients in whom combination antiretroviral treatment fails as well as those who abandon treatment or experience immune reconstitution but do not develop CMV-specific immunity.

Successful management of CMV retinitis requires not only antiretroviral regimens but also appropriate anti-CMV therapy. The inclusion of anti-CMV therapy is particularly important, given that CMV retinitis itself confers a twofold increased risk in mortality among patients with a $CD4^+$ T-cell count below 100 cells/μL (an effect not observed with counts ≥100 cells/μL) as well as the clear mortality benefit associated with systemic anti-CMV therapy. Resistant CMV infection is further associated with increased mortality among patients with HIV/AIDS being treated for CMV retinitis. Options for systemic coverage include high-dose induction with either intravenous ganciclovir (5 mg/kg twice daily) or foscarnet (90 mg/kg twice daily) for 2 weeks followed by low-dose daily maintenance therapy or oral valganciclovir (900 mg twice daily) for 3 weeks followed by maintenance therapy (900 mg/day). Intravitreal injection of ganciclovir or foscarnet is highly effective in treating intraocular disease and may be a useful alternative in patients who cannot tolerate intravenous systemic therapy because of myelotoxicity; however, it leaves extraocular systemic CMV and the fellow eye untreated. Combination treatment with oral valganciclovir may obviate this limitation and be particularly effective for patients with vision-threatening, posteriorly located retinitis. In patients with CMV retinitis who are on antiretroviral regimens and experience sustained immune recovery ($CD4^+$ T lymphocytes ≥100 cells/μL for 3–6 months), systemic anti-CMV maintenance therapy may be safely discontinued. Antiretroviral therapy–naive patients may require only 6 months of anti-CMV therapy with good immune reconstitution, whereas antiretroviral therapy–experienced patients may require long-term maintenance therapy. Moreover, aggressive anti-CMV therapy initiated at the same time as antiretroviral treatment may decrease the incidence of immune recovery uveitis. Despite immune recovery, patients with a history of CMV retinitis who discontinue maintenance anti-CMV therapy remain at risk for recurrence and should be monitored at 3-month intervals.

Among immunocompetent adults, CMV infection may produce a chronic or recurrent unilateral anterior uveitis associated with ocular hypertension, corneal edema, and variable degrees of sectoral iris atrophy. This association is based on the demonstration of CMV DNA by PCR analysis and of intraocular antibodies directed against CMV by enzyme-linked immunosorbent assay (ELISA)—together with corresponding negative study results for HSV and VZV upon aqueous analysis. CMV anterior uveitis requires specific, prolonged, systemic anti-CMV treatment, most often with valganciclovir, as relapses are common after discontinuation of therapy. Consultation with a specialist in infectious diseases may be appropriate.

Chee SP, Bascal K, Jap A, Se-Thoe SY, Cheng CL, Tan BH. Clinical features of cytomegalovirus anterior uveitis in immunocompetent patients. *Am J Ophthalmol.* 2008;145(5): 834–840.

Jabs DA, Holbrook JT, Van Natta ML, et al; Studies of Ocular Complications of AIDS Research Group. Risk factors for mortality in patients with AIDS in the era of highly active antiretroviral therapy. *Ophthalmology.* 2005;112(5):771–779.

Jabs DA, Martin BK, Forman MS; Cytomegalovirus Retinitis and Viral Resistance Research Group. Mortality associated with resistant cytomegalovirus among patients with cytomegalovirus retinitis and AIDS. *Ophthalmology.* 2010;117(1):128–132.

Kedhar SR, Jabs DA. Cytomegalovirus retinitis in the era of highly active antiretroviral therapy. *Herpes.* 2007;14(3):66–71.

Epstein-Barr virus

Epstein-Barr virus (EBV) is a ubiquitous double-stranded DNA virus with a complex capsid and envelope; it belongs to the subfamily Gammaherpesvirinae. It is the viral agent commonly associated with infectious mononucleosis (IM) and has been implicated in the pathogenesis of Burkitt lymphoma (especially among African children), nasopharyngeal carcinoma, Hodgkin disease, and Sjögren syndrome. EBV has a tropism for B lymphocytes, the only cells known to have surface receptors for the virus.

Ocular manifestations may arise as a consequence of either congenital EBV infection or, much more commonly, during primary infection in the context of IM. Cataract has been reported in association with congenital EBV infection; a mild, self-limiting follicular conjunctivitis, usually appearing early in the course of the disease, is most common with acquired IM. Other, less frequently reported anterior ocular manifestations of acquired IM include epithelial or stromal keratitis; episcleritis; bilateral, granulomatous anterior uveitis; dacryoadenitis; and less frequently, cranial nerve palsies and Parinaud oculoglandular syndrome.

A variety of posterior segment manifestations have been reported in association with EBV infection, including isolated optic disc edema and optic neuritis, macular edema, retinal hemorrhages, retinitis, punctate outer retinitis, choroiditis, multifocal choroiditis and panuveitis (MCP), pars planitis and vitritis, progressive subretinal fibrosis, uveitis, and secondary choroidal neovascularization (CNV) (Fig 7-11). ARN has also been reported. Evidence for an association between these ocular findings and the presence of antibodies against a variety of EBV-specific capsid antigens indicative of active or persistent EBV infection is not well established, especially given the very high seroprevalence of EBV (90%) in the adult population.

Most ocular disease is self-limiting and does not require treatment; however, the presence of anterior uveitis may necessitate the use of topical corticosteroids and cycloplegia; systemic corticosteroids may be required to treat posterior segment inflammation. The efficacy of systemic antiviral therapy for EBV infection has not been established in controlled studies but should be considered for the management of necrotizing retinitis/ARN.

Matoba AY. Ocular disease associated with Epstein-Barr virus infection. *Surv Ophthalmol.* 1990;35(2):145–150.

Peponis VG, Chatziralli IP, Parikakis EA, Chaira N, Katzakis MC, Mitropoulos PG. Bilateral Multifocal Chorioretinitis and Optic Neuritis due to Epstein-Barr Virus: A Case Report. *Case Rep Ophthalmol.* 2012;3(3):327–332.

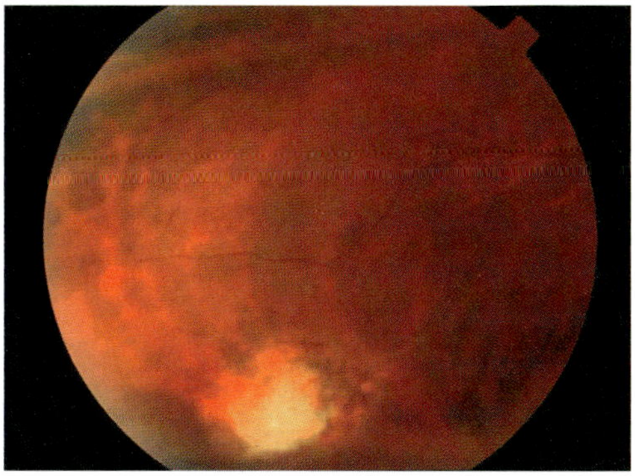

Figure 7-11 Fundus photograph of Epstein-Barr virus–related retinitis and vasculitis. *(Reproduced with permission from Vitale AT, Foster CS. Uveitis affecting infants and children: infectious causes. In: Hartnett ME, Trese M, Capone A, Keats B, Steidl SM, eds.* Pediatric Retina. *Philadelphia, PA: Lippincott Williams & Wilkins; 2004:269; courtesy of Albert T. Vitale, MD.)*

Rubella

The rubella virus is the prototypical teratogenic viral agent. It consists of single-stranded RNA surrounded by a lipid envelope, or "toga"; hence its inclusion in the Togaviridae family. Although rubella remains an important cause of blindness in resource-limited regions and nations, the epidemic pattern of the disease was interrupted in the United States by introduction of the vaccine in 1969. The peak age incidence shifted from 5–9 years (young children) in the prevaccine era to 15–19 years (older children) and more recently to 20–24 years (young adults). Approximately 5%–25% of women of childbearing age are susceptible to primary infection. Rubella may involve the retina as part of the congenital rubella syndrome (CRS) or during acquired infection (German measles).

The fetus is infected with the rubella virus transplacentally, secondary to maternal viremia during the course of primary infection. The frequency of fetal infection is highest during the first 10 weeks and the final month of pregnancy, with the rate of congenital defects varying inversely with gestational age. Although obvious maternal infection during the first trimester of pregnancy may end in spontaneous abortion, stillbirth, or severe fetal malformations, seropositive asymptomatic maternal rubella may also result in severe fetal disease.

The classic features of CRS include cardiac malformations (patent ductus arteriosus, interventricular septal defects, and pulmonic stenosis), ocular findings (chorioretinitis, cataract, corneal clouding, microphthalmia, strabismus, and glaucoma), and deafness (Fig 7-12). Hearing loss is the most common systemic finding. Individuals with CRS are at greater risk for diabetes mellitus and subsequent diabetic retinopathy later in life.

A unilateral or bilateral pigmentary retinopathy is the most common ocular manifestation of CRS (25%–50%), followed by cataract (15%) and glaucoma (10%). The pigmentary disturbance, often described as "salt-and-pepper" fundus, shows considerable variation, ranging from finely stippled, bone spicule–like, small, black, irregular masses to gross pigmentary irregularities with coarse, blotchy mottling (Fig 7-13). It can be stationary or progressive. Despite loss of the foveal light reflex and prominent pigmentary changes, neither vision nor electroretinogram results are typically affected. Congenital (nuclear) cataracts and microphthalmia are the most frequent causes of poor visual acuity and, rarely, CNV. Unless otherwise compromised by glaucoma, the optic nerve and the retinal vessels are typically normal in appearance.

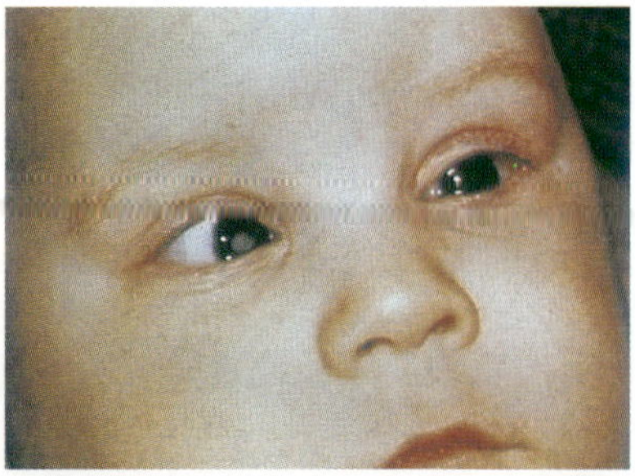

Figure 7-12 Patient with congenital rubella syndrome who exhibited cataract, esotropia, cognitive impairment, congenital heart disease, and deafness. *(Courtesy of John D. Sheppard, Jr, MD.)*

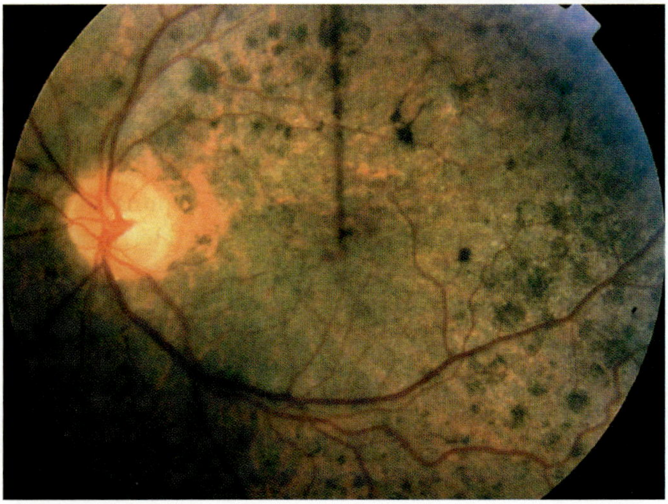

Figure 7-13 Fundus photograph of congenital rubella syndrome with diffuse retinal pigment epithelial mottling showing "salt-and-pepper" appearance. *(Courtesy of Albert T. Vitale, MD.)*

Histologic studies of the lens reveal retained cell nuclei in the embryonic nucleus as well as anterior and posterior cortical degeneration. Poor development of the pupil dilator muscle, necrosis of the iris pigment epithelium, and chronic nongranulomatous inflammation may be present in the iris. The RPE displays alternating areas of atrophy and hypertrophy. The anterior chamber angle appears similar to that of congenital glaucoma. Although the mechanism of rubella embryopathy is not known at a cellular level, it is thought that the virus inhibits cellular multiplication and establishes a chronic, persistent infection during organogenesis. The persistence of viral replication after birth, with ongoing tissue damage, is central to the pathogenesis of CRS and may explain the appearance of hearing and neurologic and/or ocular deficits long after birth.

Acquired infection (German measles) presents with a prodrome of malaise and fever in adolescents and adults before onset of the rubella exanthem. An erythematous, maculopapular rash appears first on the face, spreads toward the hands and feet, involves the entire body within 24 hours, and disappears by the third day. Although the rash is not always prominent and the occurrence of fever is variable, lymphadenopathy is invariably present.

The most frequent ocular complication of postnatally acquired rubella is conjunctivitis (70%), followed by the infrequent occurrence of epithelial keratitis and retinitis. Acquired rubella retinitis has been described in adults presenting with acute-onset decreased vision and multifocal chorioretinitis, with large areas of bullous neurosensory detachment, underlying pigment epithelial detachment involving the entire posterior pole, anterior chamber and preretinal vitreous cells, dark gray atrophic lesions of the RPE, normal appearance of the retinal vessels and optic nerve, and absence of retinal hemorrhage. The neurosensory detachments resolve spontaneously, and visual acuity returns to normal. Chronic rubella virus infection has been implicated in the pathogenesis of Fuchs heterochromic uveitis, as evidenced by the presence of rubella-specific intraocular antibody production and the intraocular persistence of the virus.

The pigmentary retinal changes and associated systemic findings, together with a history of maternal exposure to rubella suggest the diagnosis of CRS. Serologic criteria for rubella infection include a fourfold increase in rubella-specific IgG in paired sera 1–2 weeks apart or the new appearance of rubella-specific IgM. Because the fetus is capable of mounting an immune response to the rubella virus, specific IgM or IgA antibodies to rubella in the cord blood confirm the diagnosis.

The differential diagnosis of congenital rubella retinitis consists of entities constituting the TORCH syndrome (*t*oxoplasmosis, *o*ther agents, *r*ubella, *c*ytomegalovirus, and *h*erpesviruses). See also BCSC Section 6, *Pediatric Ophthalmology and Strabismus,* for additional discussion of congenital rubella. Other viral illnesses, such as mumps, exanthema subitum, postvaccination encephalitis, and infections with HSV, VZV, and CMV, should be considered and ruled out by appropriate serologic tests. There is no specific antiviral therapy for congenital rubella, and treatment is supportive. Similarly, uncomplicated acquired rubella does not require specific therapy; however, rubella retinitis and postvaccination optic neuritis may respond well to systemic corticosteroids.

Arnold JJ, McIntosh ED, Martin FJ, Menser MA. A fifty-year follow-up of ocular defects in congenital rubella: late ocular manifestations. *Aust N Z J Ophthalmol.* 1994;22(1):1–6.

Givens KT, Lee DA, Jones T, Ilstrup DM. Congenital rubella syndrome: ophthalmic manifestations and associated systemic disorders. *Br J Ophthalmol.* 1993;77(6):358–363.

Quentin CD, Reiber H. Fuchs heterochromic cyclitis: rubella virus antibodies and genome in aqueous humor. *Am J Ophthalmol.* 2004;138(1):46–54.

Lymphocytic Choriomeningitis Virus

Lymphocytic choriomeningitis virus (LCMV) is an under-recognized fetal teratogen that should probably be listed among the "other agents" in the TORCH group of congenital infections. The microbe is a single-stranded RNA virus of the Arenaviridae family; rodents are the natural hosts and reservoir. Transmission is thought to be airborne, from contamination of food by infected rodent excreta, or possibly from the bite of an infected animal. Symptomatic maternal illness occurs in approximately two-thirds of cases, with vertical transmission to the fetus occurring during episodes of maternal viremia. As with other congenital infections, transmission earlier in gestation results in more serious sequelae.

Systemic findings include macrocephaly, hydrocephalus, and intracranial calcifications. Neurologic abnormalities, seizures, and mild cognitive impairment are not uncommon. Ocular findings include macular and chorioretinal peripheral scarring, similar in morphology and distribution to that of congenital toxoplasmosis. Other findings include optic atrophy, strabismus, and nystagmus.

LCMV infection is differentiated from congenital toxoplasmosis by serologic testing of the mother and the infant and by the pattern of intracerebral calcifications, which tend to be diffuse in toxoplasmosis compared with a more periventricular distribution in congenital LCMV disease. Immunofluorescent antibody tests, Western blot, and ELISA are available for detecting the IgM and IgG antibodies that, together with the clinical findings, establish the diagnosis.

Mets MB, Barton LL, Khan AS, Ksiazek TG. Lymphocytic choriomeningitis virus: an underdiagnosed cause of congenital chorioretinitis. *Am J Ophthalmol.* 2000;130(2):209–215.

Measles (Rubeola)

Congenital and acquired measles infection is caused by a single-stranded RNA virus of the genus *Morbillivirus* in the Paramyxoviridae family. The virus is highly contagious and is transmitted either directly or via aerosolization of nasopharyngeal secretions to the mucous membranes of the conjunctiva or respiratory tract of susceptible individuals, or transplacentally from a pregnant woman to her fetus.

Despite the existence of a safe, effective, and inexpensive vaccine for more than 40 years, measles remains a leading cause of mortality worldwide among young children; in the United States, however, measles is now quite rare.

Ocular manifestations of congenital measles infection include cataract, optic nerve head drusen, and bilateral diffuse pigmentary retinopathy involving the posterior pole and retinal periphery. The retinopathy may also be associated with normal or attenuated retinal vessels, retinal edema, and macular star formation. Electroretinographic results and visual acuity are typically normal.

The most common ocular manifestations of measles are keratitis and a mild, papillary, nonpurulent conjunctivitis. Although keratitis and conjunctivitis both resolve without sequelae in the vast majority of cases in the United States, postmeasles blindness, a severe visual impairment arising specifically as a consequence of the corneal complications of the disease, is a significant problem worldwide. Measles retinopathy is more common in acquired than in congenital disease, presenting with profound loss of vision 6–12 days after the appearance of the characteristic exanthem; it may be accompanied by encephalitis. Measles retinopathy is characterized by attenuated arterioles, diffuse retinal edema, macular star formation, scattered retinal hemorrhages, blurred disc margins, and clear media. With resolution of systemic symptoms and of the acute retinopathy, further sequelae may evolve, including arteriolar attenuation with or without perivascular sheathing, optic disc pallor, and a secondary pigmentary retinopathy with either a bone spicule or salt-and-pepper appearance.

The electroretinogram is usually extinguished during the acute phase of measles retinopathy, but activity may return with improved vision as the inflammation resolves. Visual field testing may reveal severe constriction, ring scotomata, or small peripheral islands of vision. Resolution of acquired measles retinopathy over a period of weeks to months is generally associated with the return of useful vision, although the extended visual prognosis is guarded because of the possibility of permanent visual field constriction.

The differential diagnosis of congenital measles retinopathy includes the entities comprising the TORCH syndrome, atypical retinitis pigmentosa, and neuroretinitis; for acquired measles retinopathy, considerations include central serous chorioretinopathy, Vogt-Koyanagi-Harada (VKH) syndrome, retinitis pigmentosa, syphilis neuroretinitis, and other viral retinopathies.

The diagnosis of measles and its attendant ocular sequelae is made clinically by means of an accurate history and review of systems; observation of the sequence of signs, symptoms, and lesion progression; and results of serologic testing. The virus may be recovered from the nasopharynx, conjunctiva, lymphoid tissues, respiratory mucous membranes, urine, and blood for a few days before and several days after appearance of the rash. Leukopenia is frequently present during the prodromal phase. A variety of tests are available for serologic confirmation of measles infection, including complement fixation, ELISA, and immunofluorescent and hemagglutination inhibition assays.

Supportive treatment of the systemic manifestations of measles is normally sufficient because the disease is usually self-limiting. In certain high-risk populations, including pregnant women, children younger than age 1 year, and immunocompromised individuals, infection may be prevented by prophylactic treatment with gamma globulin, 0.25 mL/kg, administered within 5 days of exposure. Likewise, the ocular manifestations of measles are treated symptomatically, with topical antivirals or antibiotics to prevent secondary infections in patients with keratitis or conjunctivitis. The use of systemic corticosteroids should be considered in cases of acute measles retinopathy.

Foxman SG, Heckenlively JR, Sinclair SH. Rubeola retinopathy and pigmented paravenous retinochoroidal atrophy. *Am J Ophthalmol.* 1985;99(5):605–606.

Yoser SL, Forster DJ, Rao NA. Systemic viral infections and their retinal and choroidal manifestations. *Surv Ophthalmol.* 1993;37(5):313–352.

Subacute sclerosing panencephalitis

Subacute sclerosing panencephalitis (SSPE) is a rare, late complication of acquired measles infection that arises most often in unvaccinated children 6–8 years after the primary infection. Children infected with measles before the age of 1 year carry a 16 times greater risk than those infected at age 5 years or later. Onset is usually in late childhood or adolescence and is characterized by the insidious appearance of visual impairment, behavioral disturbances, and memory impairment, followed by myoclonus and progression to spastic paresis, dementia, and death within 1–3 years.

Ocular findings are reported in up to 50% of patients with SSPE and may precede the neurologic manifestations by several weeks to 2 years. The most consistent finding is a maculopathy, consisting of focal retinitis and RPE changes, occurring in 36% of patients (Fig 7-14). Retinitis may progress within several days to involve the posterior pole and peripheral retina. Other ophthalmoscopic findings include disc swelling and papilledema, optic atrophy, macular edema, macular pigment epithelial disturbances, small intraretinal hemorrhages, gliotic scar, whitish retinal infiltrates, serous macular detachment, drusen, preretinal membranes, macular hole, cortical blindness, hemianopsia, horizontal

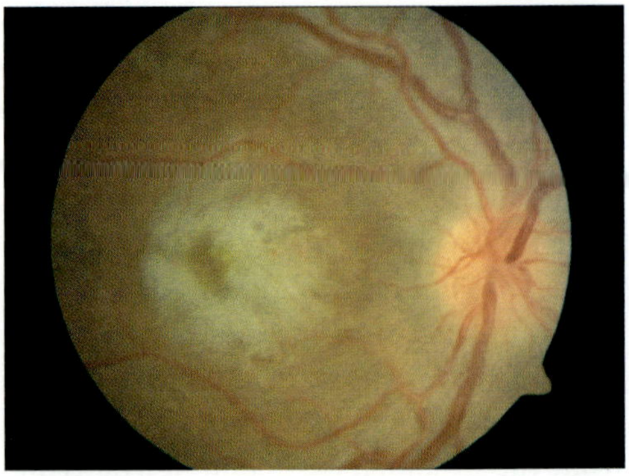

Figure 7-14 Fundus photograph of subacute sclerosing panencephalitis (SSPE) macular retinitis. *(Courtesy of Emad B. Abboud, MD.)*

nystagmus, and ptosis. Characteristically, there is little, if any, vitritis. Mottling and scarring of the RPE occurs as the retinitis resolves.

The diagnosis is made on the basis of clinical manifestations; the presence of characteristic, periodic electroencephalographic discharges; the demonstration of raised IgG antibody titer against measles in the plasma and cerebrospinal fluid (CSF); and/or histologic findings suggestive of panencephalitis on brain biopsy.

The differential diagnosis of the posterior segment findings associated with SSPE includes necrotizing viral retinitis caused by HSV, VZV, and CMV infection as well multiple sclerosis (MS). Unlike SSPE, MS is not a panencephalitis; magnetic resonance imaging (MRI) shows focal periventricular white matter lesions in MS. Furthermore, CME and retinal vasculitis are prominent features of MS but have not been found in patients with SSPE.

Definitive treatment of SSPE remains undetermined. A combination of oral isoprinosine and intraventricular interferon alpha appears to be the most effective treatment; patients whose disease responds to this regimen require lifelong therapy.

Garg RK. Subacute sclerosing panencephalitis. *Postgrad Med J.* 2002;78(916):63–70.

Robb RM, Watters GV. Ophthalmic manifestations of subacute sclerosing panencephalitis. *Arch Ophthalmol.* 1970;83(4):426–435.

West Nile Virus

West Nile virus (WNV) is a single-stranded RNA virus of the family Flaviviridae; it belongs to the Japanese encephalitis virus serocomplex and is endemic to Europe, Australia, Asia, and Africa. WNV first appeared in the United States in 1999 in an outbreak in New York City and subsequently spread westward across the country, southward into Central America, and northward into Canada. WNV is maintained in an enzootic cycle; birds are the natural host of the virus, which is transmitted from them to humans and other vertebrates through the bite of an infected mosquito of the *Culex* genus. The peak onset of the disease occurs in late summer, but it can occur anytime between July and December. The incubation period ranges from 3 to 14 days, and the vast majority of WNV infections are subclinical (80%) or present as a febrile illness (20%) often accompanied by myalgia, arthralgia, headache, conjunctivitis, lymphadenopathy, and a maculopapular or roseolar rash. Severe neurologic disease (meningitis or encephalitis), frequently found in association with diabetes mellitus and advanced age, was initially reported to occur in only 1 of 150 infections, but the severity of WNV infection has increased over time.

Presenting ocular symptoms include pain, photophobia, conjunctival hyperemia, and blurred vision. A characteristic multifocal chorioretinitis is present in the majority of patients, together with nongranulomatous anterior uveitis and vitreous cellular infiltration. Chorioretinal lesions vary in size (200–1000 μm) and number; they are distributed throughout the midperiphery, frequently (80%) in linear arrays, following the course of retinal nerve fibers, with or without involvement of the posterior pole (Fig 7-15). Active chorioretinal lesions appear whitish to yellow, are flat and deep, and evolve with varying degrees of pigmentation and atrophy. Fluorescein angiography (FA) reveals central hypofluorescence with late staining of active lesions, and early hyperfluorescence with late staining of inactive lesions. Many inactive lesions exhibit a targetlike appearance angiographically, with central hypofluorescence caused by blockage from pigment and peripheral hyperfluorescence due to atrophy (Fig 7-16). Indocyanine green (ICG) angiography reveals hypofluorescent spots, more numerous than those apparent on FA or funduscopy. Other findings include anterior uveitis, vitritis, intraretinal hemorrhages, disc edema, optic atrophy, and, less commonly, focal retinal vascular sheathing and occlusion, cranial

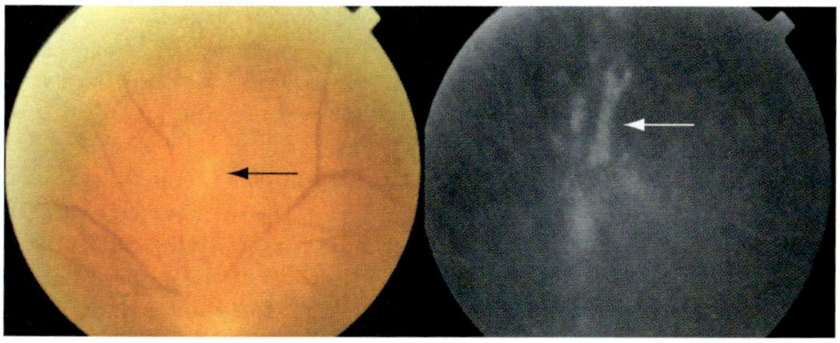

Figure 7-15 West Nile virus chorioretinitis. Fundus photograph with corresponding fluorescein angiogram of active chorioretinitis with lesions distributed in a linear array *(arrows)*. *(Reproduced with permission from Garg S, Jampol LM. Systemic and intraocular manifestations of West Nile virus infection.* Surv Ophthalmol. *2005;50(1):8.)*

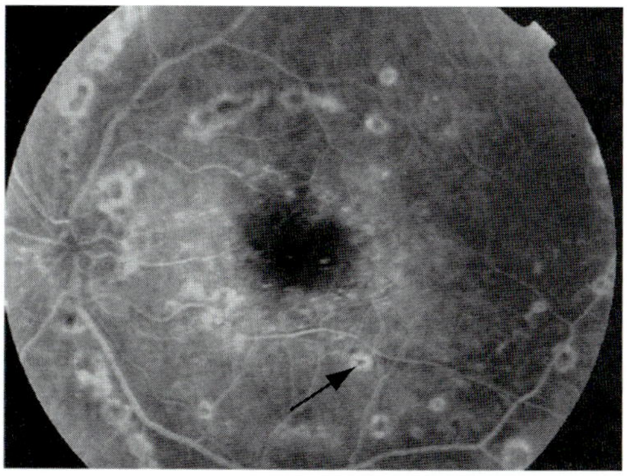

Figure 7-16 West Nile virus chorioretinitis. Midphase fluorescein angiogram showing chorioretinal lesions with central hypofluorescence and peripheral hyperfluorescence *(arrow)*. Capillary leakage is present from underlying diabetic maculopathy. *(Reproduced with permission from Khairallah M, Ben Yahia S, Ladjimi A, et al. Chorioretinal involvement in patients with West Nile virus infection.* Ophthalmology. *2004;111(11):2068.)*

nerve VI palsy, and nystagmus. Congenital WNV infection has been reported in an infant presenting without intraocular inflammation but with chorioretinal scarring in each eye.

In the majority of patients, intraocular inflammation associated with WNV infection has a self limiting course, with a return of visual acuity to baseline after several months. Loss of vision may occur because of CNV, foveal scar, ischemic maculopathy, vitreous hemorrhage, tractional retinal detachment, optic nerve pathology, and retrogeniculate damage. Diabetes mellitus has been implicated as a risk factor for WNV-related death and has been observed with significantly increased frequency, together with nonproliferative retinopathy, among patients with WNV-associated ocular involvement.

The pattern of multifocal chorioretinal lesions in patients with systemic symptoms suggestive of WNV infection can help establish the diagnosis while serologic test results are pending. Conversely, a systemic ocular evaluation including dilated funduscopy and FA may be very helpful in suggesting the diagnosis of WNV infection in patients presenting with meningoencephalitis. The most commonly used laboratory method for diagnosis is demonstration of IgM antibody to the virus using IgM antibody-capture ELISA, which can be confirmed by plaque-reduction neutralization testing (PRNT). The differential diagnosis includes syphilis, MCP, histoplasmosis, sarcoidosis, and tuberculosis.

There is currently no proven treatment for WNV infection, and patients with severe disease receive supportive therapy. Treatment of anterior uveitis with topical corticosteroids is certainly indicated, but the efficacy of systemic and periocular corticosteroids for chorioretinal manifestations is unknown. Public health strategies directed at prevention are the mainstays of WNV infection control.

Chan CK, Limstrom SA, Tarasewicz DG, Lin SG. Ocular features of West Nile virus infection in North America: a study of 14 eyes. *Ophthalmology.* 2006;113(9):1539–1546.

Garg S, Jampol LM. Systemic and intraocular manifestations of West Nile virus infection. *Surv Ophthalmol.* 2005;50(1):3–13.

Khairallah M, Ben Yahia S, Attia S, et al. Indocyanine green angiographic features in multifocal chorioretinitis associated with West Nile virus infection. *Retina.* 2006;26(3): 358–359.

Khairallah M, Ben Yahia S, Attia S, Zaouali S, Ladjimi A, Messaoud R. Linear pattern of West Nile virus–associated chorioretinitis is related to retinal nerve fibres organization. *Eye (Lond).* 2007;21(7):952–955.

Khairallah M, Yahia SB, Letaief M, et al. A prospective evaluation of factors associated with chorioretinitis in patients with West Nile virus infection. *Ocul Immunol Inflamm.* 2007;15(6):435–439.

Rift Valley Fever

Rift Valley fever (RVF) is an acute, epizootic, febrile viral illness caused by arthropod-borne Bunyaviridae of the *Phlebovirus* genus. Primarily affecting domestic animals (sheep, goats, camels, and cattle), the disease may be transmitted to humans, most often through direct contact with the blood or organs of infected animals or by the inhalation of aerosols released during their slaughter. Humans may also acquire RVF by ingesting the unpasteurized milk of infected animals or via bites from infected mosquitoes. The incubation period in humans ranges from 3 to 7 days followed by 1 of 3 clinical syndromes: an uncomplicated, febrile, influenza-like illness; hemorrhagic fever; or neurologic involvement with encephalitis, which carries a mortality rate of 1%.

Ocular disease has been reported to occur in up to 20% of individuals with RVF; visual symptoms appear within 2 weeks of disease onset. Bilateral macular or paramacular retinitis was identified in all affected eyes at the time of initial assessment during an outbreak in Saudi Arabia (Fig 7-17). Additional posterior segment manifestations included intraretinal hemorrhages (40%), vitritis (26%), optic nerve edema (15%), and retinal vasculitis (7%); an anterior uveitis was observed in 31% of patients. Fluorescein angiography revealed delayed filling of the retinal and choroidal circulation with early hypofluorescence and late staining of the inflammatory retinal lesions. Spontaneous resolution of RVF retinitis, retinal hemorrhages, and vitritis was observed within 10–12 weeks, leaving in its wake optic atrophy, ischemic retina, and attenuated, occluded retinal vessels. Although glaucoma, posterior synechiae, and cataract were uncommon complications, macular (60%) or paramacular (9%) scarring, vascular occlusion (23%), and optic atrophy (20%) were important causes of ocular morbidity and permanent vision loss. Visual acuity was profoundly reduced at presentation (less than 20/200 in 80% of affected eyes); visual acuity remained the same or deteriorated in 87%.

The diagnosis of RVF is made clinically and serologically, with the demonstration of antibodies, either IgM in a single serum sample or by a rising IgG titer in samples from acutely ill and convalescent patients. The RVF virus may be isolated from the blood in the acute phase of the illness or detected in either serum or tissue by reverse transcription PCR testing.

The differential diagnosis includes other viral entities such as measles, rubella, influenza, dengue fever, and WNV infection as well as bacterial illnesses such as brucellosis, Lyme disease, toxoplasmosis, cat-scratch disease, and rickettsial diseases. In most instances, these diseases can be differentiated from RVF by clinical history and serologic testing.

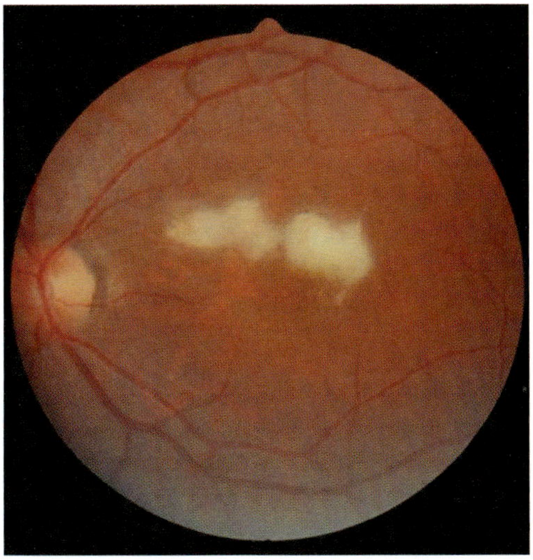

Figure 7-17 Rift Valley fever. Fundus photograph of a 44-year-old male farmer from Saudi Arabia who presented with decreased vision and macular retinitis sparing the fovea; he had a history of fever and contact with animal abortus. *(Courtesy of Albert T. Vitale, MD.)*

Whereas topical steroids may be helpful in the treatment of anterior uveitis, the role of systemic antiviral and anti-inflammatory therapy for the retinal manifestations of RVF is unknown. An inactivated vaccine has been developed for human use but is still experimental and not commercially available. Public health measures including mosquito control, increased disease awareness among residents and visitors to endemic areas, and education regarding modes of disease transmission are essential for the control and prevention of RVF outbreaks.

Al-Hazmi A, Al-Rajhi AA, Abboud EB, et al. Ocular complications of Rift Valley fever outbreak in Saudi Arabia. *Ophthalmology.* 2005;112(2):313–318.

Human T-Lymphotropic Virus Type 1

Human T-lymphotropic virus type 1 (HTLV-1), a retrovirus of the Oncovirinae subfamily, is endemic in Japan, the Caribbean islands, and parts of Central and South America; it accounts for approximately 1% of uveitis cases in Japan. It is transmitted transplacentally, by sexual contact and blood transfusion, and through breast feeding. The diagnosis of HTLV-1 infection is made by serologic testing with confirmatory Western blot analysis. Molecular analysis of selected tissue specimens for HTLV-1–related disease employing microdissection and PCR may be diagnostic in selected cases.

The major target cell of HTLV-1 is the $CD4^+$ T cell. HTLV-1 infection is the established cause of adult T-cell leukemia/lymphoma (ATL), HTLV-1–associated myelopathy/tropical spastic paralysis (HAM/TSP), and HTLV-1 uveitis (HU), defined as uveitis of undetermined origin in an HTLV-1 carrier. Additional ocular manifestations of HTLV-1 infection include retinal infiltrates caused by secondary ATL, retinal degeneration, optic neuropathy, and keratopathy, as well as keratoconjunctivitis sicca in patients with HAM/TSP.

Most cases of HU (75%) are classified anatomically as an intermediate uveitis. Women are affected more often than men, although the mean age of onset is earlier in men (35 years) than in women (48 years). Patients present with blurred vision and floaters caused by a mild granulomatous anterior uveitis (20%), unilateral vitritis (60%), membranous vitreous opacities, and/or "snowballs." Retinal vasculitis (60%), exudative retinal lesions (25%), optic disc abnormalities (20%), and CME (3%) may also be observed. Retinal vasculitis noted clinically and on FA is exquisitely responsive to corticosteroid therapy. For cases that progress despite adequate therapy, the clinician must consider a masquerade syndrome, as both retinal infiltration caused by ATL and retinal degeneration associated with HAM/TSP have been shown to mimic HU. ICG angiography of patients with HU suggests choroidal inflammatory involvement in addition to retinal vasculitis. HTLV-1–associated keratopathy has been described in Brazilian and Caribbean patients with HTLV-1 infection but has not been found among Japanese patients. Previously referred to as *HTLV-1–related chronic interstitial keratitis,* these corneal lesions are uniformly asymptomatic and do not affect vision. They result most likely from asymptomatic lymphoplasmacytic infiltrates.

Although many cases of HU respond to topical, periocular, or systemic steroid therapy and resolve completely within 1–2 months, up to one-half of patients experience recurrent disease. HU can be associated with sight-threatening ocular complications including cataract and epiretinal membrane formation, glaucoma, persistent vitreous opacification, retinal vascular occlusion, retinochoroidal degeneration, and optic atrophy; these complications may occur in up to one-third of cases, with poor visual outcomes in up to 10% of affected eyes.

Buggage RR. Ocular manifestations of human T-cell lymphotropic virus type 1 infection. *Curr Opin Ophthalmol.* 2003;14(6):420–425.

Goto H, Mochizuki M, Yamaki K, Kotake S, Usui M, Ohno S. Epidemiological survey of intraocular inflammation in Japan. *Jpn J Ophthalmol.* 2007;51(1):41–44.

Dengue Fever

Dengue fever is the most common mosquito-borne viral disease in humans; it is caused by a member of the Flaviviridae family and transmitted by the *Aedes aegypti* mosquito. It is endemic to more than 100 countries in the tropical and subtropical regions of the globe. Systemic signs and symptoms include fever, headache, myalgia, purpuric rash, and other bleeding manifestations secondary to thrombocytopenia. The most common ocular manifestation is petechial subconjunctival hemorrhage, although a maculopathy involving both the retinal and choroidal vessels may develop in approximately 10% of patients 1 month after the onset of systemic disease, presenting with a sudden decrease in vision and central scotoma. The maculopathy associated with dengue fever is bilateral (73%), albeit asymmetric; mean visual acuity is 20/40 in the affected eye. Intraretinal hemorrhages, usually in combination with periphlebitis, are observed most frequently (45%), followed by yellow subretinal dots (28%), RPE mottling (17%), foveal changes (16%), disc hyperemia (14%) and edema (11%), and arteriolar sheathing (4%). A variable degree of anterior chamber and vitreous cells are also observed. Fluorescein angiography demonstrates venous occlusive disease in 25% of eyes as well as arteriolar and/or venular leakage; ICG angiography reveals more numerous hypofluorescent spots corresponding to yellow subretinal lesions not visualized by FA or observed on clinical examination. Optical coherence tomography (OCT) is valuable in identifying foveal changes as the cause of decreased visual acuity in eyes with no apparent lesions on examination and is helpful for monitoring clinical progress. The diagnosis is made on the basis of the presence of typical clinical findings together with positive IgM results indicative of dengue. Although topical, periocular, and systemic steroids and immunoglobulins have been employed with variable success, the optimal treatment modality is unknown, as the disease may be self-limiting.

Bacsal KE, Chee SP, Cheng CL, Flores JV. Dengue-associated maculopathy. *Arch Ophthalmol.* 2007;125(4):501–510.

Chikungunya Fever

Chikungunya fever is a potentially fatal illness resembling dengue fever that is caused by an arthropod-borne *Alphavirus* in the family Togaviridae. In addition to fever, patients present with headache, fatigue, nausea, vomiting, myalgia, arthralgia, and skin rash. The ocular manifestations in a 2006 epidemic in India included, most commonly, both anterior uveitis and retinitis, and less frequently, nodular episcleritis; each had a typically benign course. The bilateral anterior uveitis may be granulomatous or nongranulomatous and associated with diffuse pigmented KPs, iris pigment release, elevated IOP, and, infrequently, posterior synechiae. Chikungunya retinitis may resemble herpetic retinitis in an immunocompetent host, in that both appear several weeks after the primary illness. However, Chikungunya retinitis is characterized by focal, multifocal, or confluent retinochoroiditis in the posterior pole with retinal hemorrhage, edema, and minimal vitritis, whereas herpetic retinitis includes peripheral retinal involvement and a more intense vitreous reaction.

The diagnosis is suggested when individuals from endemic areas present with a history of fever and arthralgia as well as anterior uveitis with pigmented KPs or posterior pole retinochoroiditis or neuroretinitis. Diagnosis may be confirmed serologically by the demonstration of Chikungunya-specific IgM antibodies, virus isolation, or results of reverse transcription PCR analysis. Although confluent retinitis has been treated with systemic acyclovir and prednisone, there is no evidence to suggest that such therapy improves visual outcome or affects the clinical course. Topical steroids and antihypertensive drugs are useful in the treatment of anterior uveitis and elevated IOP.

Mahendradas P, Ranganna SK, Shetty R, et al. Ocular manifestations associated with Chikungunya. *Ophthalmology.* 2008;115(2):287–291.

Other Viral Diseases

Acute anterior uveitis may also occur with other viral infectious entities. The uveitis observed with influenza, adenovirus infection, and IM is mild and transient. Synechiae and ocular damage seldom occur. Uveitis associated with adenovirus infection is usually secondary to corneal disease (see BCSC Section 8, *External Disease and Cornea*).

Fungal Uveitis

Ocular Histoplasmosis Syndrome

Ocular histoplasmosis syndrome (OHS) is a multifocal chorioretinitis presumed to be caused by infection with *Histoplasma capsulatum,* a dimorphic fungus with yeast and filamentous forms early in life. The yeast form is thought to be the cause of both systemic and ocular disease; primary infection occurs after inhalation of the fungal spores into the lungs. Ocular disease is thought to arise as a consequence of hematogenous dissemination of the organism. Acquired histoplasmosis is usually asymptomatic or may result in a benign illness, typically during childhood.

OHS is most frequently found in endemic areas of the United States such as the Ohio and Mississippi River valleys, where 60% of individuals react positively to histoplasmin skin testing. However, OHS has also been reported in nonendemic areas in the United States (Maryland) and sporadically throughout Europe (the United Kingdom and Netherlands). Although no serologic confirmation of histoplasmosis infection in patients with OHS has been reported, a causal relationship is strongly suggested by epidemiologic evidence linking an increased prevalence of ocular disease among patients who live or formerly resided in endemic areas. Furthermore, *H capsulatum* DNA has been detected in chronic choroidal lesions of a patient with OHS, and individuals with disciform scars are more likely than control subjects to react positively to histoplasmin skin testing. Men and women are affected equally, and the vast majority of patients are of northern European descent.

The diagnosis of OHS is based on the clinical triad of multiple white, atrophic choroidal scars (so-called *histo spots*); peripapillary pigment changes; and a maculopathy caused by CNV in the absence of vitreous cells. Histo spots may appear in the macula or periphery, are discrete and punched out (arising from a variable degree of scarring in the choroid and adjacent outer retina), and are typically asymptomatic (Fig 7-18). Approximately 1.5% of patients from endemic areas exhibit typical peripheral histo spots, first appearing during adolescence. Linear equatorial streaks are present in 5% of patients (Fig 7-19). In contrast, metamorphopsia and a profound reduction in central vision herald macular involvement from CNV and bring the patient to the attention of the ophthalmologist. The mean age of patients presenting with vision-threatening maculopathy is 41 years. Funduscopy of active neovascular lesions reveals a yellow-green subretinal membrane typically surrounded by a pigment ring; overlying neurosensory detachment;

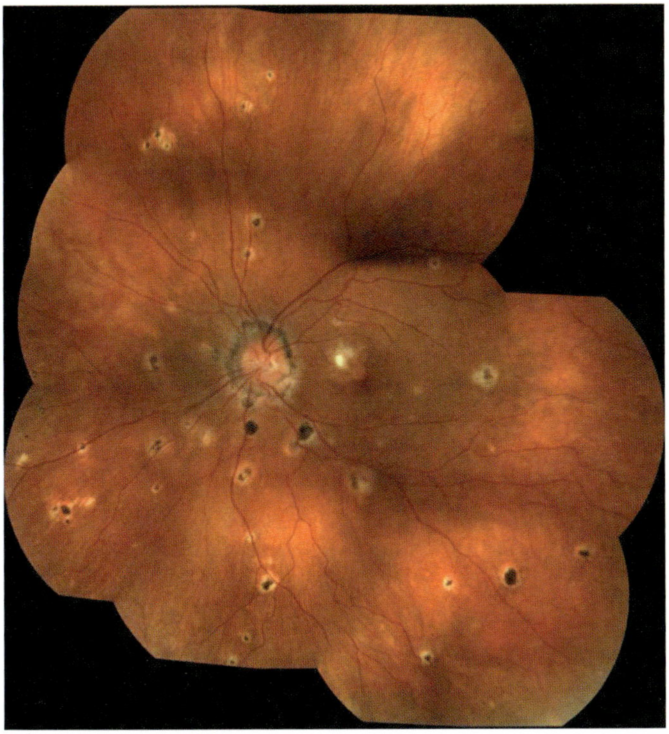

Figure 7-18 Fundus photograph from a patient with ocular histoplasmosis, showing peripapillary pigmentary scarring; midperipheral chorioretinal scars, or "histo spots" (some pigmented and fibrotic); and spontaneously regressed, nasal, juxtafoveal choroidal neovascular membrane in the absence of vitreous cells. Visual acuity, 20/25. *(Courtesy of Ramana S. Moorthy, MD.)*

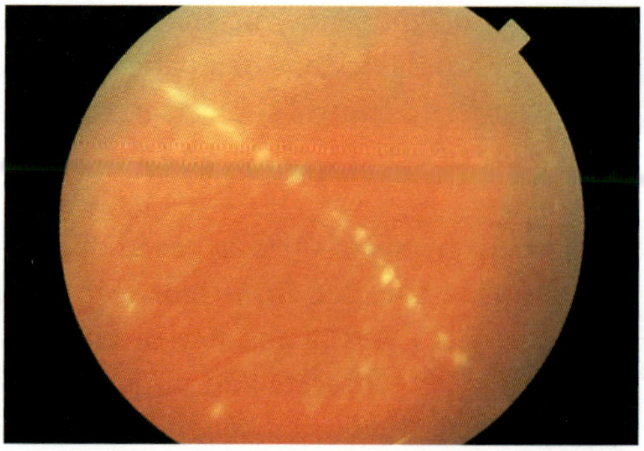

Figure 7-19 Ocular histoplasmosis fundus photograph: linear equatorial streaks. *(Courtesy of E. Mitchel Opremcak, MD.)*

and subretinal hemorrhage, frequently arising at the border of a histo scar in the disc–macula area. Cicatricial changes characterize advanced disease, with subretinal fibrosis and disciform scarring of the macula.

The pathogenesis of OHS is thought to involve a focal infection of the choroid at the time of initial systemic infection. This choroiditis may subside and leave an atrophic scar and depigmentation of the RPE, or it may result in disruption of the Bruch membrane, choriocapillaris, and RPE, as well as subsequent proliferation of subretinal vessels originating from the choroid. Lacking tight junctions, these neovascular complexes leak fluid, lipid, and blood, resulting in loss of macular function. The initiating stimulus for the growth of new subretinal vessels is unknown; however, immune mechanisms in patients with an underlying genetic predisposition for the development of this disease have been implicated. HLA-DRw2 is twice as common among patients with histo spots alone, whereas both HLA-B7 and HLA-DRw2 are 2–4 times more common among patients with disciform scars caused by OHS than among control subjects. Similarly, HLA-DR2 was absent in a group of patients with MCP, a disease that simulates OHS in many respects, whereas the antigen was present among those with CNV due to OHS.

The differential diagnosis includes entities other than age-related macular degeneration (AMD) that are frequently associated with CNV, including angioid streaks, choroidal rupture, idiopathic CNV, MCP, punctate inner choroidopathy, and granulomatous fundus lesions that may mimic the scarring of OHS (toxoplasmosis, tuberculosis, coccidioidomycosis, syphilis, sarcoidosis, and toxocariasis). The atrophic spots and maculopathy of myopic degeneration and disciform scarring in AMD may also be confused with OHS.

Over time, new choroidal scars develop in more than 20% of patients; however, only 3.8% of these cases progress to CNV. If histo spots appear in the macular area, the patient has a 15% chance of developing CNV within 5 years; if no spots are observed, the chances fall to 5%. Massive subretinal exudation and hemorrhagic retinal detachments may occur and result in permanent loss of macular function. Although some cases have been reported of spontaneous resolution with a return to normal vision, the visual prognosis of untreated OHS-associated CNV is poor, with 75% of eyes reaching a final visual acuity of 20/100 or worse over a 3-year period.

The early, acute granulomatous lesions of OHS are rarely observed but may be treated with oral or regional (periocular) corticosteroids (Fig 7-20). In the early stages of an FA

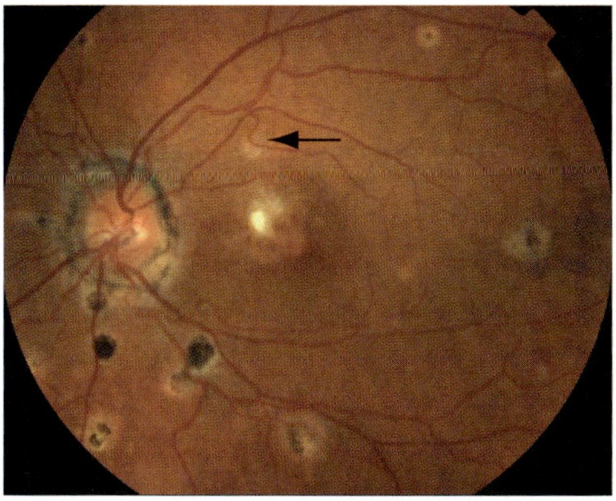

Figure 7-20 Ocular histoplasmosis fundus photograph: macular choroiditis *(arrow)* with multiple yellow elevated lesions. *(Courtesy of Ramana S. Moorthy, MD.)*

study, foci of active choroiditis block the dye and appear hypofluorescent; later in the study, these lesions stain, becoming hyperfluorescent. In contrast, areas of active CNV appear hyperfluorescent early in the angiogram and leak later in the study. Choroidal neovascular membranes may arise outside the vascular arcades, but they typically do not reduce vision and may be safely managed with observation only.

Treatment options for vision-threatening juxtafoveal or subfoveal CNV include thermal laser photocoagulation (Fig 7-21), photodynamic therapy (PDT) using verteporfin with or without intravitreal triamcinolone, submacular surgery for membrane removal, and intravitreal injection of anti–vascular endothelial growth factor (anti-VEGF) drugs. Thermal laser photocoagulation is rarely used in the treatment of subfoveal CNV associated with OHS, given the profound and immediate loss of central vision that results from the destructive effects of this modality. Based on results of small, prospective, uncontrolled case series, PDT with verteporfin has been advocated for the treatment of subfoveal OHS-associated CNV. A number of anti-VEGF drugs currently being used in the management of neovascular AMD are available for off-label treatment of OHS-associated CNV. Intravitreal anti-VEGF therapy has been shown to be superior to PDT in patients with neovascular AMD in visual acuity outcome, but no such randomized, prospective study comparing these modalities has been conducted in OHS-associated CNV. As for neovascular AMD, combination approaches using PDT and intravitreal corticosteroids or anti-VEGF drugs may prove fruitful, especially in treating entities with an underlying inflammatory etiology.

Surgical removal of subretinal neovascular membranes may be accomplished by modern vitreoretinal techniques. The submacular surgery trials (SST) examined this surgical approach to subretinal membranes. Long-term follow-up revealed recurrence rates approaching 50% and—coupled with complications of surgery including retinal breaks, retinal detachment, and cataract formation—the enthusiasm for such an approach has waned. In selected cases of extensive peripapillary CNV associated with OHS, surgical removal may provide a more definitive vision benefit with low recurrence rates, and it may be preferable to photoablation, given the likelihood of repeat PDT and anti-VEGF treatments. See BCSC Section 12, *Retina and Vitreous,* for further detail about thermal laser

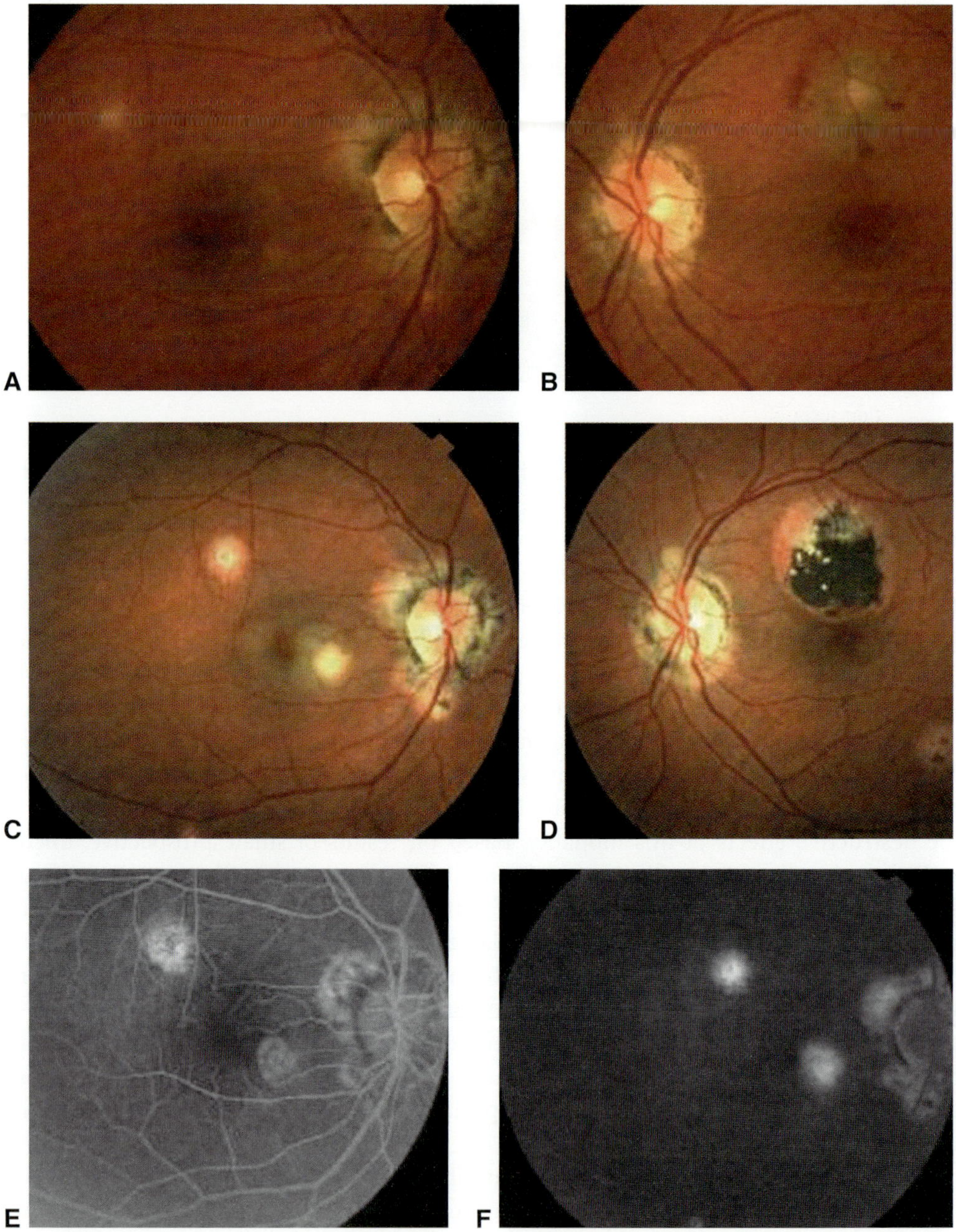

Figure 7-21 Ocular histoplasmosis. **A, B,** Color fundus photographs showing peripapillary scarring in both eyes. **A,** Punched-out chorioretinal scars present in the right eye. **B,** Active choroidal neovascularization superior to the fovea of the left eye. **C,** New choroidal neovascular membrane adjacent to a punched-out chorioretinal scar in the right eye. **D,** Chorioretinal scar after laser treatment to the choroidal neovascular membrane in the left eye. Early-phase **(E)** and late-phase **(F)** fluorescein angiography images of the right eye. *(Courtesy of David J. Browning, MD, PhD.)*

photocoagulation, PDT, anti-VEGF drugs, intravitreal corticosteroids, and submacular surgery for the treatment of CNV.

For discussions of the ocular manifestations of candidiasis, aspergillosis, cryptococcosis, and coccidioidomycosis as well as their treatments, please see Chapter 8 in this volume.

Almony A, Thomas MA, Atebara NH, Holekamp NM, Del Priore LV. Long-term follow-up of surgical removal of extensive peripapillary choroidal neovascularization in presumed ocular histoplasmosis syndrome. *Ophthalmology.* 2008;115(3):540–545.

Brown DM, Kaiser PK, Michels M, et al; ANCHOR Study Group. Ranibizumab versus verteporfin for neovascular age-related macular degeneration. *N Engl J Med.* 2006; 355(14):1432–1444.

Ehrlich R, Ciulla TA, Maturi R, et al. Intravitreal bevacizumab for choroidal neovascularization secondary to presumed ocular histoplasmosis syndrome. *Retina.* 2009;29(10): 1418–1423.

Hawkins BS, Bressler NM, Bressler SB, et al; Submacular Surgery Trials Research Group. Surgical removal vs observation for subfoveal choroidal neovascularization, either associated with the ocular histoplasmosis syndrome or idiopathic: I. Ophthalmic findings from a randomized clinical trial. Submacular Surgery Trials (SST) Group H trial: SST report no. 9. *Arch Ophthalmol.* 2004;122(11):1597–1611.

Macular Photocoagulation Study Group. Five-year follow-up of fellow eyes of individuals with ocular histoplasmosis and unilateral extrafoveal or juxtafoveal choroidal neovascularization. *Arch Ophthalmol.* 1996;114(6):677–688.

Saperstein DA, Rosenfeld PJ, Bressler NM, et al. Verteporfin therapy for CNV secondary to OHS. *Ophthalmology.* 2006;113(12):2371.e1–3.

Spencer WH, Chan CC, Shen DF, Rao NA. Detection of *Histoplasma capsulatum* DNA in lesions of chronic ocular histoplasmosis syndrome. *Arch Ophthalmol.* 2003;121(11): 1551–1555.

Protozoal Uveitis

Toxoplasmosis

Toxoplasmosis is the most common cause of infectious posterior uveitis in adults and children. It is caused by the parasite *Toxoplasma gondii,* a single-cell obligate intracellular apicomplexan parasite with a worldwide distribution (Fig 7-22). Felines are the definitive hosts of *T gondii,* and humans and a variety of other animals serve as intermediate hosts. *T gondii* has a complex life cycle and exists in 3 major forms:

1. the oocyst, or soil form (10–12 μm), which contains sporozoites
2. the tachyzoite, or infectious form (4–8 μm)
3. the tissue cyst, or latent form (10–200 μm), which contains as many as 3000 bradyzoites

Transmission of *T gondii* to humans and other animals may occur with all 3 forms of the parasite through a variety of vectors. The oocysts, which are the result of sexual

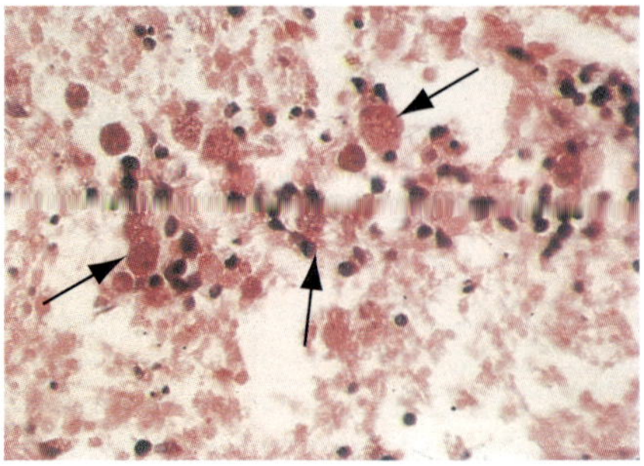

Figure 7-22 Histology of *Toxoplasma gondii* infection of the retina. Note the cysts *(arrows)* in the necrotic retina.

reproduction in the intestinal mucosa of the definitive host, are shed in infected cats' feces in large numbers, contaminating the environment. After maturation in the soil, these oocysts may then be ingested by intermediate hosts or reingested by cats. Tachyzoites, the proliferative form of the parasite, are found in the circulatory system and may invade nearly all host tissue. In an immunocompetent host, replication of tachyzoites eventually ceases, with some microorganisms persisting as dormant bradyzoites within intercellular tissue cysts.

Recent studies have identified 3 main, distinct clonal lineages of *T gondii* in humans and in animals that vary in their virulence but are antigenically similar. These 3 genotypes, designated types I, II, and III, plus recombinant atypical genotypes, can be distinguished serologically. Most human infections in North America and Europe have been attributed to type II parasites, which are less virulent than type I parasites and the atypical recombinant genotypes in animal models. In the United States, the prevalence of *T gondii* infection is 22.5% among the general population, whereas that of ocular toxoplasmosis among infected persons is estimated to be only 2%. In contrast, an estimated 80% of the population in southern Brazil is infected with *T gondii,* and up to 18% of these individuals may manifest evidence of retinochoroiditis. Some studies have demonstrated a greater heterogeneity of parasites in Brazil than in North America. It is postulated that variance in disease severity and ocular involvement in different regions around the world for both acquired and congenital infections may be due at least partly to genotypic differences of the infecting parasite, with more severe disease and higher rates of ocular involvement related to the presence of type I alleles or atypical genotypes.

Human infection by *T gondii* may be either acquired or congenital. The principal modes of transmission include

- ingestion of undercooked, infected meat containing tissue cysts
- ingestion of contaminated water, fruit, or vegetables with oocysts
- inadvertent contact with cat feces, cat litter, or soil containing oocysts
- transplacental transmission with primary infection during pregnancy
- blood transfusion or organ transplantation

At least a dozen outbreaks of toxoplasmosis have been reported from around the world. Five of the epidemics that occurred between 1979 and 2003 have been well studied, and contaminated water supplies or inhaled/ingested sporulated oocysts in dirt were implicated as sources of infection.

The reported seropositivity rates among healthy adults vary considerably throughout the world, ranging from 3% to 10.8% in the United States to between 50% and 80% in

France. Among patients with HIV infection in the United States, the reported seroprevalence of *T gondii* varies from 15% to 40%.

It has been estimated that between 70% and 80% of women of childbearing age in the United States lack antibodies to *T gondii*, which places them at risk for contracting the disease; however, the incidence of toxoplasmosis acquired during pregnancy is only 0.2%–1%. In southeastern Brazil, where the prevalence of toxoplasmosis is extremely high, the prevalence of congenital infection was reported as 1 in 770 live births, with a correspondingly high prevalence of ocular involvement.

Overall, 40% of primary maternal infections result in congenital infection; transplacental transmission is highest during the third trimester. The risk of severe disease developing in the fetus is inversely proportional to gestational age: disease acquired early in pregnancy may result in spontaneous abortion, stillbirth, or severe congenital disease, whereas that acquired later in gestation may produce an asymptomatic, normal-appearing infant with latent infection. Chronic or recurrent maternal infection during pregnancy is not thought to confer a significant risk of congenital toxoplasmosis because maternal immunity protects against fetal transmission.

Pregnant women without serologic evidence of *T gondii* infection should be advised to take the following precautions:

- Avoid ingestion of raw/undercooked meat (freezing at –20°C/–4°F overnight also destroys tissue cysts).
- Drink only well-filtered or boiled water.
- Carefully wash vegetables and fruits before consumption.
- Use gloves and wash hands and kitchen utensils well after handling meat or soil.
- Avoid contact with felines and their feces (including in soil or litter boxes).

Periodic serologic screening of susceptible women during pregnancy is also highly recommended in endemic areas.

The classic presentation of congenital toxoplasmosis includes retinochoroiditis, hydrocephalus or microcephaly, intracranial calcifications, and cognitive impairment (Sabin's tetrad), occurring in less than 10% of infected children. Retinochoroidal lesions, which can be found in up to 80% of cases, are the most common abnormality in patients with congenital toxoplasmosis; they are bilateral in approximately 85% of affected individuals and carry a predilection for the posterior pole and macula (Fig 7-23). Posterior segment involvement may be subclinical and chronic. As many as 85% of infected children develop retinochoroiditis after a mean of 3.7 years, and 25% of these become blind in 1 or both eyes. Most experts recommend antiparasitic therapy for newborns with congenital toxoplasmosis during the first year of life to reduce disease burden, regardless of the presence of ocular and/or systemic signs.

Although toxoplasmosis after infancy was previously considered to be exclusively the result of reactivation of congenital disease, acquired infection is now thought to play an important role in the development of ocular toxoplasmosis in children and adults. In one study, acquired postnatal infection was thought to represent up to two-thirds of cases of toxoplasmic ocular disease. A recent report of epidemic toxoplasmosis from India confirmed previous observations suggesting that postnatally acquired *T gondii* infection occurs in all age groups, including children, and that ocular disease can arise after infection

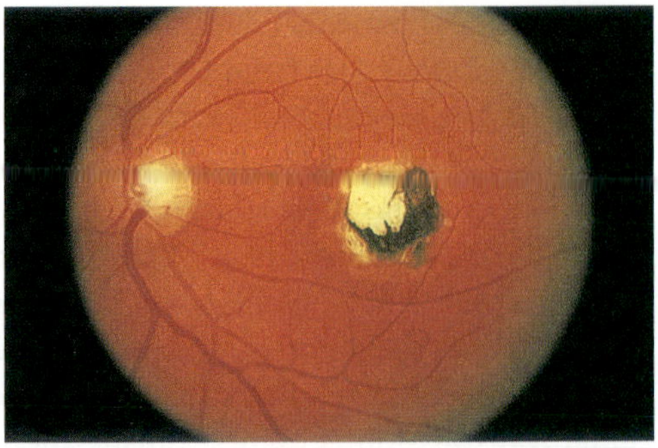

Figure 7-23 Fundus photograph of quiescent, partially pigmented, congenital toxoplasmic macular scar. Patient has 20/400 visual acuity. *(Courtesy of John D. Sheppard, Jr, MD.)*

without concurrent systemic signs or symptoms. This finding has significant public health implications with respect to primary prevention strategies, which must target not only pregnant women but also children and adults at risk for acquiring the disease. In the United States, previous studies indicated that toxoplasmosis may account for up to 38% of all cases of posterior uveitis, although this figure appears to be decreasing and varies with geography and referral bias.

Although dependent on the location of the lesion, presenting symptoms frequently include unilateral blurred or hazy vision and floaters. A mild to moderate granulomatous anterior uveitis is often observed, and up to 20% of patients have acutely elevated IOP at presentation. Classically, ocular toxoplasmosis appears as a focal, white retinochoroiditis, with overlying moderate vitreous inflammation ("headlight in the fog"), often adjacent to a pigmented retinochoroidal scar (Figs 7-24, 7-25). These lesions occur more commonly in the posterior pole but are occasionally found immediately adjacent to or directly involving the optic nerve; they are sometimes mistaken for optic neuritis. Retinal vessels in the vicinity of an active lesion may show perivasculitis with diffuse venous sheathing and segmental arterial plaques (Kyrieleis arteriolitis). Vascular occlusions

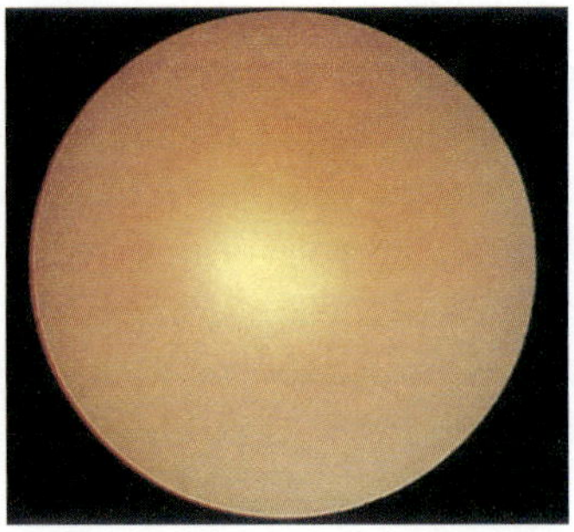

Figure 7-24 Toxoplasmic retinochoroiditis: fundus photograph showing intense focal retinitis with dense overlying vitritis, producing a "headlight in the fog" appearance.

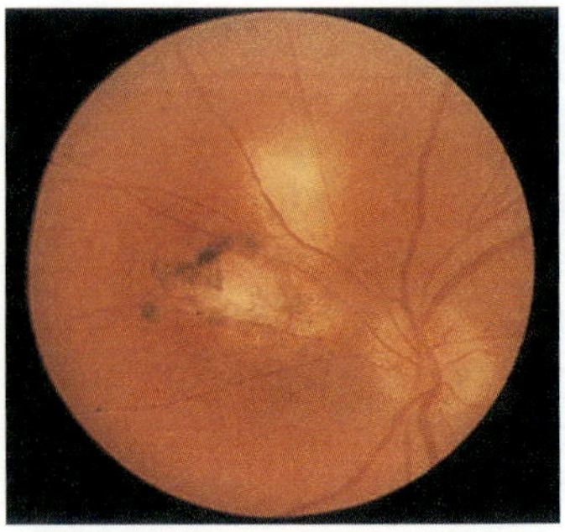

Figure 7-25 Toxoplasmosis: fundus photograph showing satellite retinochoroiditis around an old scar.

may also be present. Additional ocular complications include cataract, persistent vitreous opacities, CME, retinal detachment, epiretinal membranes, optic atrophy, and CNV (Fig 7-26). Focal retinochoroiditis in the absence of retinochoroidal scarring should raise the suspicion of recently acquired disease or of another etiology (Fig 7-27), even though remote toxoplasmic infection often cannot be excluded.

Retinochoroiditis developing in immunocompromised and older patients may present with atypical findings, including large, multiple, and/or bilateral lesions, with or without associated retinochoroidal scars. This more severe clinical picture can also occur in patients receiving steroids without concomitant antiparasitic therapy (Fig 7-28). Other atypical presentations include neuroretinitis, punctate outer retinal toxoplasmosis (PORT), unilateral pigmentary retinopathy simulating retinitis pigmentosa, and other forms of intraocular inflammation in the absence of retinochoroiditis. PORT is characterized by small, multifocal lesions at the level of the outer retina, with exudation to subretinal space and scant overlying vitreal inflammation (Fig 7-29).

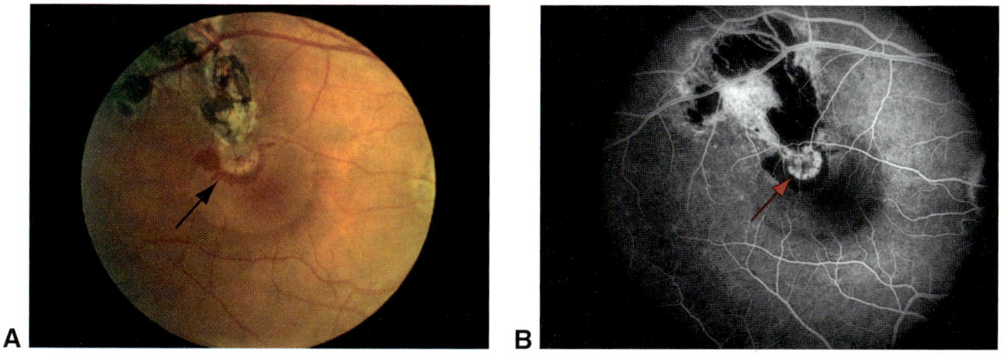

Figure 7-26 Toxoplasmic retinochoroiditis–associated choroidal neovascularization. **A,** Fundus photograph showing a choroidal neovascular membrane (CNVM) with intraretinal hemorrhage and subretinal fluid adjacent to an old toxoplasmic scar *(arrow)*. **B,** Early-phase fluorescein angiogram showing blocked fluorescence associated with scar and lacy hyperfluorescence that corresponds to CNVM *(arrow)*. *(Courtesy of Albert T. Vitale, MD.)*

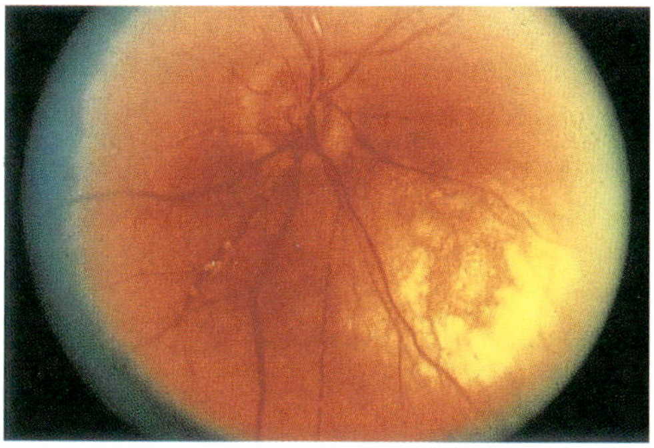

Figure 7-27 Fundus photograph of large, nonpigmented, inactive acquired toxoplasma retinal scar. *(Courtesy of John D. Sheppard, Jr, MD.)*

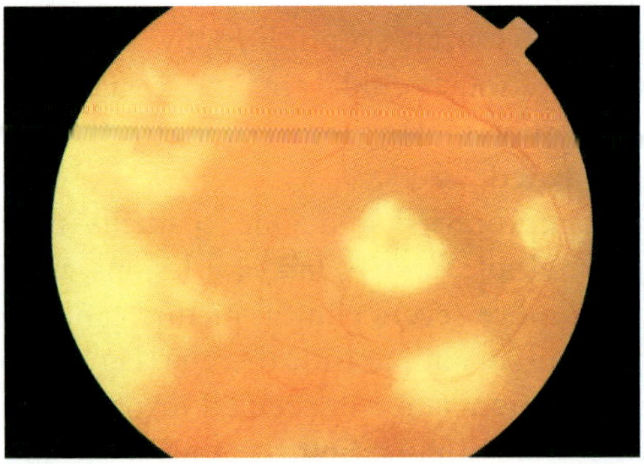

Figure 7-28 Toxoplasmosis: fundus photograph showing widespread retinal necrosis following periocular corticosteroid injection. *(Courtesy of E. Mitchel Opremcak, MD.)*

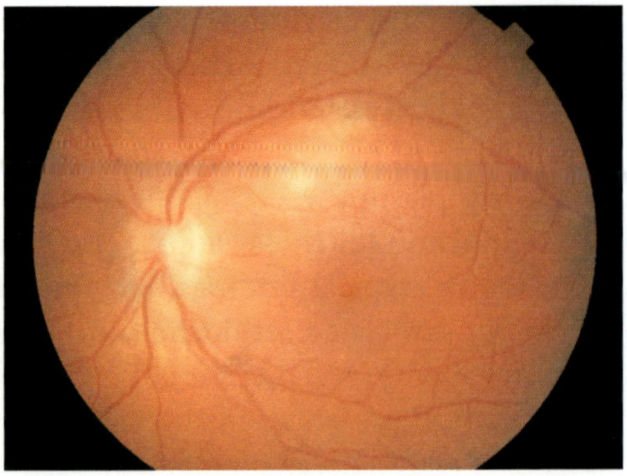

Figure 7-29 Fundus photograph showing punctate outer retinal toxoplasmosis (PORT). *(Courtesy of E. Mitchel Opremcak, MD.)*

Diagnosis

In most instances, the diagnosis of toxoplasmic retinochoroiditis is made clinically, on the basis of the appearance of the characteristic lesion on indirect ophthalmoscopy. Serologic evaluation using indirect fluorescent antibody and ELISA tests to detect specific anti–*T gondii* antibodies is commonly used to confirm exposure to the parasite. IgG antibodies appear after the first 2 weeks of infection, typically remain detectable for life at variable levels, and cross the placenta. IgM antibodies, however, increase in number early during the acute phase of the infection, typically remain detectable for less than 1 year, and do not cross the placenta. The presence of anti–*T gondii* IgG antibodies supports the diagnosis of toxoplasmic retinochoroiditis in the appropriate clinical context, whereas a negative antibody titer essentially rules out the diagnosis. The presence of IgM in newborns confirms congenital infection and is indicative of acquired disease when present in adults. Measurement of IgA antibody titers may also be useful in a diagnosis of congenital toxoplasmosis in a fetus or newborn; during this period, IgM production is often weak and the presence of IgG antibodies may indicate passive transfer of maternal antibodies in utero. IgA antibodies, however, usually disappear by 7 months. Intraocular production of specific anti-*Toxoplasma* antibodies may be computed using the GW coefficient, as described earlier in the chapter. A ratio of greater than 3 is considered diagnostic of local antibody production. Highly sensitive and specific PCR-based techniques have been used to detect *T gondii* DNA in the aqueous humor and vitreous fluid of patients with ocular toxoplasmosis; these techniques are of particular value in cases with atypical presentations.

Treatment

Ocular toxoplasmosis is a progressive and recurrent disease; new lesions may occur at the margins of old scars as well as elsewhere in the fundus, and toxoplasmic cysts may be present in a normal-appearing retina. In the immunocompetent patient, the disease has a self-limiting course; the borders of the lesions become sharper and less edematous over a 6–8-week period without treatment, and RPE hypertrophy occurs gradually over a period of months. In the immunocompromised patient, the disease tends to be more severe and progressive. Treatment is aimed at shortening the duration of the parasitic replication, which leads to more rapid cicatrization of the lesions and thereby limits retinochoroidal scarring and progression. Treatment also may reduce the frequency of inflammatory recurrences and minimize structural complications associated with intraocular inflammation.

Numerous medications have been used to treat toxoplasmosis over the years, but no single drug or combination can be applied categorically to every patient, and there is no consensus as to the most efficacious regimen. There is, in fact, little firm evidence that antimicrobial therapy alters the natural history of toxoplasmic retinochoroiditis in immunocompetent patients. In these patients, the decision to treat is influenced by the number, size, and location of the lesions relative to the macula and optic disc, as well as the severity and duration of the vitreous inflammation. Some clinicians may elect to observe small lesions in the retinal periphery that are not associated with a significant decrease in vision or vitritis; others treat virtually all patients in an effort to reduce the number of subsequent recurrences. Relative treatment indications include

- lesions threatening the optic nerve or fovea
- decreased visual acuity
- lesions associated with moderate to severe vitreous inflammation
- lesions greater than 1 disc diameter in size
- persistence of disease for more than 1 month
- presence of multiple active lesions

Treatment is indicated in immunocompromised patients (those with HIV/AIDS, with neoplastic disease, or undergoing IMT), patients with congenital toxoplasmosis, and pregnant women with recently acquired disease.

The classic regimen for the treatment of ocular toxoplasmosis consists of triple therapy: pyrimethamine (loading dose, 50–100 mg; treatment dose, 25–50 mg/day), sulfadiazine (treatment dose, 1 g, 4 times/day), and prednisone (treatment dose, 0.5–1 mg/kg/day, depending on the severity of the inflammation). Because sulfonamides and pyrimethamine inhibit folic acid metabolism, folinic acid (15 mg every day) is added to prevent myelosuppression (leukopenia and/or thrombocytopenia), which may result from pyrimethamine therapy. Leukocyte and platelet counts should be monitored weekly. Potential adverse effects of sulfa compounds include skin rash, gastrointestinal intolerance, crystalluria, kidney stones, and Stevens-Johnson syndrome. Some clinicians advocate adding clindamycin to this regimen as "quadruple" therapy or in the instance of sulfa allergy. Clindamycin, either alone or in combination with other drugs, has been effective in managing acute lesions, but pseudomembranous colitis is a potential complication of its use.

Systemic corticosteroids are generally begun either at the time of antimicrobial therapy or within 48 hours in immunocompetent patients. The use of systemic corticosteroids without appropriate antimicrobial coverage or the use of long-acting periocular and intraocular corticosteroid formulations such as triamcinolone acetonide is contraindicated because of the potential for severe, uncontrollable intraocular inflammation and loss of the eye (see Fig 7-28). Topical corticosteroids, however, are used liberally in the presence of prominent anterior segment inflammation. In general, treatment lasts from 5 to 6 weeks, at which time inflammation begins to subside and the retinal lesion shows signs of consolidation. This period may be extended if there is persistent disease activity.

Many ophthalmologists have begun to use trimethoprim-sulfamethoxazole (treatment dose, 160 mg/800 mg twice daily) and prednisone as an alternative to the classic therapy for reasons of cost, the frequent unavailability of sulfadiazine, and the presumption that trimethoprim-sulfamethoxazole has a better safety profile. A small, prospective randomized trial of trimethoprim-sulfamethoxazole versus pyrimethamine and sulfadiazine in the treatment of ocular toxoplasmosis showed no major differences in efficacy between the 2 regimens and did not convincingly demonstrate that trimethoprim-sulfamethoxazole had a superior safety profile. Azithromycin (250 mg/day) has been used successfully to treat ocular toxoplasmosis in immunocompetent patients in combination with pyrimethamine (50 mg/day). This regimen's efficacy was considered similar to that of the standard treatment of pyrimethamine and sulfadiazine in a small study, which also found it to be better tolerated and have fewer adverse effects.

Newborns with congenital toxoplasmosis are commonly treated with pyrimethamine and sulfonamides (plus folinic acid) for 1 year, in consultation with a specialist in pediatric infectious diseases.

In cases of newly acquired toxoplasmosis during pregnancy, treatment is given to prevent infection of the fetus and limit fetal damage if infection has already occurred, as well as to limit the destructive sequelae of intraocular disease in the mother. Spiramycin (treatment dose, 400 mg 3 times daily) reduces the rate of tachyzoite transmission to the fetus and may be used safely without undue risk of teratogenicity. Because this drug is commonly unavailable in the United States, alternative medications may be needed; options include azithromycin, clindamycin, and atovaquone (treatment dose, 750 mg every 6 hours). Sulfonamides may be used safely in the first 2 trimesters of pregnancy. Alternatively, local treatment involving intraocular injections of clindamycin and short-acting periocular corticosteroids (eg, dexamethasone) has been advocated in pregnant women in an effort to reduce systemic adverse effects.

Patients with HIV/AIDS require extended systemic treatment given the frequent association of ocular disease with cerebral involvement (56%) and the frequency of recurrent ocular disease when antitoxoplasmic medication is discontinued (Fig 7-30). The best regimen for secondary prophylaxis remains to be determined; however, atovaquone acts synergistically with pyrimethamine and sulfadiazine and thus may be useful for reducing the dose and toxicity of these drugs in the treatment of patients with AIDS and toxoplasmosis. The management of ocular toxoplasmosis in association with HIV/AIDS is also covered in Chapter 11.

Long-term intermittent trimethoprim-sulfamethoxazole treatment (160 mg/800 mg 3 times per week) was shown to decrease the risk of reactivation among patients with recurrent toxoplasmic retinochoroiditis observed over a 20-month period. A similar strategy may be useful as prophylaxis in patients with ocular toxoplasmosis and HIV/AIDS.

Similarly, the utility of prophylactic antimicrobial treatment shortly before and after intraocular surgery in patients with inactive toxoplasmic scars—particularly scars that

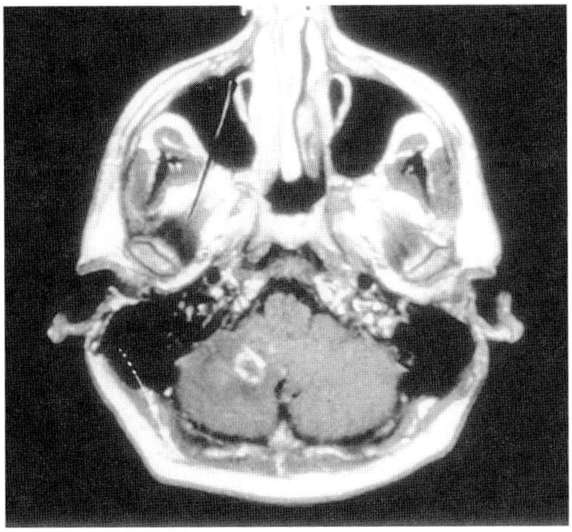

Figure 7-30 Enhanced computed tomography scan revealing a cerebellar lesion caused by central nervous system toxoplasmosis in a patient with AIDS who presented with ataxia. *(Courtesy of John D. Sheppard, Jr, MD.)*

threaten the optic disc or fovea—was raised by a report that describes an association between cataract surgery and an increased risk of reactivation of otherwise inactive toxoplasmic retinochoroiditis. There is, however, no consensus with respect to this treatment approach or to the optimal antibiotic regimen in this clinical situation.

Holland GN. Ocular toxoplasmosis: a global reassessment. Part I: epidemiology and course of disease. *Am J Ophthalmol.* 2003;136(6):973–988.

Holland GN. Ocular toxoplasmosis: a global reassessment. Part II: disease manifestations and management. *Am J Ophthalmol.* 2004;137(1):1–17.

Khan A, Jordan C, Muccioli C, et al. Genetic divergence of *Toxoplasma gondii* strains associated with ocular toxoplasmosis, Brazil. *Emerg Infect Dis.* 2006;12(6):942–949.

Kim SJ, Scott IU, Brown GC, et al. Interventions for toxoplasma retinochoroiditis: a report by the American Academy of Ophthalmology. *Ophthalmology.* 2013;120(2):371–378.

Kishore K, Conway MD, Peyman GA. Intravitreal clindamycin and dexamethasone for toxoplasmic retinochoroiditis. *Ophthalmic Surg Lasers.* 2001;32(3):183–192.

Kump LI, Androudi SN, Foster CS. Ocular toxoplasmosis in pregnancy. *Clin Experiment Ophthalmol.* 2005;33(5):455–460.

Montoya JG, Parmley S, Liesenfeld O, Jaffe GJ, Remington JS. Use of the polymerase chain reaction for diagnosis of ocular toxoplasmosis. *Ophthalmology.* 1999;106(8):1554–1563.

Silveira C, Belfort R Jr, Muccioli C, et al. The effect of long-term intermittent trimethoprim/sulfamethoxazole treatment on recurrences of toxoplasmic retinochoroiditis. *Am J Ophthalmol.* 2002;134(1):41–46.

Soheilian M, Sadoughi MM, Ghajarnia M, et al. Prospective randomized trial of trimethoprim/sulfamethoxazole versus pyrimethamine and sulfadiazine in the treatment of ocular toxoplasmosis. *Ophthalmology.* 2005;112(11):1876–1882.

Vasconcelos-Santos DV. Ocular manifestations of systemic disease: toxoplasmosis. *Curr Opin Ophthalmol.* 2012;23(6):543–550.

Vasconcelos-Santos DV, Machado Azevedo DO, Campos WR, et al; UFMG Congenital Toxoplasmosis Brazilian Group. Congenital toxoplasmosis in southeastern Brazil: results of early ophthalmologic examination of a large cohort of neonates. *Ophthalmology.* 2009;116(11):2199–2205.

Helminthic Uveitis

Toxocariasis

Ocular toxocariasis is an uncommon disease of children and young adults that may produce significant loss of vision. Non-Hispanic whites are affected most commonly; there is no sex predilection. The prevalence was recently estimated to be 1% of a large uveitic population treated at tertiary care centers in northern California. Estimates are that approximately 14% of the US population is seropositive and that the US rate is 1 in 1000 persons. Ocular involvement has been reported to occur in <1% of all seropositive children in Spain.

Human toxocariasis results from tissue invasion by the second-stage larvae of *Toxocara canis* or *T cati,* roundworm parasites that complete their life cycles in the small intestines of dogs and cats, respectively. Transmission occurs through ingestion of soil or contaminated food, or the fecal–oral route. The eating disorder pica and contact with puppies or kittens are common among children with toxocariasis. Playgrounds and sandboxes are common sources of the parasite. The organisms grow in the small intestine, enter the portal circulation, disseminate throughout the body by hematogenous and lymphatic routes, and ultimately reside in target tissues, including the eye. Maturation of the adult worm does not occur in humans; consequently, ova are not shed in the alimentary tract, rendering stool analysis for larvae unproductive. Ocular toxocariasis (OT) and the systemic disease visceral larvae migrans (VLM) rarely present contemporaneously. VLM typically affects children younger than age 3 years, possibly because of an increased rate of pica among this group; whereas OT is found most often in older children or young adults. Finally, there is a direct relationship between the degree of peripheral eosinophilia and the parasitic burden in the systemic disease but not in OT.

A large survey of ophthalmic subspecialists in the United States showed that the median age of patients with OT was 11.5 years (range, 1–66). The disorder was more likely to affect non-Hispanic white males, and almost half lived in the southern region of the United States; the majority suffered permanent vision loss.

Patients with OT present with unilateral decreased vision that may be accompanied by pain, photophobia, floaters, strabismus, or leukocoria. Bilateral disease is exceedingly rare. The anterior segment is typically white and quiet. However, nongranulomatous anterior inflammation and posterior synechiae may be present in severe disease. Posterior segment findings include 3 recognizable ocular syndromes:

1. leukocoria resulting from moderate to severe vitreous inflammation and chronic endophthalmitis: 25% of cases
2. localized macular granuloma: 25% of cases (Fig 7-31)
3. peripheral granuloma: 50% of cases (Fig 7-32)

Uncommon variants include unilateral pars planitis with diffuse peripheral inflammatory exudates and granulomas involving the optic nerve. Table 7-2 lists the characteristics of each presentation.

Determinants of the visual prognosis are multifactorial and include the degree of intraocular inflammation and the location of the inflammatory foci with respect to the foveal center; the presence or absence of CME; and the development of tractional

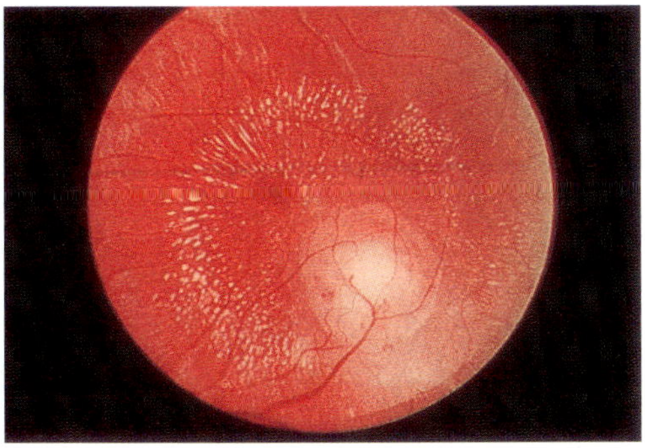

Figure 7-31 Toxocariasis: fundus photograph showing macular granuloma.

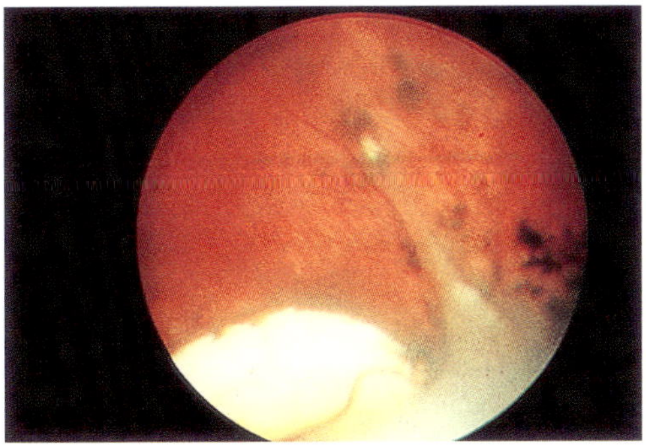

Figure 7-32 Toxocariasis: fundus photograph of peripheral granuloma.

Table 7-2 Patterns of Manifestation of Ocular Toxocariasis

Syndrome	Age of Onset, y	Characteristic Lesion
Chronic endophthalmitis	2–9	Chronic unilateral uveitis, cloudy vitreous cyclitic membrane
Localized granuloma	6–14	Present in the macula and peripapillary region Solitary, white, elevated in the retina: minimal reaction; 1–2 disc diameters in size
Peripheral granuloma	6–40	Peripheral hemispheric masses with dense connective tissue strands in the vitreous cavity that may connect to the disc Rarely bilateral

membranes involving the optic nerve, macula, and ciliary body. In the absence of foveal involvement, vision at presentation is usually best when the granulomas are located in the posterior pole, as these eyes are less likely than are eyes with peripheral granulomas to have macular traction. Eyes with endophthalmitis have the worst vision at presentation.

The diagnosis of OT is essentially clinical, and is made on the basis of the characteristic lesion morphology, supportive laboratory data, and findings on imaging studies. The serum ELISA titer of 1:8 is 91% sensitive and 90% specific for prior exposure to the organism; however, any positive titer should be considered significant in the appropriate clinical context. On the other hand, the absence of serum antibodies does not rule out the diagnosis, as up to one-third of patients with OT may have negative ELISA results. In these cases, examination of intraocular fluids with ELISA may reveal specific *T canis* antibodies and results leading to a positive GW coefficient, providing evidence of primary ocular involvement. *Toxocara* larvae have been recovered from the vitreous during pars plana vitrectomy (Fig 7-33). PCR testing of vitreous has not been successful. Finally, B-scan ultrasonography and computed tomography (CT) are useful in the presence of media opacity; they may reveal vitreous membranes and tractional retinal detachment and confirm the absence of calcium, a characteristic finding in retinoblastoma.

The most important differential diagnostic consideration is that of sporadic unilateral retinoblastoma. Factors that may be helpful in making this distinction include the

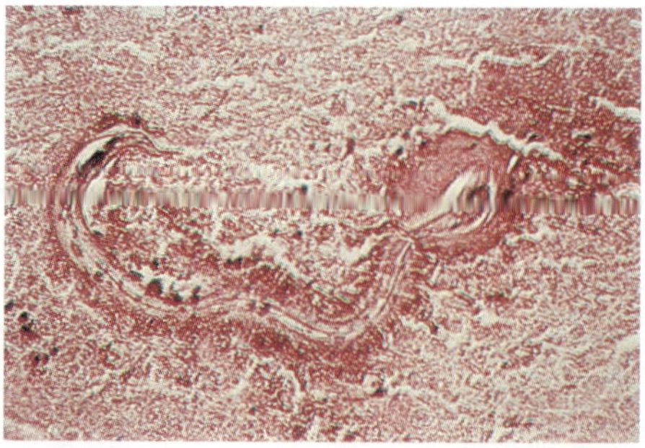

Figure 7-33 Toxocariasis: histopathology of an eosinophilic vitreous abscess. The organism is in the center of the abscess.

noticeably younger age at presentation, the paucity of inflammatory stigmata, and the demonstration of lesion growth in children with retinoblastoma. Other differential diagnostic entities include infectious endophthalmitis, toxoplasmosis, and pars planitis, as well as congenital retinovascular abnormalities such as retinopathy of prematurity, persistent fetal vasculature, Coats disease, and familial exudative vitreoretinopathy.

Although there is no uniformly satisfactory treatment for OT, medical therapy with periocular and systemic corticosteroids is aimed at reducing the inflammatory response in an effort to prevent structural complications. The utility of antihelminthic therapy has not been established, although albendazole or thiabendazole can be used in concert with corticosteroids. Vitreoretinal surgical techniques have been used successfully to manage tractional and rhegmatogenous complications. Laser photocoagulation of the larvae may be considered if identified on clinical examination and may be used to treat the rare occurrence of CNV arising in association with inactive *Toxocara* granulomas.

Centers for Disease Control and Prevention. Ocular toxocariasis—United States, 2009–2010. *MMWR.* 2011;60(22):734–736.

Schneier AJ, Durand ML. Ocular toxocariasis: advances in diagnosis and treatment. *Int Ophthalmol Clin.* 2011;51(4):135–144.

Stewart JM, Cubillan LD, Cunningham ET Jr. Prevalence, clinical features, and causes of vision loss among patients with ocular toxocariasis. *Retina.* 2005;25(8):1005–1013.

Woodhall D, Starr MC, Montgomery SP, et al. Ocular toxocariasis: epidemiologic, anatomic, and therapeutic variations based on a survey of ophthalmic subspecialists. *Ophthalmology.* 2012;119(6):1211–1217.

Cysticercosis

Cysticercosis is the most common ocular tapeworm infection; it occurs especially in underdeveloped areas where hygiene is poor. Human infection is caused by *Cysticercus cellulosae,* the larval stage of the cestode *Taenia solium,* which is endemic to Mexico, Africa, Southeast Asia, eastern Europe, Central and South America, and India. Although the eye is more commonly affected than any other organ, neural cysticercosis is associated with significant morbidity and a mortality of 40%.

Human cysticercosis is caused by ingestion of water or foods contaminated by the pork tapeworm. The eggs mature into larvae, penetrate the intestinal mucosa, and spread hematogenously to the eye via the posterior ciliary arteries into the subretinal space in the region of the posterior pole. Larvae within the subretinal space may cause an exudative retinal detachment or may perforate the retina, causing a retinal break and gain access to the vitreous cavity.

Ocular cysticercosis is a disorder of the young, occurring most frequently between the ages of 10 and 30 years, without sex predilection. The disease is mostly unilateral. Although cysticercosis may involve any structure of the eye and its adnexae, the posterior segment is involved most often, with the subretinal space harboring the parasite more often than the vitreous. Depending on the location of the cyst, patients may present asymptomatically with relatively good vision or may complain of floaters, moving sensations, ocular pain, photophobia, redness, and very poor visual acuity. Epileptiform seizures may be the first sign of cerebral cysticercosis. Both anterior chamber and vitreous may demonstrate inflammatory activity; vitreous inflammation is more pronounced during the early stages of the disease. Larvae death produces a severe inflammatory reaction characterized by zonal granulomatous inflammation surrounding necrotic larvae on histologic examination.

Larvae may be observed in the vitreous or subretinal space in up to 46% of infected patients. The characteristic clinical appearance is that of a globular or spherical, translucent, white cyst with a head, or scolex, that undulates in response to the examining light within the vitreous or subretinal space. The cyst itself varies in size from 1.5 to 6 disc diameters. RPE atrophy may be observed surrounding the presumptive entry site of the cysticercus into the subretinal space; retinal detachment has been observed with high frequency in some series.

The characteristic appearance of a motile cysticercus in the anterior chamber, vitreous, or subretinal space is pathognomonic (Figs 7-34, 7-35). Anticysticercus antibodies are detected by ELISA in approximately 50% and 80% of patients with ocular and neural cysticercosis, respectively. Anterior chamber paracentesis may reveal a large number of eosinophils; peripheral eosinophilia may also be present. If a patient is a definitive host, with an adult tapeworm in the gastrointestinal tract, stool examination may find the eggs of *T solium*. B-scan ultrasonography may also be helpful diagnostically in the presence of intraocular cysticerci, revealing a characteristic picture of a sonolucent zone with a well-defined anterior and posterior margin. A central echo-dense, curvilinear, highly reflective structure within the cyst is suggestive of a scolex, further narrowing the diagnosis. OCT can also help identify the cyst; CT may reveal intracerebral calcification or hydrocephalus in patients with neural cysticercosis.

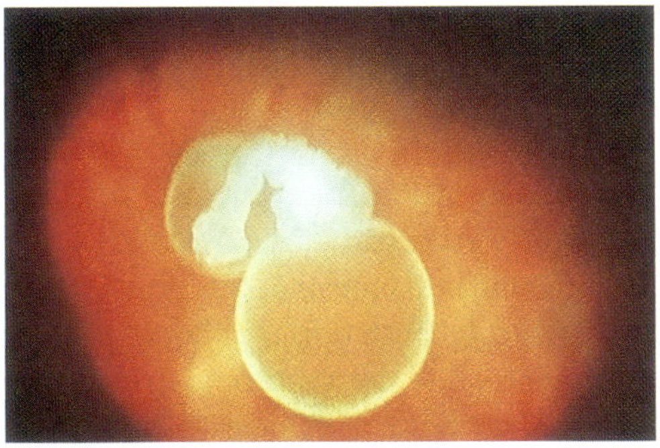

Figure 7-34 Fundus photograph showing intraocular cysticercus.

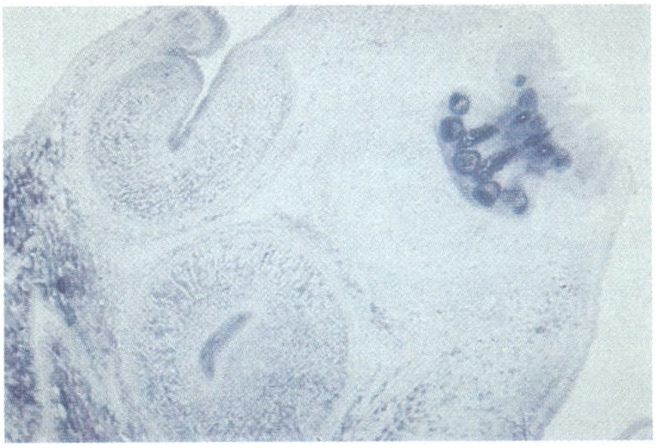

Figure 7-35 Histopathology image of cysticercus, showing the protoscolex, or head, of the larva.

The differential diagnosis includes conditions associated with leukocoria (retinoblastoma, Coats disease, retinopathy of prematurity, persistent fetal vasculature, toxocariasis, and retinal detachment) and diffuse unilateral subacute neuroretinitis (see the following section).

Left untreated, intravitreal or subretinal cysticercosis can cause blindness, retinal atrophy, and phthisis within 3–5 years. Antihelminthic drugs such as praziquantel and albendazole have been used successfully in the medical management of active neural cysticercosis; however, these drugs are generally not effective for intraocular disease. They are frequently used in combination with systemic corticosteroids because larvae death is accompanied by worsening of the ocular disease and panuveitis. Similarly, laser photocoagulation has been advocated for small subretinal cysticerci; however, most authors report poor results when the dead parasite is allowed to remain within the eye. For this reason, early removal of the larvae from the vitreous cavity or subretinal space with vitreoretinal surgical techniques has been advocated and successfully employed.

Sinha S, Takkar B, Venkatesh P, Khanduja S. High-resolution Fourier-domain optical coherence tomography findings in subretinal cysticercosis. *Retina.* 2012;32(3):643–644.

Wender JD, Rathinam SR, Shaw RE, Cunningham ET Jr. Intraocular cysticercosis: case series and comprehensive review of the literature. *Ocul Immunol Inflamm.* 2011;19(4):240–245.

Diffuse Unilateral Subacute Neuroretinitis

Diffuse unilateral subacute neuroretinitis (DUSN) is an uncommon but important disease believed to be caused by nematode infection. It should be considered in the differential diagnosis of posterior uveitis occurring among otherwise healthy, young patients (mean age, 14 years; range, 11–65 years) because early recognition and prompt treatment may preserve vision. Evidence to date suggests that DUSN is caused by solitary nematodes of 2 different sizes, apparently related to geographic region, that migrate through the subretinal space. The smaller worm, measuring 400–1000 μm in length, has been proposed to be either *Ancylostoma caninum* (the dog hookworm) or *T canis,* though the latter has never been reported to be isolated from an eye with DUSN. The larger worm is believed to be *Baylisascaris procyonis* (the raccoon roundworm), which measures 1500–2000 μm in length and has been found in the northern midwestern United States and Canada. DUSN has also been reported outside North America.

The clinical course of DUSN is characterized by the insidious onset of unilateral loss of vision from recurrent episodes of focal, multifocal, and diffuse inflammation of the retina, RPE, and optic nerve. The early stages of the disease are marked by moderate to severe vitritis; optic disc swelling; and multiple, focal, gray-white lesions in the postequatorial fundus that vary in size from 1200 μm to 1500 μm (Fig 7-36). These lesions are evanescent and may be associated with overlying serous retinal detachment. It is in the early stages that the worms are most easily visualized in the subretinal space. Differential diagnosis at this phase of the disease includes sarcoidosis-associated uveitis, MCP, acute posterior multifocal placoid pigment epitheliopathy (APMPPE), multiple evanescent white dot syndrome (MEWDS), serpiginous choroidopathy, Behçet disease, OT, OHS, nonspecific optic neuritis, and papillitis. The later disease stages are typified by retinal arteriolar narrowing, optic atrophy, diffuse pigment epithelial degeneration, and abnormal electroretinographic results (Fig 7-37).

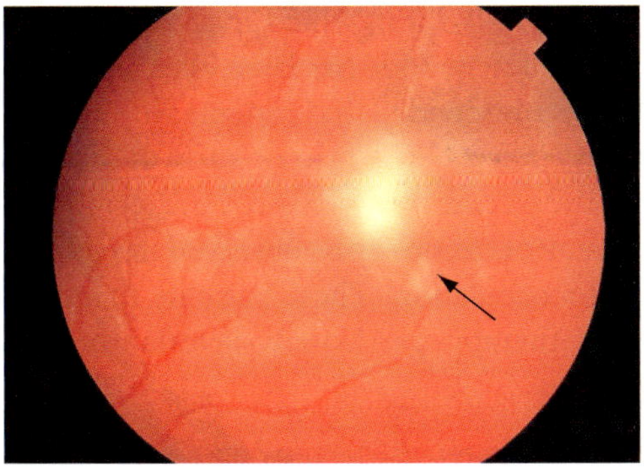

Figure 7-36 Fundus photograph of diffuse unilateral subacute neuroretinitis (DUSN). Note the multiple, white retinal lesions and the S-shaped nematode in the subretinal space *(arrow)*. *(Courtesy of E. Mitchel Opremcak, MD.)*

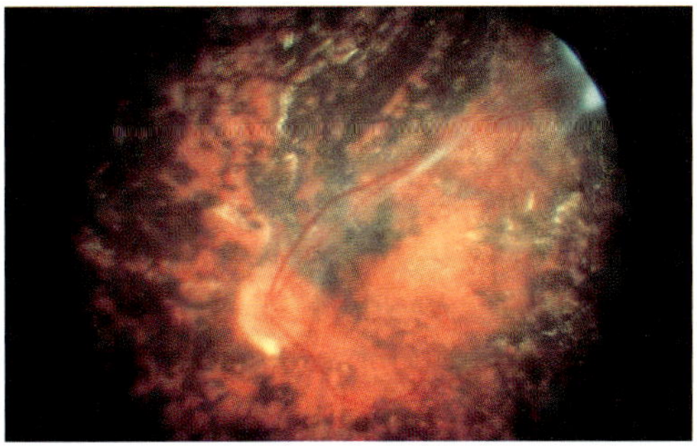

Figure 7-37 Fundus photograph of DUSN, or "unilateral retinal wipeout syndrome." *(Courtesy of E. Mitchel Opremcak, MD.)*

These findings may be confused with posttraumatic chorioretinopathy, occlusive vascular disease, toxic retinopathy, and retinitis pigmentosa. Although highly unusual, bilateral cases have been reported, as have cases of DUSN associated with neurologic disease (neural larvae migrans).

The diagnosis is made according to the aforementioned clinical picture and is most strongly supported by the observation of a worm in the subretinal space (Video 7-1). Results of systemic and laboratory evaluations are typically negative for patients with DUSN. Electroretinographic abnormalities may be present even when the test is performed early in the disease course.

Direct laser photocoagulation of the worm in the early phases of the disease may be highly effective in halting progression of the disease and improving visual acuity; it has not been associated with a significant exacerbation of inflammation (Fig 7-38). Medical therapy with corticosteroids may achieve transient control of the inflammation, but that is followed by recurrence of symptoms and progression of vision loss. Although initial experience with antihelminthic therapy was disappointing, successful treatment has been reported with oral thiabendazole (22 mg/kg twice daily for 2–4 days with a maximum

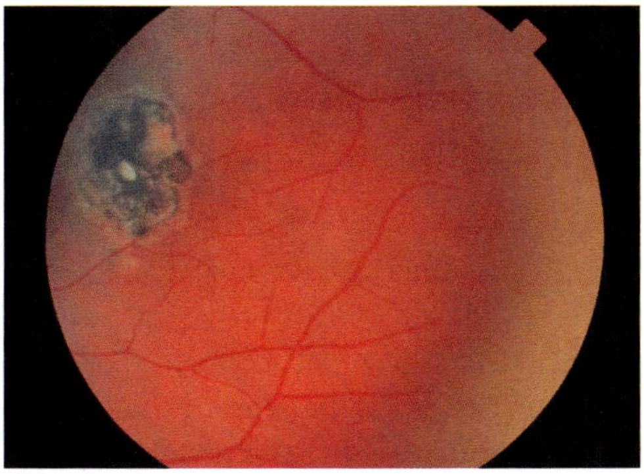

Figure 7-38 Fundus photograph showing a retinal scar following laser photocoagulation of a nematode in a patient with DUSN. *(Courtesy of E. Mitchel Opremcak, MD.)*

dose of 3 g) and albendazole (200 mg twice daily for 30 days), which may be a better-tolerated alternative. Immobilization of the subretinal nematode has been observed after systemic antihelminthic therapy; thus, it has been recommended that patients with DUSN in whom the worm cannot be initially identified undergo a course of such therapy to maximize the chance of identifying and treating the offending organism. Furthermore, a second nematode, presumably from reinfection, may occasionally be observed in patients who have undergone a successful previous photocoagulation. These patients may also benefit from a course of systemic antihelminthic therapy, particularly if inflammation does not abate promptly after laser photocoagulation.

VIDEO 7-1 How to find a live worm in diffuse unilateral subacute neuroretinitis (07:05).
Courtesy of Carlos AA Garcia, MD.
Scan the QR code or access the video at www.aao.org/bcscvideo_section09.

Cortez R, Denny JP, Muci-Mendoza R, Ramirez G, Fuenmayor D, Jaffe GJ. Diffuse unilateral subacute neuroretinitis in Venezuela. *Ophthalmology.* 2005;112(12):2110–2114.

de Amorim Garcia Filho CA, Gomes AH, de A Garcia Soares AC, de Amorim Garcia CA. Clinical features of 121 patients with diffuse unilateral subacute neuroretinitis. *Am J Ophthalmol.* 2012;153(4):743–749.

Souza EC, Casella AM, Nakashima Y, Monteiro ML. Clinical features and outcomes of patients with diffuse unilateral subacute neuroretinitis treated with oral albendazole. *Am J Ophthalmol.* 2005;140(3):437–445. [Erratum appears in *Am J Ophthalmol.* 2006;141(4):795–796.]

Onchocerciasis

A leading cause of blindness in the world, onchocerciasis is endemic in many areas of sub-Saharan Africa and in isolated foci in Central and South America. It is rarely encountered or diagnosed in the United States. Worldwide, at least 18 million people are infected, of whom almost 300,000 are blind. In hyperendemic areas, everyone over the age of 15 years is infected, and half will become blind before they die.

Humans are the only host for *Onchocerca volvulus,* the filarial parasite that causes the disease. The larvae of *O volvulus* are transmitted through the bite of female black flies of the *Simulium* genus. The flies breed in fast-flowing streams; hence, the disease is commonly called *river blindness.* The larvae develop into mature adult worms that form subcutaneous nodules. The adult female releases millions of microfilariae that migrate throughout the body, particularly to the skin and the eye. Microfilariae probably reach the eye by various routes:

- direct invasion of the cornea from the conjunctiva
- penetration of the sclera, both directly and through the vascular bundles
- hematogenous spread (possibly)

Live microfilariae are usually well tolerated, but dead microfilariae initiate a focal inflammatory response.

Anterior segment signs of onchocerciasis are common. Microfilariae can be observed swimming freely in the anterior chamber. Live microfilariae can be seen in the cornea; dead microfilariae cause a small stromal punctate inflammatory opacity that clears with time. Mild uveitis and limbitis are common, but severe anterior uveitis may also occur and lead to synechiae, secondary glaucoma, and cataract. Chorioretinal changes are also common and vary widely in severity. Early disruption of the RPE is typical, with pigment dispersion and focal areas of atrophy. Later, severe chorioretinal atrophy occurs, predominantly in the posterior pole. Optic atrophy is common in advanced disease (Fig 7-39).

Diagnosis is made according to the clinical appearance and a history of pathogen exposure in an endemic area and confirmed by finding microfilariae in small skin biopsies or in the eye. Ivermectin, a macrolytic lactone and the treatment of choice for onchocerciasis, safely kills the microfilariae but does not have a permanent effect on the adult worms. Although not approved for sale in the United States, ivermectin is available on a compassionate use basis for individual treatment. A single oral dose of 150 μg/kg should be repeated annually, probably for 10 years. Topical corticosteroids can be used to control any anterior uveitis.

Although annual ivermectin treatment reduces the microfilarial load in the anterior chamber and the development of new anterior chamber lesions, it does not reduce the macrofilarial load even at doses as high as 1600 μg/kg. Ivermectin does not appear to prevent the development of new chorioretinal lesions or resolve existing lesions, although it does appear to slow progression of visual field loss and optic atrophy, even in advanced disease. Nodules containing adult worms can be removed surgically, but this approach does not usually cure the disease because many nodules are deeply buried and cannot be found. The adult worm is infected with the parasitic bacterium *Wolbachia,* an organism crucial to the sexual development of the worm. Targeting Wolbachia with a 6-week course of doxycycline, in addition to ivermectin, has become the treatment of choice because the organism can cause long-term sterilization of adult worms and early worm death.

Ejere HO, Schwartz E, Wormald R, Evans JR. Ivermectin for onchocercal eye disease (river blindness). *Cochrane Database Syst Rev.* 2012;8:CD002219.

Winthrop KL, Furtado JM, Silva JC, Resnikoff S, Lansingh VC. River blindness: an old disease on the brink of elimination and control. *J Glob Infect Dis.* 2011;3(2):151–155.

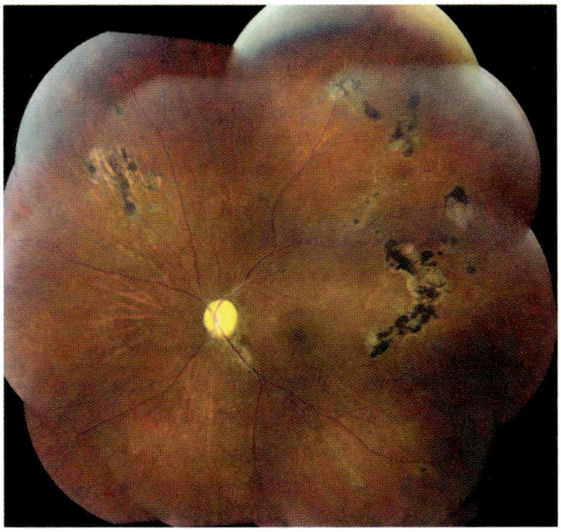

Figure 7-39 Fundus photograph montage showing extensive chorioretinal scars involving both the periphery and the posterior pole as well as optic nerve pallor secondary to onchocerciasis. *(Courtesy of H. Nida Sen, MD.)*

Bacterial Uveitis

Syphilis

Syphilis is a multisystem, chronic bacterial infection caused by the spirochete *Treponema pallidum* that is associated with numerous ocular manifestations in both the acquired and congenital forms of the disease. Transmission occurs most often through sexual contact; however, transplacental infection of the fetus may occur after the tenth week of pregnancy. Having reached an all-time low in the year 2000 in the United States, the incidence rate of syphilis at any disease stage is rising; in 2010, it was 14.9 cases per 100,000 persons (2010 rate for primary and secondary syphilis, 4.5 in 100,000) per year and is still increasing, especially among men, particularly men who have sex with men, and African Americans, for whom the rate is 5 times greater than among non-Hispanic whites. The total number of US cases of syphilis increased 2.2% during the period 2009–2010. In contrast, the rate of congenital syphilis was reported to be 8.7 in 100,000 live births in 2010, down from 14.3 in 2000, reflecting sharp declines in both primary and secondary syphilis among women over the past decade.

Although syphilis is thought to be responsible for less than 2% of all uveitis cases, it is one of the great masqueraders of medicine and should always be considered in the differential diagnosis of any intraocular inflammatory disease. It is one of the few entities that can be cured with appropriate antimicrobial therapy, even in patients with HIV/AIDS. Delay in the diagnosis of syphilitic uveitis may lead not only to permanent vision loss but also to significant neurologic and cardiac morbidity, which may have been averted with early treatment.

Centers for Disease Control and Prevention. *Sexually Transmitted Disease Surveillance 2010.* Atlanta: US Department of Health and Human Services; 2011. Available at www.cdc.gov/STD/stats10/default.htm. Accessed August 14, 2014.

Congenital syphilis

Congenital syphilis persists in the United States largely because a significant number of women do not receive serologic testing until late in pregnancy, if at all, which is related to absent or late prenatal care. Primary or secondary syphilis in the mother is more likely to be transmitted to the baby than is latent syphilis; the longer the mother had syphilis, the less likely is the transmission. Systemic findings in patients with early congenital syphilis (age 2 years or younger) include hepatosplenomegaly, characteristic changes of the long bones on radiographic examination, abdominal distention, desquamative skin rash, low birth weight, pneumonia, and severe anemia. Late manifestations (age 3 years or older) result from scarring during early systemic disease and include Hutchinson teeth, Mulberry molars, abnormal facies, cranial nerve VIII deafness, bony changes such as saber shins and perforations of the hard palate, cutaneous lesions such as rhagades, and neurosyphilis. Cardiovascular complications are unusual in late congenital syphilis. For further discussion of congenital syphilis, see the chapter Ocular Manifestations of Systemic Disease in BCSC Section 6, *Pediatric Ophthalmology and Strabismus.*

Ocular inflammatory signs of congenital syphilis may present at birth or decades later and include uveitis, interstitial keratitis, optic neuritis, glaucoma, and congenital cataract. A multifocal chorioretinitis and, less commonly, retinal vasculitis are the most frequent uveitic manifestations of early congenital infection. They may result in a bilateral salt and pepper fundus, which affects the peripheral retina, posterior pole, or a single quadrant. These changes are not progressive, and the patient may have normal vision. A less commonly described funduscopic variation is that of a bilateral secondary degeneration of the RPE, which may mimic retinitis pigmentosa with narrowing of the retinal and choroidal vessels, optic disc pallor with sharp margins, and morphologically variable deposits of pigment.

Nonulcerative stromal interstitial keratitis, often accompanied by anterior uveitis, is the most common inflammatory sign of untreated late congenital syphilis, occurring in up to 50% of cases, most commonly in girls (Fig 7-40). Keratouveitis is thought to be an allergic response to *T pallidum* in the cornea. Symptoms include intense pain and photophobia. Blood vessels invade the cornea, and late stages show deep "ghost" (nonperfused) stromal vessels and corneal opacities. Left untreated, the corneal inflammation may regress but leave the cornea diffusely opaque, with reduced vision, even to the level of light perception only. Anterior uveitis accompanying interstitial keratitis may be difficult to observe because of corneal haze. Glaucoma may also occur. The constellation of interstitial keratitis, cranial nerve VIII deafness, and Hutchinson teeth is called the *Hutchinson triad.*

Acquired syphilis

The natural history of untreated acquired syphilis has been well described. *Primary syphilis* follows an incubation period of approximately 3 weeks and is characterized by a chancre, a painless, solitary lesion that originates at the site of inoculation, resolving spontaneously within 12 weeks regardless of treatment. The central nervous system (CNS) may be seeded with treponemes during this period, although there is an absence of neurologic findings.

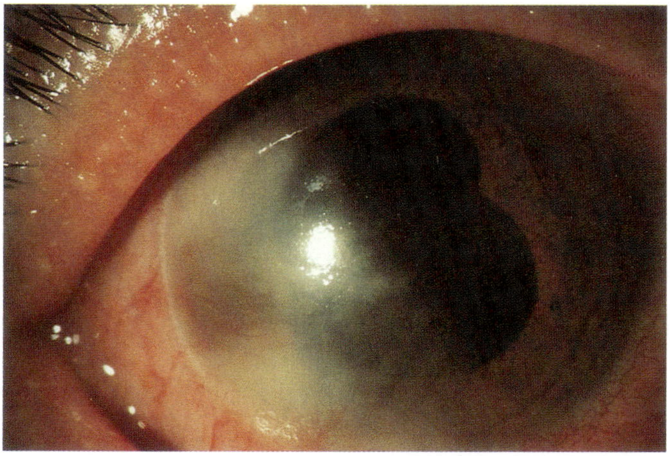

Figure 7-40 Active syphilitic interstitial keratitis.

Secondary syphilis occurs 6–8 weeks later and is heralded by the appearance of lymphadenopathy and a generalized maculopapular rash that may be prominent on the palms and soles. Uveitis occurs in approximately 10% of cases. This phase is followed by a latent period ranging from 1 year (early latency) to decades (late latency). Approximately one-third of untreated patients incur *tertiary syphilis,* which may be further subcategorized as benign tertiary syphilis (the characteristic lesion being gumma, most frequently found on the skin and mucous membranes but also in the choroid and iris), cardiovascular syphilis, and neurosyphilis. Although uveitis may occur in up to 5% of patients whose disease has progressed to tertiary syphilis, it can occur at any stage of infection, including primary disease. Because the eye is an extension of the CNS, ocular syphilis is best regarded as a variant of neurosyphilis, a notion that has important diagnostic and therapeutic implications.

The ocular manifestations of syphilis are protean and affect all structures, including the conjunctiva, sclera, cornea, lens, uveal tract, retina, retinal vasculature, optic nerve, cranial nerves, and pupillomotor pathways. Patients present with pain, redness, photophobia, blurred vision, and floaters. Intraocular inflammation may be granulomatous or nongranulomatous, unilateral or bilateral, and it may affect the anterior, intermediate, or posterior segments. Anterior segment findings can include iris roseola, vascularized papules (iris papulosa), larger red nodules (iris nodosa), and gummata. Interstitial keratitis, posterior synechiae, lens dislocation, and iris atrophy can also occur.

Posterior segment findings of acquired syphilis include vitritis, chorioretinitis, focal retinitis, necrotizing retinitis, retinal vasculitis, exudative retinal detachment, isolated papillitis, and neuroretinitis. A focal or multifocal chorioretinitis, usually associated with a variable degree of vitritis, is the most common manifestation (Fig 7-41). These lesions are typically small, grayish yellow, and located in the postequatorial fundus, but they may become confluent. Retinal vasculitis and disc edema, with exudates appearing around the disc and the retinal arterioles, together with serous retinal detachment, may accompany

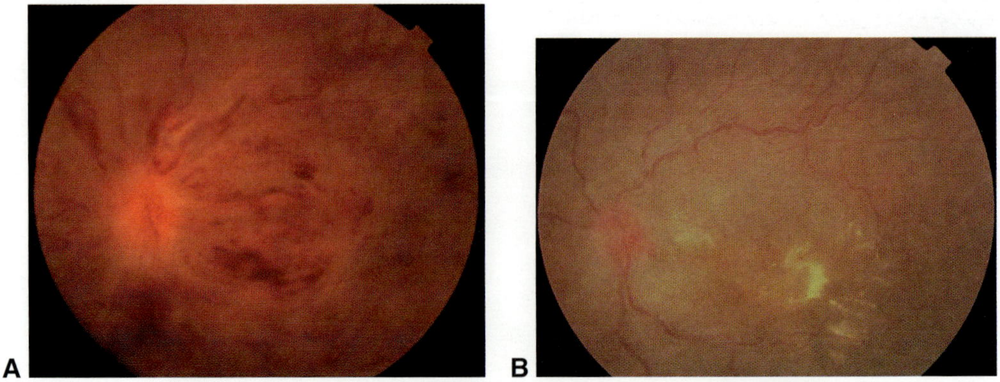

Figure 7-41 **A,** Fundus photograph of acute syphilitic chorioretinitis. Note diffuse edema of the disc, retina, and choroid in the posterior pole. **B,** Fundus photograph showing healing chorioretinitis after 2 weeks of intravenous penicillin therapy. Note the subretinal hard exudate that is organizing, as well as the reduction in disc edema and choroidal inflammation. *(Courtesy of Ramana S. Moorthy, MD.)*

the chorioretinitis. A syphilitic posterior placoid chorioretinitis has been described, the clinical appearance and angiographic characteristics of which are thought to be pathognomonic of secondary syphilis (Fig 7-42). Solitary or multifocal, macular or papillary, placoid, yellowish gray lesions at the level of the RPE, often with accompanying vitritis, display corresponding early hypofluorescence and late staining, along with retinal perivenous staining on FA. ICG shows hypofluorescent spots corresponding to lesions.

Less common posterior segment involvement includes focal retinitis, periphlebitis, and, infrequently, exudative retinal detachment. Syphilis may present as a focal retinitis (Fig 7-43) or as a peripheral necrotizing retinitis that may resemble ARN or PORN. Punctate inner retinal infiltrates have also been described (Fig 7-44). Although the foci of retinitis may become confluent and are frequently associated with retinal vasculitis,

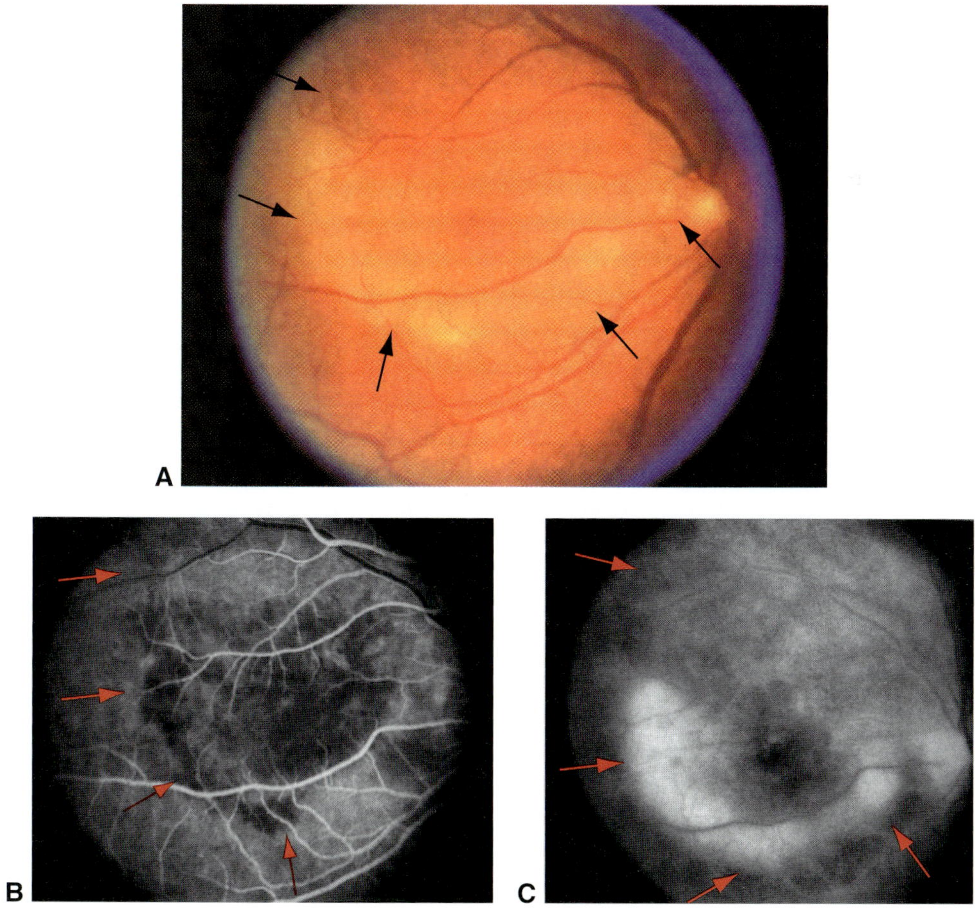

Figure 7-42 Syphilitic posterior placoid chorioretinitis. **A,** Fundus photograph of the right eye showing a large, geographic lesion involving the central macula *(arrows)*. **B,** Fluorescein angiogram disclosing early, irregular hypofluorescence *(arrows)* followed by **(C)** late staining at the level of the pigment epithelium *(arrows)*. *(Reproduced with permission from Gass JDM, Braunstein RA, Chenoweth RG. Acute syphilitic posterior placoid chorioretinitis.* Ophthalmology. *1990;97(10):1289–1290.)*

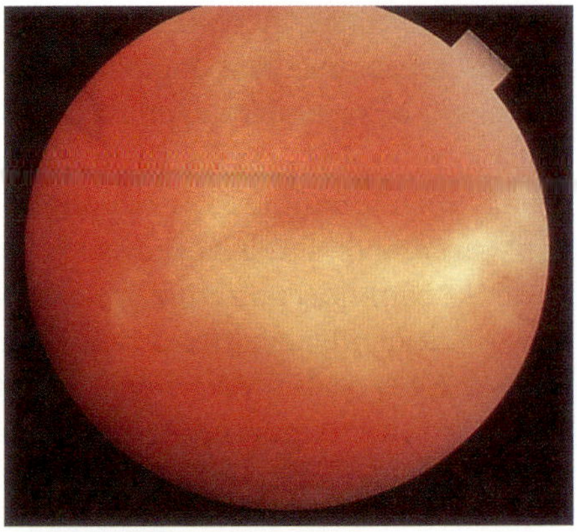

Figure 7-43 Fundus photograph of acute syphilitic retinitis.

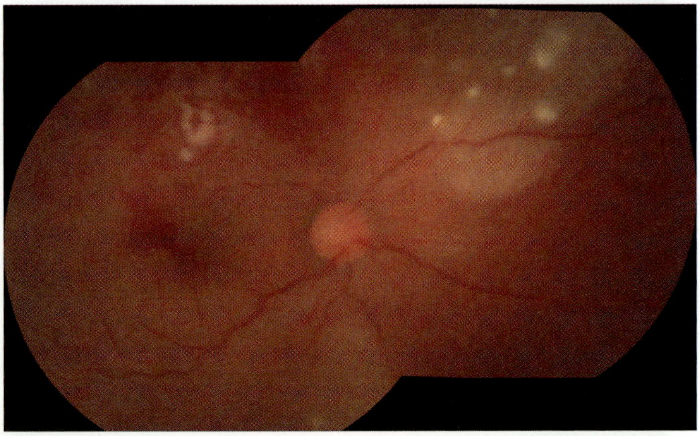

Figure 7-44 Fundus photograph of the right eye of a patient with syphilitic posterior uveitis, disclosing punctate inner retinal infiltrates overlying an area of retinal edema superonasally. *(Courtesy of Daniel Vitor Vasconcelos-Santos, MD, PhD.)*

syphilitic retinitis is more slowly progressive and responds dramatically to therapy with intravenous penicillin, often with a good visual outcome. Isolated retinal vasculitis that affects the retinal arterioles, capillaries, and larger arteries or veins (or both) is another feature of syphilitic intraocular inflammation that may best be appreciated on FA. Focal retinal vasculitis may masquerade as a branch retinal vein occlusion.

Syphilis is an important entity to consider in the differential diagnosis of patients with neuroretinitis and papillitis who present with macular star formation. Patients with syphilis who are immunocompromised or who have HIV/AIDS may have atypical or more fulminant ocular disease patterns. Optic neuritis and neuroretinitis are more common in the initial presentation of these patients, and disease recurrences are noted even after appropriate antibacterial therapy.

Neuro-ophthalmic manifestations of syphilis include the Argyll Robertson pupil, ocular motor nerve palsies, optic neuropathy, and retrobulbar optic neuritis, all of which appear most often in patients with tertiary syphilis or in neurosyphilis. (See BCSC Section 5, *Neuro-Ophthalmology,* for a more complete discussion.)

Diagnosis

The diagnosis of syphilitic uveitis is usually made according to the history and clinical presentation and is supported by serologic testing. Primary syphilis may be diagnosed by direct visualization of spirochetes with dark-field microscopy and by direct fluorescent antibody tests of lesion exudates or tissue. Serodiagnosis is based on the results of both nontreponemal and treponemal antigen tests. Nontreponemal tests include the Venereal Disease Research Laboratory (VDRL) and rapid plasma reagin (RPR) evaluations; treponemal tests include the fluorescent treponemal antibody absorption (FTA-ABS) assay and the microhemagglutination assay for *T pallidum* antibodies (MHA-TP).

Nontreponemal antibody titers correlate with disease activity, generally increasing during primary or secondary syphilis and decreasing when the spirochetes are not active, such as during latent syphilis or after adequate antibiotic treatment. They are useful barometers for monitoring therapy for both systemic and ocular disease. Results of treponemal tests become positive during the secondary stage of syphilis and remain positive, with rare exceptions, throughout the patient's life; as such, they are not useful in assessing therapeutic response.

Testing for HIV infection should be performed in all patients with syphilis, given the high frequency of coinfection. As a result of the passive transfer of immunoglobulin G (IgG) across the placenta, the VDRL and FTA-ABS IgG test results are positive among infants born to mothers with syphilis. For this reason, serodiagnosis of congenital syphilis is made using the IgM FTA-ABS test, which indicates infection in the infant.

False-positive nontreponemal test results occur in a variety of medical conditions, including systemic lupus erythematosus (SLE), leprosy, advanced age, intravenous drug abuse, bacterial endocarditis, tuberculosis, vaccinations, infectious mononucleosis, HIV infection, atypical pneumonia, malaria, pregnancy, rickettsial infections, and other spirochetal infections (eg, Lyme disease). False-positive treponemal test results are rare (1%–2%) and may occur with other spirochetal infections (Lyme disease, leptospirosis), autoimmune disease (SLE, primary biliary cirrhosis, and rheumatoid arthritis), leprosy, malaria, and advanced age. Although nontreponemal tests are appropriate for screening large populations with a relatively lower risk for syphilis, specific treponemal tests, such as FTA-ABS, have a higher predictive value in patients with uveitis and should be used in conjunction with nontreponemal tests in diagnosing and treating ocular syphilis. Both the false-positive and false-negative rates of serologic testing may be greater in HIV-infected patients. A lumbar puncture with examination of CSF is warranted in every case of syphilitic uveitis. A positive CSF VDRL result is diagnostic for neurosyphilis, but it may be nonreactive in some cases of active CNS involvement. Although less specific, the CSF FTA-ABS test is highly sensitive and may be useful in excluding neurosyphilis. Follow-up for patients with chorioretinitis and abnormal CSF findings requires spinal fluid examination every 6 months until the cell count, protein, and VDRL results return to normal. Finally, specific ELISA- and PCR-based DNA amplification techniques are being used with increasing frequency in the serodiagnosis of syphilis. Given their high sensitivity and specificity, these techniques, particularly PCR analysis of intraocular and/or cerebrospinal fluids, may be valuable in confirming the diagnosis in atypical cases.

Van Gelder RN. Diagnostic testing in uveitis. *Focal Points: Clinical Modules for Ophthalmologists.* San Francisco: American Academy of Ophthalmology; 2013, module 4.

Treatment

Parenteral penicillin G is the preferred treatment for all stages of syphilis (Table 7-3). Although the formulation, dose, route of administration, and duration of therapy vary with the stage of the disease, patients with syphilitic uveitis should be considered as having a CNS disease, requiring neurologic dosing regimens regardless of immune status. The current CDC recommendation for the treatment of neurosyphilis is 18–24 million units (MU) of aqueous crystalline penicillin G per day, administered as 3–4 MU intravenously every 4 hours or as a continuous infusion for 10–14 days. This may be supplemented with intramuscular benzathine penicillin G, 2.4 MU weekly for 3 weeks. Alternatively, neurosyphilis may be treated with 2.4 MU/day of intramuscular procaine penicillin plus probenecid 500 mg 4 times a day, both for 10–14 days.

The recommended treatment regimen for congenital syphilis in infants during the first months of life is intravenous aqueous crystalline penicillin G, 100,000–150,000 units/kg/day, administered intravenously as 50,000 units/kg/dose every 12 hours during the first 7 days of life and every 8 hours thereafter, for a total of 10 days. Alternatively, procaine penicillin G, 50,000 units/kg/dose, may be administered intramuscularly in a single daily dose for 10 days.

Table 7-3 Treatment of Syphilis in Adults

Stage of Disease	Primary Treatment Regimen	Alternative Treatment Regimen
Primary, secondary, or early latent disease	Benzathine penicillin G 2.4 million U intramuscularly as a single dose	Doxycycline 100 mg orally 2 times per day for 2 weeks or tetracycline 500 mg orally 4 times per day for 2 weeks
Late latent or latent syphilis of uncertain duration, tertiary disease in the absence of neurosyphilis	Benzathine penicillin G 2.4 million U intramuscularly, weekly for 3 doses	Doxycycline 100 mg orally 2 times per day for 4 weeks or tetracycline 500 mg orally 4 times per day for 4 weeks
Neurosyphilis	Aqueous penicillin G 18–24 million U/day given intravenously as 3–4 million U every 4 hours or continuous infusion, for 10–14 days	Procaine penicillin 2.4 million U/day intramuscularly *plus* probenecid 500 mg orally 4 times per day, both for 10–14 days

U = units.

Adapted from Centers for Disease Control and Prevention. *Sexually Transmitted Disease Surveillance 2010.* Atlanta: US Department of Health and Human Services; 2011. Available at www.cdc.gov/STD/stats10/default.htm. Accessed August 14, 2014.

There are no proven alternatives to penicillin for the treatment of neurosyphilis, congenital infection, or disease in pregnant women or patients coinfected with HIV; for that reason, patients with penicillin allergy require desensitization and then treatment with penicillin. Alternative treatments in penicillin-allergic patients who show no signs of neurosyphilis and who are HIV-seronegative include doxycycline or tetracycline. Ceftriaxone and chloramphenicol have been reported to be effective alternatives in patients with ocular syphilis who are penicillin allergic and HIV coinfected.

Patients should be monitored for the development of the Jarisch-Herxheimer reaction, a hypersensitivity response of the host to treponemal antigens that are released in large numbers as spirochetes are killed during the first 24 hours of treatment. Patients present with constitutional symptoms, such as fever, chills, hypotension, tachycardia, and malaise, but they may also experience a concomitant increase in the severity of ocular inflammation that may require local and/or systemic corticosteroids. In the vast majority of cases, however, supportive care and observation are sufficient.

Topical, periocular, and/or systemic corticosteroids, under appropriate antibiotic cover, may be useful adjuncts for treating the anterior and posterior segment inflammation associated with syphilitic uveitis. According to the Centers for Disease Control and Prevention (CDC), syphilis is designated a nationally "notifiable" disease; thus, appropriate health authorities should be notified according to local regulations. Finally, the sexual contacts of the patient must be identified and treated, as a high percentage of these individuals are at risk for acquiring and transmitting this disease.

Amaratunge BC, Camuglia JE, Hall AJ. Syphilitic uveitis: a review of clinical manifestations and treatment outcomes of syphilitic uveitis in human immunodeficiency virus–positive and negative patients. *Clin Experiment Ophthalmol.* 2010;38(1):68–74.

Eandi CM, Neri P, Adelman RA, Yannuzzi LA, Cunningham ET Jr; International Syphilis Study Group. Acute syphilitic posterior placoid chorioretinitis: report of a case series and comprehensive review of the literature. *Retina.* 2012;32(9):1915–1941.

Jumper JM, Randhawa S. Imaging syphilis uveitis. *Int Ophthalmol Clin.* 2012;52(4):121–129.

Lyme Disease

Lyme disease (LD) is the most common tick-borne illness in the United States. It has protean systemic and ocular manifestations and is caused by the spirochete *Borrelia burgdorferi.* Animal reservoirs include deer, horses, cows, rodents, birds, cats, and dogs. The spirochete is transmitted to humans through the bite of infected ticks, *Ixodes scapularis* in the northeast, mid-Atlantic, and midwestern United States and *I pacificus* in the western United States. In 2011, the national incidence rate of confirmed or probable LD was 10.8 cases per 100,000 persons per year (7.9 for confirmed; 2.8 for probable), which reflects a slight increase from 2010 although the overall number of cases remains substantially lower than in 2008 and 2009. The disease affects men (53%) slightly more often than women and has a bimodal distribution, with peaks in children aged 5–14 years and in adults aged 50–59 years. Whites are affected more commonly than are other races. There is a seasonal variation, with most cases occurring between May and August. LD may be found worldwide, but outside the United States it is caused by different species of *Borrelia,* such as *B afzelli* and *B garinii.*

Clinical features

The clinical manifestations of LD are divided into 3 stages; ocular findings vary within each stage. The most characteristic feature of stage 1, or local disease, is a macular rash known as *erythema chronicum migrans* at the site of the tick bite; it appears within 2–28 days in approximately 70% of patients. As the lesion enlarges and becomes papular, the paracentral area may clear, forming a "bull's eye" lesion, with the site of the bite marking the center (Figs 7-45, 7-46). Constitutional symptoms appear at this stage and include fever, malaise, fatigue, myalgias, and arthralgias.

Stage 2, or disseminated disease, occurs several weeks to 4 months after exposure. Spirochetes spread hematogenously to the skin, CNS, joints, heart, and eyes. A secondary erythema chronicum migrans rash may appear at sites remote from that of the tick bite. Left untreated, up to 80% of patients with erythema chronicum migrans develop joint manifestations, most commonly a monoarthritis or oligoarthritis involving the large joints, typically the knee (Fig 7-47). Joint involvement may be the only clinical manifestation of Lyme disease in children, and juvenile idiopathic arthritis (JIA) must be considered in the differential diagnosis.

Neurologic involvement, which occurs in up to 40% of patients, may include meningitis, encephalitis, painful radiculitis, or unilateral or bilateral Bell palsy. In endemic areas,

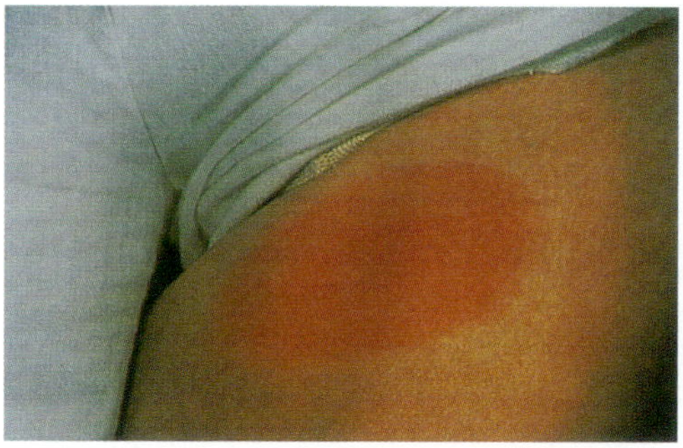

Figure 7-45 Erythema chronicum migrans in a patient with Lyme disease, demonstrating a single dense erythematous lesion. *(Courtesy of Alan B. MacDonald, MD.)*

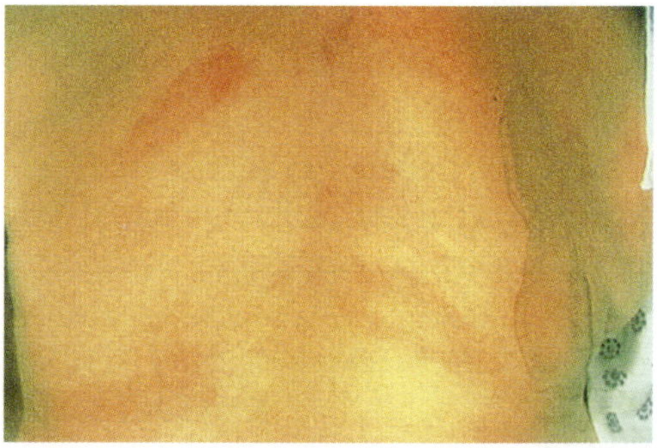

Figure 7-46 Erythema chronicum migrans: multiple bull's-eye lesions in a patient with Lyme disease. *(Courtesy of Alan B. MacDonald, MD.)*

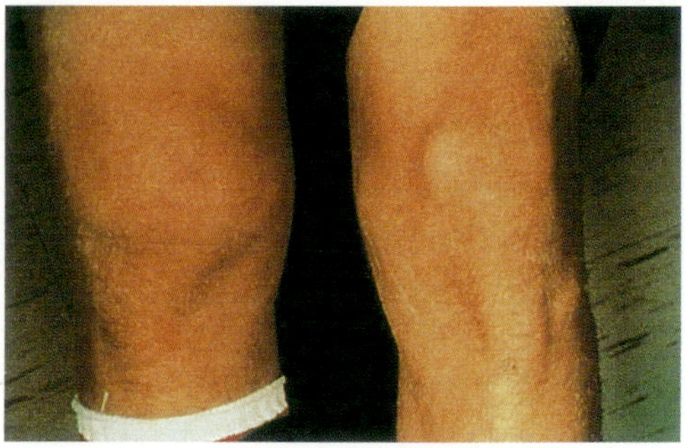

Figure 7-47 Lyme disease arthritis. *(Courtesy of Alan B. MacDonald, MD.)*

as many as 25% of new-onset cranial nerve VII palsies may be attributed to *B burgdorferi* infection.

The most frequent systemic manifestation of stage 3, or persistent disease, which occurs 5 months or more after the initial infection, is episodic arthritis that may become chronic. Chronic arthritis has been associated with the HLA-DR4 and -DR2 haplotypes in North America; individuals expressing HLA-DR4 have a poorer response to antibiotics. Acrodermatitis chronica atrophicans, a bluish red lesion on the extremities that may progress to fibrous bands and nodules, can occur in some patients, as may chronic neurologic syndromes including neuropsychiatric disease, radiculopathy, chronic fatigue, peripheral neuropathy, and memory loss.

Ocular disease

The spectrum of ocular findings in patients with LD is expanding and varies with disease stage. The most common ocular manifestation of early stage 1 disease is a follicular conjunctivitis, which occurs in approximately 11% of patients; less commonly present is episcleritis. (See BCSC Section 1, *Update on General Medicine,* and Section 8, *External Disease and Cornea,* for further discussion and the differential diagnosis.)

Intraocular inflammatory disease is reported most often in stage 2 and, less frequently, in stage 3 disease; it may manifest as anterior uveitis, intermediate uveitis, posterior uveitis, or panuveitis. Intermediate uveitis is one of the most common intraocular presentations. Vitritis may be severe and accompanied by a granulomatous anterior chamber reaction, papillitis, neuroretinitis, choroiditis, retinal vasculitis, and exudative retinal detachment (Figs 7-48, 7-49).

A distinct clinical entity of peripheral multifocal choroiditis has been described in patients with LD; it is characterized by multiple, small, round, punched-out lesions associated with vitritis, similar to those present in sarcoidosis. Choroidal involvement may lead to pigment epithelial clumping resembling the inflammatory changes that occur with syphilis or rubella. Retinal vasculitis, found in association with peripheral multifocal choroiditis or vasculitic branch retinal vein occlusion, may be more common than previously known.

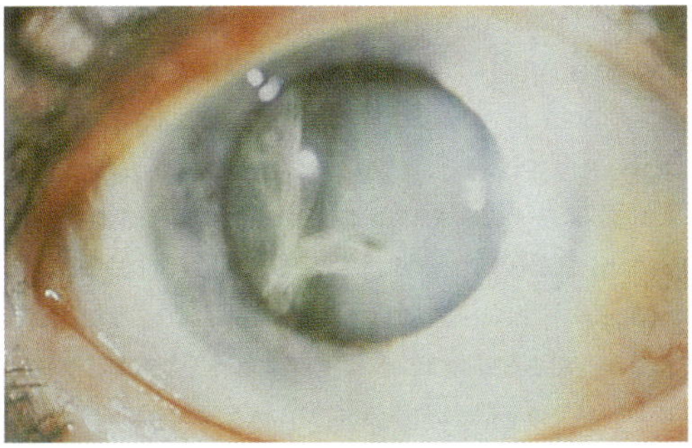

Figure 7-48 Dense anterior vitreous debris causing floaters in ocular Lyme disease. *(Courtesy of William W. Culbertson, MD.)*

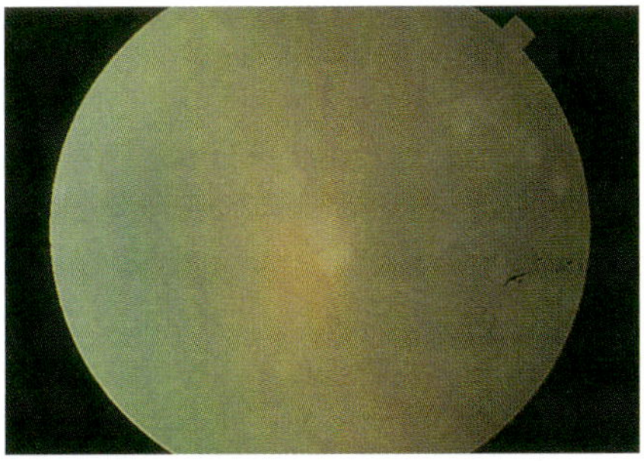

Figure 7-49 Fundus photograph revealing dense vitreous cells and haze in Lyme disease vitritis. *(Courtesy of John D. Sheppard, Jr, MD.)*

Neuro-ophthalmic manifestations include involvement of multiple cranial nerves (II, III, IV, V, VI, and, most commonly, VII) unilaterally or bilaterally, either sequentially or simultaneously. Optic nerve findings include optic neuritis, papilledema associated with meningitis, and most commonly papillitis. Horner syndrome has also been reported.

Keratitis is the most common ocular manifestation of stage 3 disease; much less common is episcleritis. Both may present months to years after the onset of infection. Typically, infiltrates are bilateral, patchy, focal, and stromal; subepithelial infiltrates with indistinct borders, peripheral keratitis with stromal edema, and corneal neovascularization can also occur. The keratitis is thought to represent an immune phenomenon rather than an infectious process because it responds to topical corticosteroids alone.

Diagnosis

The diagnosis of LD is made on the basis of history, clinical presentation, and supportive serology. In the appropriate clinical context, erythema chronicum migrans is diagnostic. However, interpreting serologic data is problematic because of the lack of standardization of the values by which a positive test result is defined—the degree of cross-reactivity with other spirochetes—thus leading to frequent false-positive and false-negative test results. The CDC recommends a 2-step protocol for the diagnosis of active disease or previous infection:

1. ELISA for IgM and IgG, followed by
2. Western immunoblot testing

PCR-based assays have been used successfully to amplify both genomic and plasmid *B burgdorferi* DNA from a variety of tissues, including ocular fluids, with the highest yields obtained from the skin.

Treatment

The current treatment recommendations for the various clinical manifestations of LD are listed in Table 7-4. For patients with ocular involvement, the route and duration of antibiotic treatment has not been established; however, as with syphilitic uveitis, intraocular inflammation associated with LD is best regarded as a manifestation of CNS involvement and warrants careful neurologic evaluation, including a lumbar puncture. Patients with severe posterior segment manifestations—and certainly those with confirmed CNS involvement—require intravenous antibiotic therapy with neurologic dosing regimens. Likewise, patients with less-severe disease that responds incompletely or relapses when oral antibiotics are discontinued should probably be treated with intravenous drugs as outlined. Patients with Lyme carditis or who have atrioventricular block should be admitted to the hospital and monitored as well as administered treatment with intravenous antibiotics.

After the initiation of appropriate antibiotic therapy, anterior segment inflammation may be treated with topical corticosteroids and mydriatics. The use of systemic corticosteroids has been described as part of the management of LD; however, the routine use of corticosteroids is controversial, as it has been associated with an increase in antibiotic treatment failures. As with syphilis, the Jarisch-Herxheimer reaction may complicate

Table 7-4 Recommended Antimicrobial Regimens for Treatment of Lyme Disease

Drug	Adult Dosage	Pediatric Dosage
Preferred oral regimens		
Amoxicillin	500 mg 3 times per day*	50 mg/kg per day in 3 divided doses (maximum, 500 mg per dose)*
Doxycycline	100 mg twice per day†	Not recommended for children aged <8 years For children aged ≥8 years, 4 mg/kg per day in 2 divided doses (maximum, 100 mg per dose)
Cefuroxime axetil	500 mg twice per day	30 mg/kg per day in 2 divided doses (maximum, 500 mg per dose)
Alternative oral regimens		
Selected macrolides‡	For recommended dosing regimens, see footnote§	For recommended dosing regimens, see footnote§
Preferred parenteral regimen		
Ceftriaxone	2 g intravenously once per day	50–75 mg/kg intravenously per day in a single dose (maximum, 2 g)
Alternative parenteral regimens		
Cefotaxime	2 g intravenously every 8 hours‖	150–200 mg/kg per day intravenously in 3–4 divided doses (maximum, 6 g per day)‖
Penicillin G	18–24 million U per day intravenously, divided every 4 h‖	200,000–400,000 U/kg per day divided every 4 hours‖ (not to exceed 18–24 million U per day)

*Although a higher dosage given twice per day might be equally as effective, in view of the absence of data on efficacy, twice-daily administration is not recommended.

†Tetracyclines are relatively contraindicated in pregnant or lactating women and in children aged <8 years.

‡Because of their lower efficacy, macrolides are reserved for patients who are unable to take or who are intolerant of tetracyclines, penicillins, and cephalosporins.

§For adult patients intolerant of amoxicillin, doxycycline, and cefuroxime axetil, azithromycin (500 mg orally per day for 7–10 days), clarithromycin (500 mg orally twice per day for 14–21 days, if the patient is not pregnant), or erythromycin (500 mg orally 4 times per day for 14–21 days) may be given. Recommended dosages for children: azithromycin 10 mg/kg per day (maximum of 500 mg per day); clarithromycin, 7.5 mg/kg twice per day (maximum of 500 mg per dose); and erythromycin, 12.5 mg/kg 4 times per day (maximum of 500 mg per dose). Patients treated with macrolides should be closely observed to ensure resolution of the clinical manifestations.

‖Dosage should be reduced for patients with impaired renal function.

Used with permission from Wormser GP, Dattwyler RJ, Shapiro ED, et al. The clinical assessment, treatment, and prevention of Lyme disease, human granulocytic anaplasmosis, and babesiosis: clinical practice guidelines by the Infectious Diseases Society of America. *Clin Infect Dis.* 2006;43(9):1089–1134.

antibiotic therapy. Patients may become reinfected with *B burgdorferi* after successful antibiotic therapy, especially in endemic areas, or they may experience a more severe or chronic course by virtue of concomitant babesiosis (an intraerythrocytic parasitic infection caused by protozoa of the genus *Babesia,* which is also transmitted by *Ixodes* species ticks) or human granulocytic anaplasmosis (previously known as *human granulocytic ehrlichiosis*) and require retreatment with antibiotics. Prevention strategies include avoiding tick-infested habitats, using tick repellents, wearing protective outer garments, removing ticks promptly, and reducing tick populations.

Centers for Disease Control and Prevention. Summary of Notifiable Diseases–United States, 2011, Lyme Disease. *MMWR.* 2012;60(53):17–97.

Mikkila E, Smith C, Sood S. The expanding clinical spectrum of ocular Lyme borreliosis. *Ophthalmology.* 2000;107(3):581–587.

Stanek G, Strle F. Lyme borreliosis. *Lancet.* 2003;15;362(9396):1639–1647.

Wormser GP, Dattwyler RJ, Shapiro ED, et al. The clinical assessment, treatment, and prevention of Lyme disease, human granulocytic anaplasmosis, and babesiosis: clinical practice guidelines by the Infectious Diseases Society of America. *Clin Infect Dis.* 2006; 43(9):1089–1134.

Leptospirosis

Leptospirosis, a zoonotic infection with a worldwide distribution, occurs most frequently in tropical and subtropical regions and is caused by the gram-negative spirochete *Leptospira interrogans.* The natural reservoirs for *Leptospira* organisms are animals, including livestock, horses, dogs, and rodents, which excrete the organism in their urine. Humans contract the disease upon exposure to contaminated soil or water; thus, groups at risk include agricultural workers, sewer workers, veterinarians, fish workers, slaughterhouse workers, military personnel, as well as swimmers, triathletes, and whitewater rafters. The disease is not known to spread from person to person, but maternal–fetal transmission may occur infrequently. It is very rare in the United States, with only 38 cases reported to the CDC in 1994. Between 1999 and 2008, 198 laboratory-confirmed cases were identified in Hawaii. Leptospirosis ceased to be a nationally notifiable disease in 1995, although it remains reportable in some states including Hawaii, where the majority of US cases occur.

Leptospirosis is frequently a biphasic disease, with the initial, or leptospiremic, phase following an incubation period of 2–4 weeks heralded by the abrupt onset of fever, chills, headache, myalgias, vomiting, and diarrhea. Severe septicemic leptospirosis, also known as *Weil disease,* is characterized by renal and hepatocellular dysfunction; it is rare (occurs in 10%) but can be fatal in 30%. Leptospires may be isolated from the blood and CSF but are cleared rapidly as the disease progresses to the second, or immune, phase of the illness, which is characterized by meningitis, leptospiruria, cranial nerve palsies, myelitis, and uveitis. The organism may persist for longer periods of time in immunologically privileged sites such as the brain and the eye.

Ocular involvement can occur in both the leptospiremic and immune phases, but there is frequently a prolonged interval between systemic and ocular disease. Circumcorneal conjunctival hyperemia is the earliest and most common sign of ocular leptospirosis and is considered pathognomonic, but the development of intraocular inflammation, which can range from mild anterior uveitis to panuveitis with retinal vasculitis (in 10%–44% of patients), is the more serious, potentially vision-threatening complication.

The differential diagnosis includes HLA-B27–associated uveitis, idiopathic pars planitis, Behçet disease, Eales disease, sarcoidosis, tuberculosis, and syphilis. Appropriate history and laboratory evaluation help distinguish these entities from leptospiral uveitis. A definitive diagnosis requires isolation of the organism from bodily fluids. A presumptive diagnosis is made on the basis of serologic assays; recently, rapid serologic assays such as ELISA and complement-fixation tests for the detection of IgM antibodies against leptospiral antigens have been developed that are highly sensitive and specific, and PCR-based assays are under evaluation. Leptospirosis may cause a false-positive result on RPR or FTA-ABS tests.

Intravenous antibiotic therapy with 1.5 MU of penicillin G every 6 hours or oral doxycycline, 100 mg twice daily for 1 week, may be used for mild or moderate cases. It is not known whether systemic antibiotic treatment is protective with respect to long-term complications such as uveitis. However, systemic antibiotic treatment should be considered for ocular disease that occurs even months after onset of the acute systemic disease. In addition, topical, periocular, or systemic corticosteroids, together with mydriatic and cycloplegic drugs, are routinely used to suppress intraocular inflammation. The visual prognosis of leptospiral uveitis is quite favorable despite severe panuveal inflammation.

Centers for Disease Control and Prevention. Summary of Notifiable Diseases–United States, 2011. *MMWR.* 2012;60(53):104–106.

Katz AR, Buchholz AE, Hinson K, Park SY, Effler PV. Leptospirosis in Hawaii, USA, 1999–2008. *Emerg Infect Dis.* 2011;17(2):221–226.

Rathinam SR. Ocular manifestations of leptospirosis. *J Postgrad Med.* 2005;51(3):189–194.

Ocular Nocardiosis

Nocardia asteroides is a gram-positive rod with partially acid-fast beaded branching filaments—a bacterium that acts like a fungus. Although ocular involvement in patients with *N asteroides* infection is rare, ocular disease may be the presenting problem in this potentially lethal but treatable systemic disease characterized by pneumonia and disseminated abscesses. The responsible organism is commonly found in soil, and initial infection occurs by ingestion or inhalation, causing an insidious inflammation. Immunocompromised individuals are more likely to be affected. Ocular involvement occurs by hematogenous spread of the bacteria, and symptoms may vary from the mild pain and redness of anterior uveitis to the severe pain and decreased vision of panophthalmitis. Nocardia infection can affect essentially any ocular structure, including periorbital tissue and the adnexae. Findings range from keratitis, necrotizing scleritis, or an isolated, unilateral choroidal or subretinal mass (abscess) with minimal vitritis to panuveitis with anterior chamber cell and flare, vitritis, and multiple choroidal abscesses with overlying retinal detachment mimicking fungal endophthalmitis.

Diagnosis can be established with a culture of the organism taken from tissue or fluid, by vitreous aspiration for Gram stain and culture, or, occasionally, by enucleation and microscopic identification of organisms. Treatment of systemic *N asteroides* infection with systemic sulfonamide (trimethoprim-sulfamethoxazole) may be required for protracted periods of time. Combination therapy with additional antibiotics may be required.

Garg P. Fungal, mycobacterial, and Nocardia infections and the eye: an update. *Eye (Lond).* 2012;26(2):245–251.

Tuberculosis

Tuberculosis (TB) was once considered the most common cause of uveitis; currently, ocular involvement caused by TB is uncommon in the United States. In 2011, the TB incidence rate in the United States was 3.4 in 100,000 persons. Worldwide, however, TB remains the most important systemic infectious disease, with more than 9.4 million new cases and 1.8 million deaths reported in 2008. Nearly one-third of the world's population is infected, and 95% of cases occur in resource-limited countries. In the United States, after many years of annual decline, the incidence of TB began to increase coincident with the AIDS epidemic, and the disease reemerged as an important public health problem. Although the frequency of ocular disease parallels the prevalence of TB in general, it remains relatively uncommon both in endemic areas and among institutionalized populations with unequivocal systemic disease. In the United States, the incidence of uveitis attributable to TB at a large tertiary care facility was only 0.6%, whereas at major referral centers in India, it ranged from 0.6% to 10% and in similar institutions in Japan and Saudi Arabia, was 7.9% and 10.5%, respectively.

Tuberculosis is caused by *Mycobacterium tuberculosis,* an acid-fast–staining, obligate aerobe most commonly transmitted by aerosolized droplets. The organism has an affinity for highly oxygenated tissues, and tuberculous lesions are commonly found in the apices of the lungs as well as in the choroid, which has the highest blood flow rate in the body. Systemic infection may occur primarily, as a result of recent exposure; in the vast majority (90%) of patients, however, it occurs secondarily from reactivation of the disease with immune compromise. Widespread hematogenous dissemination of TB, known as *miliary disease,* likewise occurs most often in immunocompromised persons. High-risk groups include health care professionals, recent immigrants from endemic areas, the indigent, immunocompromised patients (chronic disease, HIV/AIDS, or IMT), and older adults.

Pulmonary TB develops in approximately 80% of patients, whereas extrapulmonary disease occurs in about 20%, with one-half of these patients having a normal-appearing chest radiograph and up to 20% having a negative result on the purified protein derivative (PPD) skin test. Patients coinfected with HIV present more often with extrapulmonary disease, the frequency of which increases with deteriorating immune function. Only 10% of infected individuals develop symptomatic disease; one-half of these manifest illness within the first 1–2 years. The vast majority, however, remain infected but asymptomatic. The classic presentation of symptomatic disease—fever, night sweats, and weight loss—occurs in both pulmonary and extrapulmonary infection. This fact is important to keep in mind when conducting a review of systems in patients suspected of tuberculous uveitis because histologically proven intraocular TB has been found in asymptomatic patients as well as in patients with extrapulmonary disease.

Ocular disease

The ocular manifestations of TB may result from either active infection or an immunologic reaction to the organism. *Primary ocular TB* is defined as TB in which the eye is the primary portal of entry, and it manifests mainly as conjunctival, corneal, and scleral disease. *Secondary ocular TB,* of which uveitis is the most common manifestation, occurs by virtue of hematogenous dissemination or by contiguous spread from adjacent structures. External ocular and anterior segment findings include scleritis, phlyctenulosis, interstitial keratitis, corneal infiltrates, anterior chamber and iris nodules, and isolated granulomatous anterior uveitis; the last is exceedingly uncommon in the absence of posterior segment disease.

Tuberculous uveitis is classically a chronic granulomatous disease that may affect the anterior and/or posterior segments; it is replete with mutton-fat KPs, iris nodules, posterior synechiae, and secondary glaucoma, although a nongranulomatous uveitis may also occur. Patients typically experience a waxing and waning course, with accumulation of vitreous opacities and CME (Figs 7-50, 7-51).

Disseminated choroiditis is the most common presentation and is characterized by multiple deep, discrete, yellowish lesions between 0.5 mm and 3.0 mm in diameter and numbering from 5 to several hundred (Fig 7-52). These lesions, or tubercles, are located

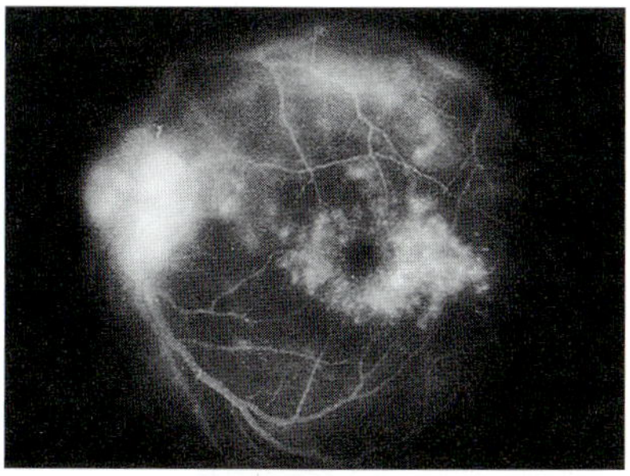

Figure 7-50 Fluorescein angiogram of chronic tuberculous uveitis with disc edema, vasculitis, periphlebitis, and cystoid macular edema (CME). *(Courtesy of John D. Sheppard, Jr, MD.)*

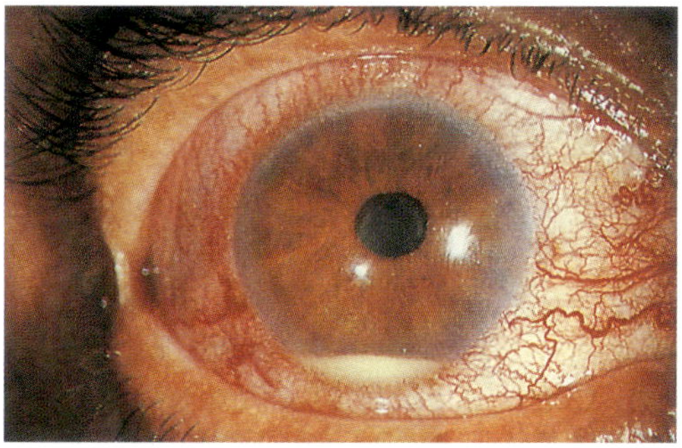

Figure 7-51 Acute tuberculous uveitis with hypopyon, posterior synechiae, vitritis, retinal vasculitis, and CME. *(Courtesy of John D. Sheppard, Jr, MD.)*

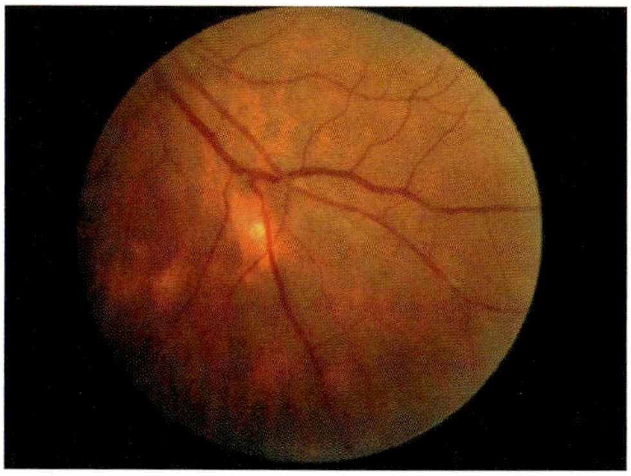

Figure 7-52 Fundus photograph showing multifocal, discrete, yellowish choroidal lesions in a patient with pulmonary tuberculosis. *(Reproduced with permission from Vitale AT, Foster CS. Uveitis affecting infants and children: infectious causes. In: Hartnett ME, Trese M, Capone A, Keats B, Steidl SM, eds.* Pediatric Retina. *Philadelphia, PA: Lippincott Williams & Wilkins; 2005:277; courtesy of Albert T. Vitale, MD.)*

predominantly in the posterior pole and may be accompanied by disc edema, nerve fiber layer hemorrhages, and varying degrees of vitritis and granulomatous anterior uveitis. Alternatively, they may present as a single, focal, large, elevated choroidal mass (tuberculoma) that varies in size from 4 mm to 14 mm and may be accompanied by neurosensory retinal detachment and macular star formation (Fig 7-53). Choroidal tubercles may be one of the earliest signs of disseminated disease and are more commonly observed among immunocompromised hosts. On FA, active choroidal lesions display early hyperfluorescence with late leakage, and cicatricial lesions show early blocked fluorescence with late staining. ICG angiography reveals early- and late-stage hypofluorescence corresponding to the choroidal lesions, which are frequently more numerous than those seen on FA or clinical examination. Other manifestations include multifocal choroiditis and a serpiginous-like choroiditis (Fig 7-54). In patients with HIV/AIDS, tuberculous choroiditis may progress despite effective antituberculous therapy.

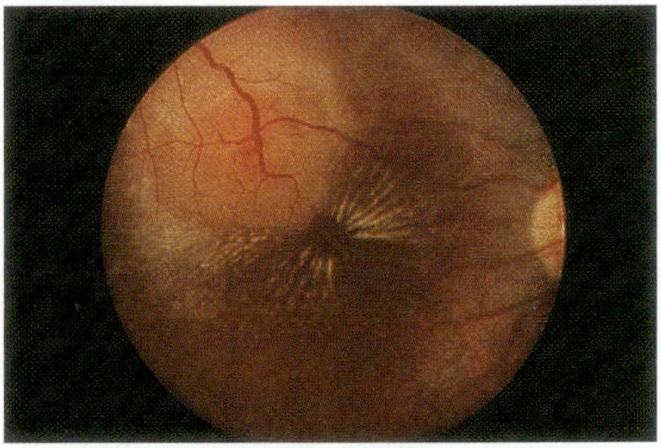

Figure 7-53 Fundus photograph of a choroidal tubercle with a macular star formation (miliary tuberculosis).

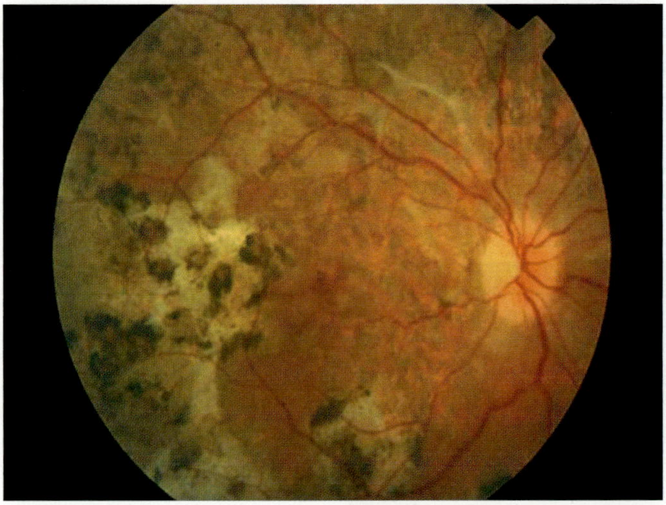

Figure 7-54 Fundus photograph showing tuberculous choroiditis masquerading as atypical serpiginous-like choroiditis. The patient showed progression and recurrence while receiving immunomodulatory drugs; however, after antituberculous treatment was begun, the patient showed improvement in vision and resolution of the vitritis without recurrences. *(Courtesy of Narsing A. Rao, MD.)*

Retinal involvement in TB is usually secondary to extension of the choroidal disease or an immunologic response to mycobacteria. Historically, Eales disease has been described as a peripheral retinal perivasculitis that presents in otherwise healthy young men aged 20–40 years with recurrent, unilateral retinal and vitreous hemorrhage and subsequent involvement of the fellow eye. A periphlebitis is most commonly observed, which may be accompanied by venous occlusion, peripheral nonperfusion, neovascularization, and the eventual development of tractional retinal detachment (Fig 7-55). The association between TB and retinal vasculitis is supported by the identification by PCR-based assays of *M tuberculosis* DNA from the aqueous, vitreous, and epiretinal membranes of patients with Eales disease. Other posterior segment findings of TB include subretinal abscess, CNV, optic neuritis, and acute panophthalmitis.

Diagnosis

Definitive diagnosis of TB requires direct evidence of mycobacteria in bodily fluids or tissues. In many cases of ocular TB, this confirmation is not possible, and the diagnosis is instead presumptive, based on indirect evidence. A positive result on a PPD test or an interferon-gamma release assay is indicative of prior exposure to TB but not necessarily of active systemic infection. In the United States, an induration of 5 mm or more, read 48–72 hours after intradermal injection of the standard 5-tuberculin-unit (5-TU), or intermediate-strength, test dose is considered a positive result in individuals with HIV infection, those exposed to active TB, or those whose radiographs are consistent with healed tuberculous lesions. An induration of 10 mm or more is considered indicative of a positive result for other high-risk individuals, including patients with diabetes mellitus or renal failure, those on IMT, health care workers, and recent immigrants from high-prevalence countries. Patients with no known risks for tuberculosis are considered to exhibit a positive test result with an induration of 15 mm or more.

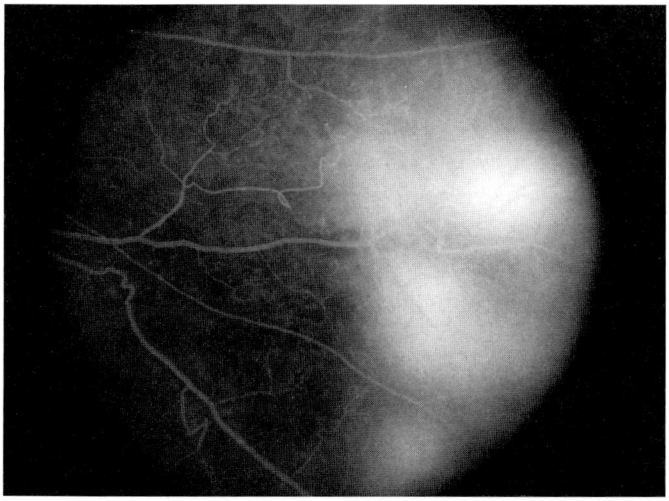

Figure 7-55 Eales disease. Fluorescein angiogram showing diffuse late leakage from peripheral retinal neovascularization. *(Courtesy of Albert T. Vitale, MD.)*

False-negative skin testing results occur at a rate of 25% because of patients with profound acute illness or immune compromise, which can stem from corticosteroid use, advanced age, poor nutrition, and sarcoidosis. False-positive results may arise from patients infected with atypical mycobacteria, immunized with BCG vaccine, and treated with intraluminal BCG injections for bladder carcinoma. Individuals recently immunized with BCG vaccine may have an induration measuring around 10 mm at presentation, but the reaction is usually not sustained and tends to decrease with time compared with the reaction following the skin test after more recent systemic TB exposure. A Bayesian analysis predicts that routine screening of uveitis patients for TB has a low probability of detecting disease in settings where the prevalence of TB is low. It is recommended, therefore, that testing be selectively used for patients in whom the index of suspicion has been heightened by a careful history, review of systems, and clinical examination. Testing for TB is of particular importance in patients being considered for treatment with tumor necrosis factor inhibitors.

A history of recent exposure to TB or a positive TB test result warrants a concerted search for systemic infection, using chest radiography, positron emission tomography scanning, and/or microbiologic analysis of sputum, urine, or gastric aspirates, or a cervical lymph node biopsy for acid-fast bacilli. Failure to demonstrate systemic disease does not, however, exclude the possibility of intraocular infection. For cases of suspected ocular TB in which the results of the above-mentioned testing for systemic infection are negative, the patient is asymptomatic, or the infection is thought to be extrapulmonary, definitive diagnosis may require intraocular fluid analysis or tissue biopsy. Nucleic acid amplification techniques, with either transcription-mediated amplification of 16S ribosomal RNA or PCR amplification of unique DNA sequences of *M tuberculosis,* have been successfully used in some cases to diagnose intraocular TB, though the yield may be low because of a thick cell wall and possibly low bacterial load in the vitreous. Chorioretinal biopsy used in conjunction with PCR testing and routine histologic examination may be necessary in atypical cases where the differential diagnosis and therapeutic options are widely divergent. Recently, antibodies against purified cord factor, the most antigenic and abundant cell wall component of tubercle bacilli, have been detected by ELISA and may be useful for rapid serodiagnosis of pulmonary TB, in addition to providing supportive data for the diagnosis of ocular infection.

Treatment

Systemic antibiotic therapy is clearly indicated for patients with uveitis whose TB test results have recently converted to positive, patients with an abnormal-appearing chest radiograph, or persons with positive bacterial culture or PCR results. Multidrug therapy is recommended because of the increasing incidence of resistance to isoniazid (INH), as well as adherence problems associated with long-term therapy. These problems, together with the extremely slow growth rate of TB, contribute to the acquisition of multidrug-resistant tuberculosis (MDRTB). Patients at risk for MDRTB include nonadherent patients receiving single-drug therapy; migrant or indigent populations; immunocompromised patients, including those with HIV infection; and recent immigrants from countries where INH and rifampin are available over the counter. In brief, treatment entails an initial 2-month induction course of INH, rifampin, and pyrazinamide administered daily, followed by a continuation phase of 4–7 months. In the event of drug resistance, another drug, such as ethambutol or streptomycin, is added to the initial triple-drug regimen, followed by a 4-month continuation of INH and rifampin. More than 95% of immunocompetent patients may be successfully treated with a full course of therapy, provided they remain adherent to this regimen. Directly observed therapy (DOT) plays a crucial role in ensuring this success and is now the standard of care in the treatment of tuberculosis. Treatment protocols have been standardized and are available from the CDC.

More difficult is the treatment approach to patients with uveitis consistent with TB, normal chest radiograph appearance, and positive TB test result. In this situation, a diagnosis of extrapulmonary TB may be entertained and treatment initiated, particularly in cases with medically unresponsive uveitis or other findings supportive of the diagnosis, such as recent exposure to or inadequate treatment of the disease, a large area of induration, or skin test result recently converted to positive. Topical and systemic corticosteroids are frequently used in conjunction with antimicrobial therapy to treat the inflammatory component of the disease. Because intensive corticosteroid treatment administered without appropriate antituberculous cover may lead to progressive worsening of ocular disease, any patient suspected of harboring TB should undergo appropriate testing before beginning such therapy. Patients with a positive TB test result or abnormal chest film appearance for whom systemic corticosteroid treatment is being considered, or patients who have received corticosteroids for longer than 2 weeks at doses greater than 15 mg/day, may benefit from prophylactic treatment with INH for 6 months to 1 year. Likewise, patients with latent TB in whom anti–tumor necrosis factor therapy is being considered should be treated with INH prophylaxis beginning at least 3 weeks before the first infusion.

Ang M, Wong WL, Li X, Chee SP. Interferon γ release assay for the diagnosis of uveitis associated with tuberculosis: a Bayesian evaluation in the absence of a gold standard. *Br J Ophthalmol.* 2013;97(8):1062–1067.

Centers for Disease Control and Prevention. Summary of Notifiable Diseases–United States, 2011, *MMWR.* 2012;60(53):98.

Diel R, Loddenkemper R, Nienhaus A. Evidence-based comparison of commercial interferon-gamma release assays for detecting active TB: a metaanalysis. *Chest.* 2010; 137(4):952–968.

Gan WL, Jones NP. Serpiginous-like choroiditis as a marker for tuberculosis in a non-endemic area. *Br J Ophthalmol.* 2013;97(5):644–647.

Gupta A, Gupta V. Tubercular posterior uveitis. *Int Ophthalmol Clin.* 2005;45(2):71–88.

Troutbeck R, Lim LL. Clinical controversy: to treat, or not to treat? That is the tuberculosis question. *Clin Experiment Ophthalmol.* 2012;40(7):653–654.

Varma D, Anand S, Reddy AR, et al. Tuberculosis: an under-diagnosed aetiological agent in uveitis with an effective treatment. *Eye (Lond).* 2006;20(9):1068–1073.

Yeh S, Sen HN, Colyer M, Zapor M, Wroblewski K. Update on ocular tuberculosis. *Curr Opin Ophthalmol.* 2012;23(6):551–556.

Ocular Bartonellosis

Bartonella henselae (formerly *Rochalimaea henselae*), a small, fastidious, gram-negative rod, initially isolated from the tissue of patients with bacillary angiomatosis of AIDS, is now known to be the principal etiologic agent of cat-scratch disease (CSD) and is associated with an expanding spectrum of ocular manifestations. CSD is a feline-associated zoonotic disease found worldwide, with an estimated annual incidence rate in the United States of 9.3 cases per 100,000 persons; the highest age-specific incidence is among children younger than 10 years of age. Cats are the primary mammalian reservoir of *B henselae* and *B quintana,* and the cat flea is an important vector for the transmission of the organism among cats. The disease follows a seasonal pattern, occurring predominantly in the fall and winter, and is most prevalent in the southern states, California, and Hawaii. The disease is transmitted to humans by the scratches, licks, and bites of domestic cats, particularly kittens.

Systemic manifestations of CSD include a mild to moderate flulike illness associated with regional adenopathy that usually precedes the ocular manifestations of the disease. An erythematous papule, vesicle, or pustule usually forms at the primary site of cutaneous injury 3–10 days after primary inoculation and 1–2 weeks before the onset of lymphadenopathy and constitutional symptoms. Less commonly, more severe and disseminated disease may develop that is associated with encephalopathy, aseptic meningitis, osteomyelitis, hepatosplenic disease, pneumonia, and pleural and pericardial effusions.

Ocular involvement, which occurs in 5%–10% of patients with CSD, includes Parinaud oculoglandular syndrome (unilateral granulomatous conjunctivitis and regional lymphadenopathy) in approximately 5% of patients and a wide array of posterior segment and neuro-ophthalmic findings. Entities to be considered in the differential diagnosis of Parinaud oculoglandular syndrome include tularemia, tuberculosis, syphilis, sporotrichosis, and acute *Chlamydia trachomatis* infection.

The most well-known posterior segment manifestation of *B henselae* infection is neuroretinitis, a constellation of findings that includes abrupt vision loss, unilateral optic disc swelling, and macular star formation, which occurs in 1%–2% of patients with CSD (focal retinochoroiditis, however, is the most common uveitic manifestation of CSD). This syndrome, formerly known as *idiopathic stellate maculopathy* and later renamed *Leber idiopathic stellate neuroretinitis,* is now known to be caused by *B henselae* infection in approximately two-thirds of cases. Table 7-5 lists other entities that may cause neuroretinitis. Visual acuity loss varies to between 20/25 and 20/200 or worse and follows the onset of constitutional symptoms by approximately 2–3 weeks. Although the presentation is most often unilateral, bilateral cases of neuroretinitis have been reported and are frequently asymmetric. Optic disc edema, associated with peripapillary serous retinal detachment, has been observed 2–4 weeks before the appearance of the macular star and may be a sign of systemic *B henselae* infection. The development of the macular star is variable and may be partial or incomplete, usually resolving in approximately 8–12 weeks (Fig 7-56).

Most patients with *Bartonella*-associated neuroretinitis exhibit some degree of anterior chamber inflammation and vitritis. Discrete, focal, or multifocal retinal and/or choroidal lesions measuring 50–300 μm are common posterior segment findings. Both arterial and venous occlusive disease, as well as localized neurosensory macular detachments, have been described in association with focal retinitis. Other posterior segment ocular complications include epiretinal membranes, inflammatory mass of the optic nerve head, peripapillary angiomatosis, intermediate uveitis, retinal white dot syndromes, orbital abscess, isolated optic disc swelling, and panuveitis.

A diagnosis of CSD is made on the basis of characteristic clinical features together with confirmatory serologic testing. The indirect fluorescent antibody assay for the

Table 7-5 Neuroretinitis: Other Associated Causes

Infectious
- Bartonellosis *(Bartonella henselae)*
- Syphilis
- Lyme disease
- Tuberculosis
- Diffuse unilateral subacute neuroretinitis (DUSN) *(Ancylostoma caninum, Baylisascaris procyonis)*
- Toxoplasmosis
- Toxocariasis
- Leptospirosis
- Salmonella
- Chickenpox (varicella)
- Mumps
- Herpes simplex
- Ehrlichiosis
- Rocky Mountain spotted fever

Noninfectious
- Sarcoidosis
- Acute systemic hypertension
- Diabetes mellitus
- Idiopathic intracranial hypertension
- Anterior ischemic optic neuropathy
- Leukemic infiltration of the optic nerve

Idiopathic
- Recurrent idiopathic neuroretintis

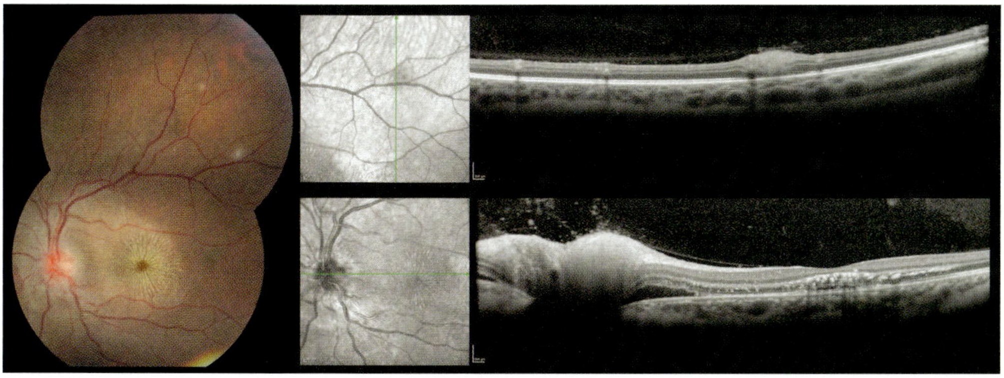

Figure 7-56 *Left,* color fundus photograph of the left eye of a patient with cat-scratch disease shows neuroretinitis with optic disc involvement associated with a macular star. Punctate retinal infiltrates are also visible superiorly. *Upper right,* spectral-domain optical coherence tomography scan delineates the inner retinal infiltrate; *lower right,* scan reveals subretinal fluid, intraretinal exudates, vitreous inflammatory infiltration, and optic disc and macular edema. *(Courtesy of Daniel Vitor Vasconcelos-Santos, MD, PhD.)*

detection of serum anti–*B henselae* antibodies is 88% sensitive and 94% specific, with titers of greater than 1:64 considered positive. Enzyme immunoassays with a sensitivity for IgG of 86%–95% and a specificity of 96%, together with Western blot analysis, have also been developed. A single positive indirect fluorescent antibody or enzyme immunoassay titer for IgG or IgM is sufficient to confirm the diagnosis of CSD. Other diagnostic approaches include bacterial cultures, which may require several weeks for colonies to become apparent; skin testing, which has a sensitivity of up to 100% and a specificity of up to 98%; and PCR-based techniques that target the bacterial 16S ribosomal RNA gene or *B henselae* DNA.

Definitive treatment guidelines have not emerged for CSD because it is a self-limiting illness in most cases, with an overall excellent systemic and visual prognosis. A variety of antibiotics, including doxycycline, erythromycin, rifampin, trimethoprim-sulfamethoxazole, ciprofloxacin, and gentamycin, have been used in the treatment of more severe systemic or ocular manifestations, despite the fact that their efficacy has not been demonstrated conclusively. A typical regimen for immunocompetent patients older than age 8 years consists of doxycycline, 100 mg orally twice daily for 2–4 weeks. For more severe infections, doxycycline may be given intravenously or used in combination with rifampin, 300 mg orally twice daily; among immunocompromised individuals, this treatment is extended for 4 months. Children with CSD may be treated with azithromycin, but the safety of ciprofloxacin in individuals younger than age 18 years has not been established. The efficacy of oral corticosteroids on the course of systemic and ocular disease is unknown. In the subset of patients with recurrent idiopathic neuroretinitis, long-term IMT may be of benefit.

Chi SL, Stinnett S, Eggenberger E, et al. Clinical characteristics in 53 patients with cat scratch optic neuropathy. *Ophthalmology.* 2012;119(1):183–187.

Roe RH, Jumper JM, Fu AD, Johnson RN, McDonald HR, Cunningham ET. Ocular bartonella infections. *Int Ophthalmol Clin.* 2008;48(3):93–105.

Suhler ED, Lauer AK, Rosenbaum JT. Prevalence of serologic evidence of cat scratch disease in patients with neuroretinitis. *Ophthalmology.* 2000;107(5):871–876.

Whipple Disease

Whipple disease is a rare multisystem disease caused by the *Tropheryma whipplei* bacterium. It is most common in middle-aged white men. Migratory arthritis occurs in 80% of cases, and gastrointestinal symptoms, including diarrhea, steatorrhea, and malabsorption, occur in 75%. Intestinal loss of protein results in pitting edema and weight loss. Cardiomyopathy and valvular disease can also occur. CNS involvement occurs in 10% of cases and results in seizures, dementia, and coma. Neuro-ophthalmic signs can include cranial nerve palsies, nystagmus, and ophthalmoplegia. Some patients develop a progressive supranuclear palsy–like condition.

Intraocular involvement is rare and occurs in less than 5% of cases. Patients can present with bilateral panuveitis and retinal vasculitis. Both anterior uveitis and moderate vitritis are present. Diffuse chorioretinal inflammation and diffuse retinal vasculitis in the perifoveal and midperipheral regions may occur. Retinal vascular occlusions and retinal hemorrhages may result from the vasculitis. Optic disc edema and, later, optic atrophy may occur. Unusual granular, crystalline deposits on the iris, capsular bag, and intraocular lens have also been reported.

The gold standard for diagnosis of Whipple disease is a duodenal biopsy that demonstrates a periodic acid–Schiff–positive bacillus in macrophages within intestinal villi. PCR analysis of peripheral blood and vitreous may show *T whipplei* DNA and confirm the diagnosis. Culturing of *T whipplei* is difficult but possible. The differential diagnosis of uveitis associated with Whipple disease includes diseases that can cause retinal vasculitis with multisystem involvement, including sarcoidosis, SLE, polyarteritis nodosa, and Behçet disease.

Untreated Whipple disease can be fatal. Systemic trimethoprim-sulfamethoxazole is the preferred treatment. Patients allergic to sulfonamides may be treated with ceftriaxone, tetracycline, or chloramphenicol. Treatment duration may vary from 1 to 3 months, but relapses occur in 30% of cases, necessitating prolonged (up to 1 year) treatment. Retinal vasculitis can resolve with treatment, but neurologic deficits become permanent.

Chan RY, Yannuzzi LA, Foster CS. Ocular Whipple's disease: earlier definitive diagnosis. *Ophthalmology.* 2001;108(12):2225–2231.

Nubourgh I, Vandergheynst F, Lefebvre P, Lemy A, Dumarey N, Decaux G. An atypical case of Whipple's disease: case report and review of the literature. *Acta Clin Belg.* 2008;63(2): 107–111.

Razonable RR, Pulido JS, Deziel PJ, Dev S, Salomão DR, Walker RC. Chorioretinitis and vitreitis due to *Tropheryma whipplei* after transplantation: case report and review. *Transpl Infect Dis.* 2008;10(6):413–418.

Touitou V, Fenollar F, Cassoux N, et al. Ocular Whipple's disease: therapeutic strategy and long-term follow-up. *Ophthalmology.* 2012;119(7):1465–1469.

Infectious Scleritis

Differentiation of infectious from noninfectious scleritis is important, as treatment regimens differ. See Chapter 6 in this volume and BCSC Section 8, *External Disease and Cornea,* for discussions of noninfectious scleritis.

Etiology

A wide variety of agents can infect the sclera, including *Pseudomonas* organisms (most common after pterygium excision), *Actinomyces* and *Nocardia* species, mycobacteria, fungi such as *Fusarium* and *Aspergillus* species, and gram-positive cocci (*Staphylococcus pneumococcus* and *Streptococcus* species). In addition, HSV and VZV can cause chronic infectious scleritis. Infectious scleritis can occur after any previous ocular surgery, including pterygium surgery (especially when beta irradiation or mitomycin C is utilized), scleral buckling, cataract surgery, and pars plana vitrectomy. Trauma with a penetrating injury contaminated by soil or vegetable matter may also result in infectious scleritis.

Clinical Features

Infectious scleritis may present in a manner similar to noninfectious scleritis, with pain, redness, and decreased vision. A precipitating surgery may be recent or remote (in rare cases, many years before). The sclera appears necrotic, thin, and avascular, with inflammation at the edges (Fig 7-57), usually at the site of a surgical or traumatic wound. A mucopurulent discharge may be present, depending on the infectious agent responsible.

Diagnostic Workup

Cultures should be obtained of the area of involvement, including the base and edges of the lesion. A lamellar scleral biopsy should be considered if the condition worsens on

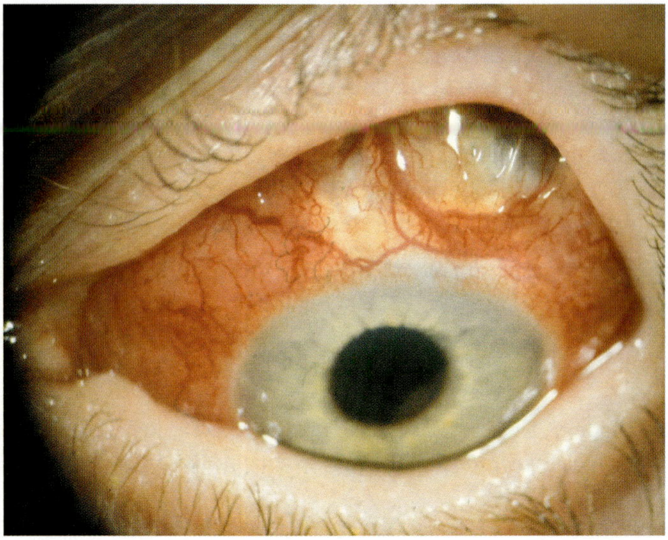

Figure 7-57 Necrotizing scleritis from a *Nocardia* species infection that followed cataract surgery. Note the violaceous hue to the sclera as well as localized avascular, necrotic sclera superiorly in the bed of the original corneoscleral contact wound. *(Courtesy of Ramana S. Moorthy, MD.)*

anti-inflammatory therapy alone. A diagnostic evaluation for noninfectious necrotizing scleritis should be performed, as detailed in Section 8, *External Disease and Cornea.*

Treatment

Both medical and surgical approaches may be needed. Debridement of infected tissues may be useful. Antibiotics can be delivered topically (including by drop or continuous lavage), subconjunctivally, or systemically and should be selected according to the suspected agent and culture results; microorganisms may be difficult to eradicate from the sclera and long-term treatment may be necessary. Corticosteroids should be avoided initially. Scleral patch grafting may be necessary if there is severe thinning, and scleral biopsy may be needed for diagnosis.

Prognosis

Infectious scleritis is difficult to treat, and numerous complications are common. If surgery is required, globe perforation may occur because of the thin necrotic sclera. Inadequate excision of infected tissues can result in disease recurrence, and an extension of the infection to the cornea may occur, as may endophthalmitis from intraocular extension.

Lin CP, Su CY. Infectious scleritis and surgical induced necrotizing scleritis. *Eye (Lond).* 2010;24(4):740.

Meallet MA. Subpalpebral lavage antibiotic treatment for severe infectious scleritis and keratitis. *Cornea.* 2006;25(2):159–163.

Raiji VR, Palestine AG, Parver DL. Scleritis and systemic disease association in a community-based referral practice. *Am J Ophthalmol.* 2009;148(6):946–950.

CHAPTER 8

Endophthalmitis

Endophthalmitis is a clinical diagnosis made when intraocular inflammation involving both the posterior and anterior chambers is attributable to bacterial or fungal infection. The retina or the choroid may be involved; occasionally there is concomitant infective scleritis or keratitis. Acute postoperative and posttraumatic endophthalmitis are covered in BCSC Section 12, *Retina and Vitreous,* and are not discussed here. Chronic postoperative (infectious) endophthalmitis occurs weeks or months after surgery (usually cataract extraction) and can be caused by a myriad of bacteria and fungi. Endogenous endophthalmitis occurs when bacteria or fungi are hematogenously disseminated into the ocular circulation. "Sterile endophthalmitis" describes cases in which infection is suspected but that return negative culture results.

Chronic Postoperative Endophthalmitis

Chronic postoperative endophthalmitis has a distinctive clinical course, with multiple recurrences of chronic indolent inflammation in an eye that had previously undergone surgery, typically cataract extraction. This recurrent indolent inflammation may occur at any point during the postoperative course, as early as 1–2 weeks after surgery, but it is often delayed by many weeks to months and sometimes years. This course is quite different from the explosive onset of acute postoperative endophthalmitis. The incidence of acute postoperative endophthalmitis varies between 0.07% and 0.1%. The incidence of chronic endophthalmitis, however, has not been well established, as the condition may often go undiagnosed. Chronic postoperative endophthalmitis can be divided into bacterial and fungal varieties. Chronic postoperative fungal endophthalmitis should be distinguished from endogenous fungal endophthalmitis, which is typically caused by *Candida* and *Aspergillus* species.

Chronic postoperative bacterial endophthalmitis is most commonly caused by *Propionibacterium acnes.* Other bacteria with limited virulence, such as *Staphylococcus epidermidis* and *Corynebacterium* species, may also cause similar chronic infection. *P acnes,* a commensal, anaerobic, gram-positive, pleomorphic rod, is commonly found on the eyelid skin or on the conjunctiva. *P acnes* may sequester itself between an intraocular lens (IOL) implant and the posterior capsule. In this relatively anaerobic environment, the organism grows and forms colonies, which manifest as whitish plaques between the posterior capsule and the IOL implant (Fig 8-1). The patient may present with slight blurring of vision and a persistent granulomatous inflammation that begins on average 3–4 months

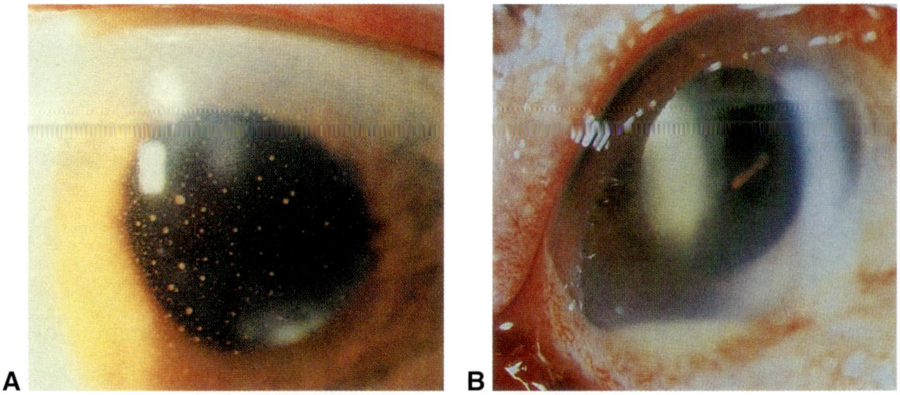

Figure 8-1 **A, B,** Two views of chronic postoperative endophthalmitis caused by *Propionibacterium acnes* infection. Note granulomatous keratic precipitates and white plaque in the capsular bag. *(Courtesy of David Meisler, MD.)*

after surgery; this infection may respond initially to topical or regional corticosteroids but often worsens or recurs when the corticosteroids are tapered. There may be vitreous inflammation, corneal decompensation, and even iris neovascularization in the most severe untreated cases. Nd:YAG capsulotomy can trigger chronic endophthalmitis by liberating the organism into the vitreous cavity, resulting in a more severe vitreous inflammation and an exacerbation of the underlying infection.

Chronic postoperative fungal endophthalmitis may present in a very similar fashion to that caused by *P acnes.* Numerous fungal organisms have been implicated in this chronic inflammatory process, including *Candida parapsilosis, Aspergillus flavus, Torulopsis candida,* and *Paecilomyces lilacinus,* as well as *Verticillium* species. Most of these cases have occurred after cataract surgery, although other kinds of surgery may predispose eyes to the development of fungal endophthalmitis. Patients may present with a delayed-onset, indolent, progressive inflammation that is not responsive to corticosteroids. Certain clinical signs may be helpful in differentiating a fungal from a bacterial etiology, including the presence of corneal infiltrate or edema, mass in the iris or ciliary body, or development of necrotizing scleritis. The presence of vitreous "snowballs" with a "string-of-pearls" appearance in the vitreous may also be indicative of a fungal infection. The intraocular inflammation may worsen after topical, periocular, or intraocular steroid therapy, which should automatically raise the suspicion of a possible infectious masquerade syndrome.

The diagnosis of chronic postoperative endophthalmitis is confirmed by obtaining aerobic, anaerobic, and fungal cultures of the aqueous, capsular plaques (if present), and undiluted vitreous at the time of therapeutic pars plana vitrectomy. Gram and Giemsa stains of undiluted specimens, capsular plaques, and vitreous snowballs should also be obtained along with polymerase chain reaction (PCR) studies of vitreous for *P acnes* or suspected fungi. The value of Gram and Giemsa stains should not be underestimated, especially in cases of fungal endophthalmitis. The bacterial and fungal stains may yield immediate information, enabling the clinician to tailor therapy and improve clinical prognosis long before the results of the cultures turn positive. Because of the slow-growing and fastidious nature of the organisms that cause chronic endophthalmitis, cultures must be retained by the microbiology laboratory for 2 or more weeks. PCR evaluation of aqueous, vitreous, and capsular plaques using pan-fungal and pan-bacterial primers is also of significant diagnostic value in these cases.

The differential diagnosis of chronic postoperative endophthalmitis includes noninfectious causes such as lens-induced uveitis from retained cortical material or retained intravitreal lens fragments, intraocular inflammation from iris chafing resulting from IOL malposition, uveitis-glaucoma-hyphema syndrome, and intraocular lymphoma masquerade syndrome.

Pars plana vitrectomy and injection of intravitreal and endocapsular vancomycin is therapeutic in many cases of chronic postoperative bacterial endophthalmitis; however, this treatment may not be completely successful in eradicating the infection, especially if equatorial lens capsule sequestrae of bacteria are present. In such cases, IOL explantation, complete capsulectomy, and intravitreal vancomycin injection is curative. The decision to explant the IOL must be based in part on the clinical course, the severity of the intraocular inflammation, and the level of vision loss; it is made on a case-by-case basis. There is no preferred method for treating this condition, but it is clear from the existing literature that more than one surgery may be necessary in some cases to completely eradicate this chronic infection. The treatment of chronic fungal endophthalmitis is more difficult and requires the use of intravitreal antifungal drugs (amphotericin and voriconazole) and, possibly, systemic antifungal drugs in the most severe cases. Multiple surgeries may be necessary. The role of systemic therapy in this chronic form of fungal endophthalmitis is not well established or proven.

Lai JY, Chen KH, Lin YC, Hsu WM, Lee SM. *Propionibacterium acnes* DNA from an explanted intraocular lens detected by polymerase chain reaction in a case of chronic pseudophakic endophthalmitis. *J Cataract Refract Surg.* 2006;32(3):522–525.

Meisler DM, Mandelbaum S. *Propionibacterium*-associated endophthalmitis after extracapsular cataract extraction. Review of reported cases. *Ophthalmology.* 1989; 96(1):54–61.

Endogenous Endophthalmitis

Endogenous Bacterial Endophthalmitis

Endogenous endophthalmitis is caused by hematogenous dissemination of bacterial organisms, resulting in intraocular infection. This entity is uncommon and accounts for less than 10% of all forms of endophthalmitis. Patients who have compromised immune systems are most at risk for endogenous endophthalmitis. Predisposing conditions include diabetes mellitus, systemic malignancy, sickle cell anemia, systemic lupus erythematosus, and human immunodeficiency virus (HIV) infection. Extensive gastrointestinal surgery, endoscopy, and dental procedures may all increase risk of endogenous endophthalmitis. Systemic immunomodulatory therapy and chemotherapy may also put patients at risk. Although the eye may be the only location where the infection can be found, there is an extraocular focus in 90% of cases. Possible sources of infection to be considered are pneumonia, urinary tract infection, bacterial meningitis, or liver abscess. A wide variety of bacteria can cause endogenous endophthalmitis. The most common gram-positive organisms are *Streptococcus* species (endocarditis), *Staphylococcus aureus* (cutaneous infections), and *Bacillus* species (from intravenous drug use). The most common gram-negative organisms are *Neisseria meningitidis, Haemophilus influenzae,* and enteric organisms such as *Escherichia coli* and *Klebsiella* species. In Asia, infection from *Klebsiella* species in liver abscesses is the most common cause of endogenous endophthalmitis. It is important to also consider endogenous endophthalmitis in newborns and infants, especially those younger than 6 months.

The clinical features of endogenous bacterial endophthalmitis are suggestive of an ongoing systemic infection and may include fever greater than 101.5°F, elevated peripheral leukocyte count, and positive bacterial cultures from extraocular sites (blood, urine, sputum). Patients are often ill and being treated for a primary underlying disease when they present with endogenous endophthalmitis. The underlying disease may include cancer treated with prolonged intravenous chemotherapy as well as other chronic infections, which may subsequently sequester in the eye. A nonocular infection serving as a nidus for bacterial dissemination to the eye may be very difficult to diagnose, especially in cases of osteomyelitis, sinusitis, or pneumonia misdiagnosed as a simple upper respiratory tract infection. In these situations, laboratory tests cannot substitute for a detailed history and review of systems, which provide the most crucial information for making the clinical diagnosis in any uveitic condition.

Clinical symptoms include acute onset of pain, photophobia, and blurred vision. Examination usually reveals severely reduced visual acuity, periorbital and eyelid edema, and fibrin in the anterior chamber; hypopyon may be present (Fig 8-2). There may be significant vitreous inflammation and vitreous cells. Sometimes, both eyes are affected simultaneously. Small microabscesses in the retina or subretinal space and white, centered retinal hemorrhages (Roth spots) may also be present.

Diagnosis is based on anterior chamber paracentesis and vitrectomy with vitreous and aqueous cultures and Gram and Giemsa stains if fungal organisms are suspected. As for cases of chronic postoperative endophthalmitis, PCR evaluation of ocular fluids with pan-bacterial or pan-fungal primers is extremely useful. Blood and other body fluid cultures should be used along with ocular culture results to confirm the diagnosis and establish therapy. Intravitreal antibiotics are administered at the time of vitrectomy; if it is not clear whether fungal organisms may be involved, treatment of both fungal and

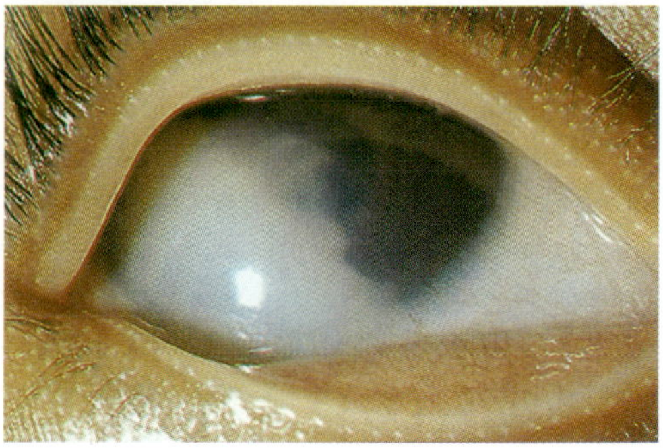

Figure 8-2 Anterior chamber involvement with a "mass effect" from endogenous endophthalmitis.

bacterial etiologies is indicated at the time of vitrectomy. In addition, intravenous antibiotic treatment is sometimes required for several weeks, depending on the organism isolated. Similarly, in patients who have endogenous fungal endophthalmitis, systemic antifungal therapy may be warranted for 6 weeks or more. Initial antimicrobial choices may be empiric and may be tailored to culture results.

The complications of endogenous endophthalmitis can be serious. If the diagnosis of systemic infection is missed, the patient may develop sepsis and even die. In severe cases, recurrent or persistent intraocular infection may require numerous surgeries and repeat injections of intravitreal antibiotics. In addition, complications such as cataract development, retinal detachment, suprachoroidal hemorrhage, vitreous hemorrhage, hypotony, and phthisis bulbi can occur in the most severe cases. The prognosis is directly related to the offending organism and the systemic status of the patient.

Okada AA, Johnson RP, Liles WC, D'Amico DJ, Baker AS. Endogenous bacterial endophthalmitis. Report of a ten-year retrospective study. *Ophthalmology.* 1994;101(5):832–838.

Endogenous Fungal Endophthalmitis

Endogenous fungal endophthalmitis develops slowly as focal or multifocal areas of chorioretinitis. Granulomatous or nongranulomatous inflammation is observed with keratic precipitates, hypopyon, and vitritis with cellular aggregates. The infection usually begins in the choroid, appearing as yellow-white lesions with indistinct borders that range in size from small cotton-wool spots to several disc diameters. It can subsequently break through into the vitreous, producing localized cellular and fungal aggregates overlying the original site(s). Iris nodules and rubeosis may also be observed in cases of severe fungal endophthalmitis.

Endogenous fungal endophthalmitis due to *Candida* (the most common cause), *Aspergillus,* and *Coccidioides* species can be considered a nonneoplastic masquerade syndrome because, in many patients, the condition is mistaken for noninfectious uveitis and treated with corticosteroids alone. This treatment usually worsens the clinical course of the disease, necessitating further investigation to establish the correct diagnosis. The condition often requires aggressive systemic and local antifungal therapy as well as surgical intervention.

Endogenous fungal endophthalmitis caused by *Histoplasma capsulatum, Cryptococcus neoformans, Sporothrix schenkii,* and *Blastomyces dermatitidis* is less common than that caused by *Candida* and *Aspergillus* species.

Gonzales CA, Scott IU, Chaudhry NA, et al. Endogenous endophthalmitis caused by *Histoplasma capsulatum* var. *capsulatum:* a case report and literature review. *Ophthalmology.* 2000;107(2):725–729.

Candida *endophthalmitis*

Candida species are an important cause of nosocomial infections and are the most common fungal organisms, causing endogenous endophthalmitis in both pediatric and adult populations. Although *Candida albicans* remains the most common pathogen, non-*albicans* species (eg, *C glabrata*) have also been identified in patients developing ocular disease. In patients with candidemia, the reported prevalence rates of intraocular candidiasis vary widely, ranging between 9% and 78%. However, when strict criteria are applied for the classification of chorioretinitis and endophthalmitis, these numbers drop precipitously; in 1 series, when patients were examined within 72 hours of a positive blood culture result, only 9% had chorioretinitis and none had endophthalmitis. Endogenous *Candida* endophthalmitis occurs in up to 37% of patients with candidemia if they are not receiving antifungal therapy. Ocular involvement drops to 3% in patients who are receiving treatment. Predisposing conditions associated with candidemia and the development of intraocular infection include hospitalization with a history of recent major gastrointestinal surgery, bacterial sepsis, systemic antibiotic use, use of indwelling catheters, hyperalimentation, debilitating diseases (eg, diabetes mellitus), immunomodulatory therapy, prolonged neutropenia, organ transplantation, or a combination of these. Hospitalized neonates and intravenous drug users are also at risk. Immunodeficiency per se does not appear to be a prominent predisposing factor, attested to by the paucity of reported cases of *Candida* chorioretinitis or endophthalmitis among patients with HIV infection or AIDS.

Patients may present with blurred or decreased vision resulting from macular chorioretinal involvement or pain arising from anterior uveitis, which may be severe. Typically, *Candida* chorioretinitis is characterized by multiple, bilateral, white, well-circumscribed lesions less than 1 mm in diameter; these lesions are distributed throughout the postequatorial fundus and associated with overlying vitreous cellular inflammation (Fig 8-3). The chorioretinal lesions may be associated with vascular sheathing and intraretinal hemorrhages; the vitreous exudates may assume a string-of-pearls appearance.

Histologically, *Candida* species are recognized as budding yeast with a characteristic pseudohyphate appearance (Fig 8-4). The organisms reach the eye hematogenously through metastasis to the choroid. Fungi may then break through the Bruch membrane, form subretinal abscesses, and secondarily involve the retina and vitreous.

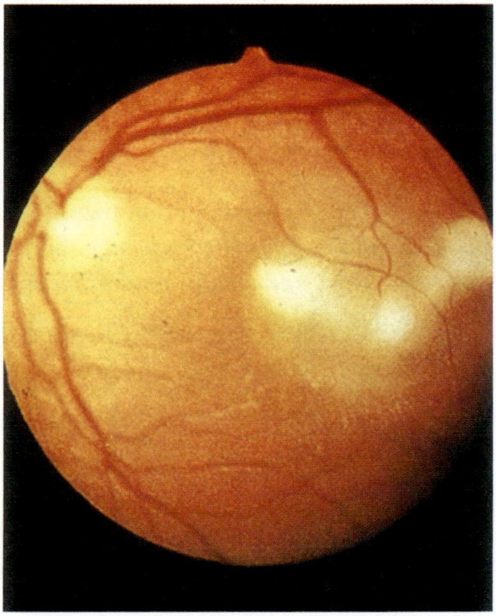

Figure 8-3 Fundus photograph of *Candida* retinitis.

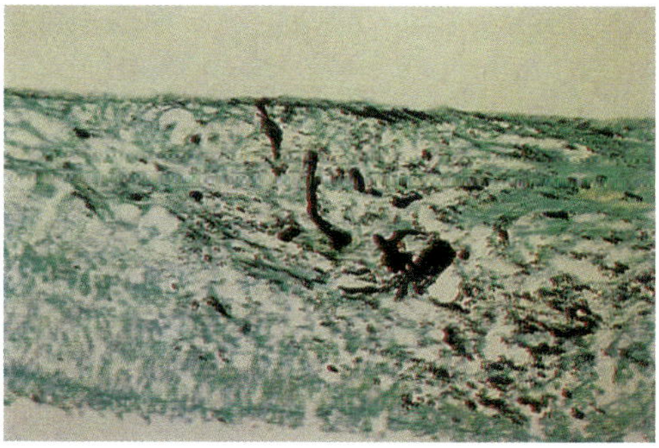

Figure 8-4 Pathology of *Candida* retinitis: fungi *(black)* are revealed in a Gomori methenamine silver stain of the retina taken from a patient diagnosed with fungal endophthalmitis.

The diagnosis of ocular candidiasis is suggested by the presence of chorioretinitis or endophthalmitis in the appropriate clinical context and confirmed by positive results on either blood or vitreous cultures. It has been suggested that all patients with candidemia undergo baseline dilated funduscopic examinations and receive monitoring for the development of metastatic ocular candidiasis for at least 2 weeks after an initial eye examination; the reasoning is that earlier treatment of candidal endophthalmitis has been associated with better visual outcomes, and patients with ocular lesions are more likely to have infection involving a greater number of organ systems than are patients without eye lesions. The presence of vitreous snowballs and endophthalmitis requires diagnostic and therapeutic vitrectomy. Giemsa stains, PCR for *Candida* species, and fungal cultures should be obtained on undiluted vitreous fluid samples.

The differential diagnosis of *Candida* endophthalmitis includes toxoplasmic retinochoroiditis, which exhibits posterior pole lesions that can appear yellow-white with fluffy borders and range in size from small cotton-wool spots to several disc diameters wide. *Candida* vitreous snowball lesions may also resemble pars planitis.

Treatment of intraocular candidiasis includes intravenous and intravitreal administration of antifungal drugs. Consultation with a specialist in infectious diseases is essential. Chorioretinal lesions not yet involving the vitreous body may be treated effectively with the oral triazole antifungal drugs fluconazole and voriconazole (200 mg, twice daily, for 2–4 weeks), with vigilant monitoring for evidence of progression. Voriconazole has good oral bioavailability, achieving therapeutic intravitreal levels with a broad spectrum of antifungal activity. Intravitreal injection of antifungal drugs (amphotericin B, 5–10 μg/0.1 mL, or voriconazole, 100 μg/0.1 mL, with or without dexamethasone, 0.4 mg/0.1 mL) should be considered when the vitreous body is involved, usually in conjunction with pars plana vitrectomy. Vitrectomy may be useful diagnostically by allowing for the analysis of intraocular fluid by microbiologic and molecular techniques, and therapeutically by debulking the pathogen load. More severe infections may require intravenous amphotericin B with or without flucytosine. Significant dose-limiting toxicities (renal, cardiac, and neurologic) associated with conventional amphotericin B therapy were greatly reduced by the development of liposomal lipid complex formulations. Finally, intravenously administered caspofungin, an antifungal drug in the echinocandin class (drugs that inhibit synthesis of glucan in the cell wall) with activity against *Candida* and *Aspergillus* species, has been successfully employed in a small number of patients with *Candida* endophthalmitis;

some treatment failures have also been reported with this drug, however. Another echinocandin, intravenous micafungin, is also available in the United States and Europe for treatment of candidiasis. Oral voriconazole, flucytosine, fluconazole, or rifampin may be administered in addition to intravenous amphotericin B or caspofungin. Prompt treatment of both peripherally located lesions and lesions not involving the macular center may salvage useful vision.

Breit SM, Hariprasad SM, Mieler WF, Shah GK, Mills MD, Grand MG. Management of endogenous fungal endophthalmitis with voriconazole and caspofungin. *Am J Ophthalmol.* 2005;139(1):135–140.

Hidalgo JA, Alangaden GJ, Eliott D, et al. Fungal endophthalmitis diagnosis by detection of *Candida albicans* DNA in intraocular fluid by use of a species-specific polymerase chain reaction assay. *J Infect Dis.* 2000;181(3):1198–1201.

Krishna R, Amuh D, Lowder CY, Gordon SM, Adal KA, Hall G. Should all patients with candidemia have an ophthalmic examination to rule out ocular candidiasis? *Eye (Lond).* 2000;14(Pt 1):30–34.

Rao NA, Hidayat AA. Endogenous mycotic endophthalmitis: variations in clinical and histopathologic changes in candidiasis compared with aspergillosis. *Am J Ophthalmol.* 2001;132(2):244–251.

Shah CP, McKey J, Spirn MJ, Maguire J. Ocular candidiasis: a review. *Br J Ophthalmol.* 2008; 92(4):466–468.

Aspergillus *endophthalmitis*

Endogenous *Aspergillus* endophthalmitis is a rare disorder associated with disseminated aspergillosis among patients with severe chronic pulmonary diseases, cancer, endocarditis, severe immunocompromise, or intravenous drug abuse. It is particularly common among patients who have undergone orthotopic liver transplantation. In rare instances, *Aspergillus* endophthalmitis may occur in immunocompetent patients with no apparent predisposing factors. Disseminated infection most commonly involves the lung, with the eye as the second most common site of infection. *Aspergillus fumigatus* and *A flavus* are the species most frequently isolated from patients with intraocular infection.

Aspergillus species are found in soils and decaying vegetation. The spores of these ubiquitous saprophytic molds become airborne and seed the lungs and paranasal sinuses of humans. Human exposure is very common, but infection is rare and depends on the virulence of the fungal pathogen and immunocompetence of the host. Ocular disease occurs via hematogenous dissemination of *Aspergillus* organisms to the choroid.

Endogenous *Aspergillus* endophthalmitis results in rapid onset of pain and loss of vision. A confluent yellowish infiltrate is often present in the macula, beginning in the choroid and subretinal space. A hypopyon can develop in the subretinal or subhyaloidal space (Fig 8-5A). Retinal hemorrhages, retinal vascular occlusions, and full-thickness retinal necrosis may occur. The infection can spread to produce a dense vitritis and variable degrees of cells, flare, and hypopyon in the anterior chamber. The macular lesions form a central atrophic scar when healed. In contrast to the lesions associated with *Candida* chorioretinitis and endophthalmitis, lesions produced by *Aspergillus* species are larger and more likely to be hemorrhagic, and they commonly invade the retinal and choroidal vessels, which may result in broad areas of ischemic infarction.

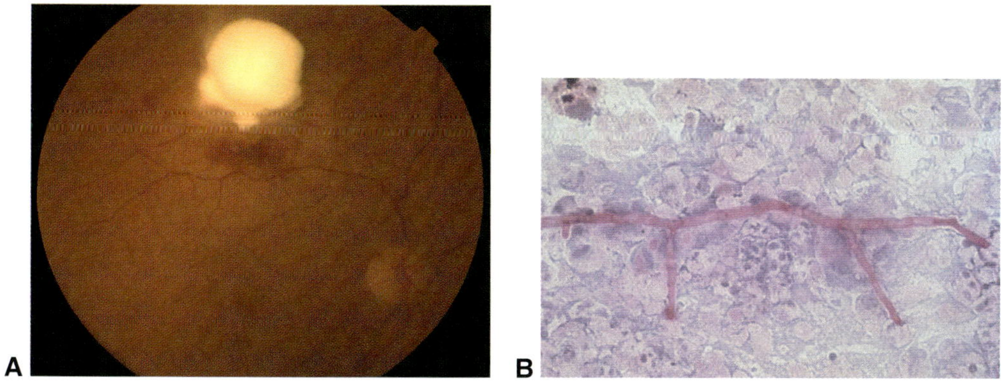

Figure 8-5 **A,** Fundus photograph of a biopsy-proven, culture-positive choroidal aspergilloma caused by endogenous *Aspergillus flavus* endophthalmitis in an immunocompetent patient with disseminated pulmonary aspergillosis. **B,** Light micrograph shows branching hyphae of *Aspergillus fumigatus* (periodic acid–Schiff × 220). *(Part A courtesy of Ramana S. Moorthy, MD. Part B reproduced with permission from Valluri S, Moorthy RS, Liggett PE, Rao NA. Endogenous* Aspergillus *endophthalmitis in an immunocompetent individual.* Int Ophthalmol. *1993;17(3):133.)*

The diagnosis of endogenous *Aspergillus* endophthalmitis is based on clinical findings combined with positive results from pars plana vitreous biopsy and cultures as well as results from Gram and Giemsa stains. Coexisting systemic aspergillosis can be a strong clue, especially among high-risk patients. The diagnosis requires a high degree of suspicion within the correct clinical context and is confirmed by the demonstration of septate, dichotomously branching hyphae on analysis of vitreous fluid specimens. *Aspergillus* organisms may be difficult to culture from the blood.

The differential diagnosis of endogenous *Aspergillus* endophthalmitis includes *Candida* endophthalmitis, cytomegalovirus retinitis, *Toxoplasma* retinochoroiditis, coccidioidomycotic choroiditis or endophthalmitis, and bacterial endophthalmitis.

Aspergillus endophthalmitis lesions are histologically angiocentric. Mixed acute (polymorphonuclear leukocytes) and chronic (lymphocytes and plasma cells) inflammatory cells infiltrate the infected areas of the choroid and retina. Hemorrhage is present in all retinal layers. Granulomas contain rare giant cells. Branching fungal hyphae may be apparent spreading on the surface of the Bruch membrane without penetrating it. Polymorphonuclear leukocytes are present in the vitreous. Fungal hyphae are often surrounded by macrophages and lymphocytes, which form small vitreous abscesses (Fig 8-5B). In *Candida* endophthalmitis, the vitreous is the prominent focus of infection, but in *Aspergillus* endophthalmitis, the principal foci are retinal and choroidal vessels and the subretinal or subretinal pigment epithelial space.

Endogenous *Aspergillus* endophthalmitis usually requires aggressive treatment with diagnostic and therapeutic pars plana vitrectomy combined with intravitreal injection of amphotericin B or voriconazole; intravitreal corticosteroids may be used in conjunction with these drugs. Because most patients with this condition have disseminated aspergillosis, systemic treatment with oral voriconazole, intravenous amphotericin B, or caspofungin is often required. Other systemic antifungal drugs, such as itraconazole, miconazole, fluconazole, and ketoconazole, may also be used. Systemic aspergillosis is best managed by an infectious diseases specialist.

Despite aggressive treatment, the visual prognosis is poor because of frequent macular involvement. Final visual acuity is usually less than 20/200.

Hariprasad SM, Mieler WF, Holz ER, et al. Determination of vitreous, aqueous, and plasma concentration of orally administered voriconazole in humans. *Arch Ophthalmol.* 2004;122(1):42–47.

Rao NA, Hidayat AA. Endogenous mycotic endophthalmitis: variations in clinical and histopathologic changes in candidiasis compared with aspergillosis. *Am J Ophthalmol.* 2001;132(2):244–251.

Cryptococcosis

Cryptococcus neoformans is a yeast found in high concentrations worldwide in contaminated soil and pigeon feces. Infection is acquired through inhalation of the aerosolized fungus. It has a predilection for the central nervous system and may produce severe disseminated disease among immunocompromised or debilitated patients. Although overall it remains an uncommon disease, cryptococcosis is the most common cause of fungal meningitis, as well as the most frequent fungal eye infection in patients with HIV infection or AIDS. The fungus probably reaches the eye hematogenously; however, the frequent association of ocular cryptococcosis with meningitis suggests that ocular infection may result from direct extension from the optic nerve. Ocular infections may occur months after the onset of meningitis or, in rare instances, before the onset of clinically apparent central nervous system disease.

The most frequent presentation of ocular cryptococcosis is multifocal chorioretinitis, which appears as solitary or multiple discrete yellow-white lesions varying markedly in size in the postequatorial fundus. Associated findings include variable degrees of vitritis, vascular sheathing, exudative retinal detachment, papilledema, and granulomatous anterior cellular inflammation. It has been hypothesized that the infection begins as a focus in the choroid, with subsequent extension and secondary involvement of overlying tissues. Severe intraocular infection progressing to endophthalmitis may be observed in the absence of meningitis or clinically apparent systemic disease.

The clinical diagnosis requires a high degree of suspicion and is supported by demonstration of the organism with India ink stains or by culture of the fungus from cerebrospinal fluid. Intravenous amphotericin B and oral flucytosine are required to halt disease progression. With optic nerve or macular involvement, the prognosis is poor for recovery of vision.

Sheu SJ, Chen YC, Kuo NW, Wang JH, Chen CJ. Endogenous cryptococcal endophthalmitis. *Ophthalmology.* 1998;105(2):377–381.

Shields JA, Wright DM, Augsburger JJ, Wolkowicz MI. Cryptococcal chorioretinitis. *Am J Ophthalmol.* 1980;89(2):210–217.

Coccidioidomycosis

Coccidioidomycosis is a disease produced by the dimorphic soil fungus *Coccidioides immitis,* which is endemic to the San Joaquin Valley of central California, certain parts of the southwestern United States, and parts of Central and South America. Infection follows inhalation of dust-borne arthrospores, most commonly resulting in pulmonary infection and secondary dissemination to the central nervous system, skin, skeleton, and eyes. Approximately 40% of infected patients are symptomatic; the vast majority present with a mild upper respiratory tract infection or pneumonitis approximately 3 weeks after exposure to the organism. Erythema nodosum or multiforme may appear from 3 days to 3 weeks after the onset of symptoms; disseminated infection is rare, occurring in less than 1% of patients with pulmonary coccidioidomycosis.

Ocular coccidioidomycosis is likewise uncommon, even with disseminated disease. Disseminated disease usually causes blepharitis, keratoconjunctivitis, phlyctenular and granulomatous conjunctivitis, episcleritis and scleritis, and extraocular nerve palsies and orbital infection. Uveal involvement is still rarer: fewer than 20 pathologically verified cases have been reported. The anterior and posterior segments are equally involved. Intraocular manifestations include unilateral or bilateral granulomatous anterior uveitis, iris granulomas (Fig 8-6), and a multifocal chorioretinitis characterized by multiple, discrete, yellow-white lesions usually less than 1 disc diameter in size located in the postequatorial fundus. These choroidal granulomas may resolve, leaving punched-out chorioretinal scars. Vitreous cellular infiltration, vascular sheathing, retinal hemorrhage, serous retinal detachment, and involvement of the optic nerve have also been reported.

Positive results of serologic testing for anticoccidioidal antibodies in the serum, cerebrospinal fluid, vitreous, and aqueous, as well as of skin testing for exposure to coccidioidin establishes the diagnosis in the correct clinical context. One-half of patients with ocular involvement have systemic disease, and complement-fixation titers are often elevated (>1:32). With isolated anterior segment involvement, an anterior chamber tap may be useful. Culturing for the organism may delay diagnosis. The material from the anterior chamber tap may also be directly examined for coccidioidal organisms using the Papanicolaou stain.

Histologically, *C immitis* evokes pyogenic, granulomatous, and mixed reactions. Intraocular lesions from the anterior segment usually demonstrate zonal granulomatous inflammation that involves the uvea and angle structure, and *Coccidioides* organisms are usually visible.

The differential diagnosis of coccidioidal uveitis includes *Candida, Aspergillus,* and *Histoplasma* species endophthalmitis and tuberculous uveitis. Coccidioidal uveitis should

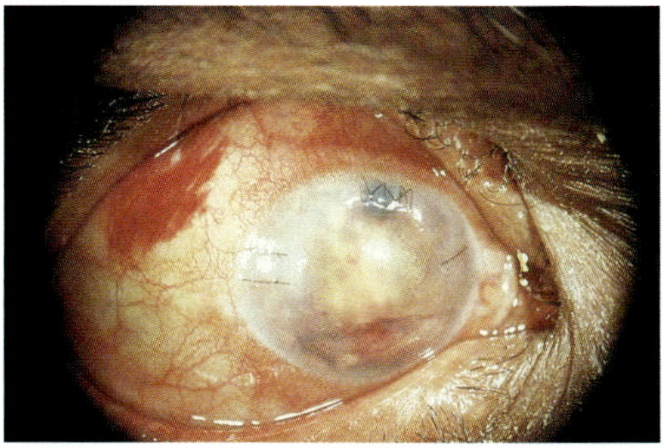

Figure 8-6 Coccidioidal iris granuloma in the pupil. This granuloma was biopsied and a peripheral iridectomy just performed because it was causing pupillary block and angle-closure glaucoma. *(Courtesy of Ramana S. Moorthy, MD.)*

be considered in the differential diagnosis of any patient with apparent idiopathic granulomatous iritis who has lived in or traveled through the southwestern United States, southern California and the San Joaquin Valley, northern Mexico, or Argentina, where the organism is endemic.

The Infectious Diseases Society of America recommends initiating treatment with an oral azole antifungal drug such as fluconazole or itraconazole. Amphotericin B treatment is usually reserved for patients with lesions that are worsening rapidly or that are located in vital sites such as the spine. The visual prognosis is variable and determined in large part by the location of the chorioretinal lesions with respect to the optic nerve and foveal center. Surgical debulking of anterior chamber granulomas, pars plana vitrectomy, and intraocular injections of amphotericin and voriconazole may be required. With systemic disease, much higher doses and a longer duration of intravenous amphotericin therapy or oral voriconazole therapy may be needed. An infectious diseases specialist is essential in the management of coccidioidomycosis.

Despite aggressive treatment, ocular coccidioidomycosis carries a poor visual prognosis, and most eyes require enucleation because of pain and blindness.

Glasgow BJ, Brown HH, Foos RY. Miliary retinitis in coccidioidomycosis. *Am J Ophthalmol.* 1987;104(1):24–27.

Moorthy RS, Rao NA, Sidikaro Y, Foos RY. Coccidioidomycosis iridocyclitis. *Ophthalmology.* 1994;101(12):1923–1928.

Vasconcelos-Santos DV, Lim JI, Rao NA. Chronic coccidioidomycosis endophthalmitis without concomitant systemic involvement: a clinicopathological case report. *Ophthalmology.* 2010;117(9):1839–1842.

CHAPTER 9

Masquerade Syndromes

Masquerade syndromes are a heterogeneous group of disorders noteworthy for mimicking immune-mediated entities and thus are difficult to diagnose. They may be divided into neoplastic and nonneoplastic conditions. At one tertiary referral center, masquerade syndromes accounted for nearly 5% of all patients who presented for evaluation of uveitis.

Neoplastic Masquerade Syndromes

Neoplastic masquerade syndromes may account for 2%–3% of all patients evaluated in tertiary uveitis referral clinics. The most common entity is intraocular primary central nervous system (CNS) lymphoma.

Primary Central Nervous System Lymphoma

Nearly all (98%) primary central nervous system lymphomas (PCNSLs) are non-Hodgkin B-lymphocyte lymphomas. Approximately 2% are T-lymphocyte lymphomas. Although the median age of onset of PCNSL is in the sixth to seventh decade of life, with a peak incidence between the ages of 75 and 84 years, PCNSL also occurs rarely in adolescents and children. The incidence of PCNSL appears to be increasing and is projected to occur in 1 of every 100,000 immunocompetent patients.

Clinical features and findings

Up to 25% of patients with PCNSL have ocular involvement (intraocular or vitreoretinal lymphoma). More than two-thirds of patients with primary intraocular lymphoma will develop CNS disease—usually within 29 months of diagnosis. Sites of ocular involvement can include the vitreous, retina, subretinal pigment epithelium (sub-RPE), and any combination thereof. The most common presenting symptoms are decreased vision and floaters.

Examination reveals a variable degree of vitritis and anterior chamber cells. Posterior segment involvement can appear as creamy yellow subretinal infiltrates with overlying RPE detachments (Fig 9-1) and discrete white lesions that may mimic acute retinal necrosis, toxoplasmosis, "frosted branch" angiitis, or retinal arteriolar obstruction with co-existing multifocal chorioretinal scars and retinal vasculitis. The lesions vary in thickness from approximately 1 mm to 2 mm. Treatment with anti-inflammatory medication can improve the vitreous cellular infiltration, but the effect is not long-lasting.

CNS signs may be present and vary in nature. Behavioral changes appear to be the most frequent sign because of the periventricular location of many of the CNS lesions.

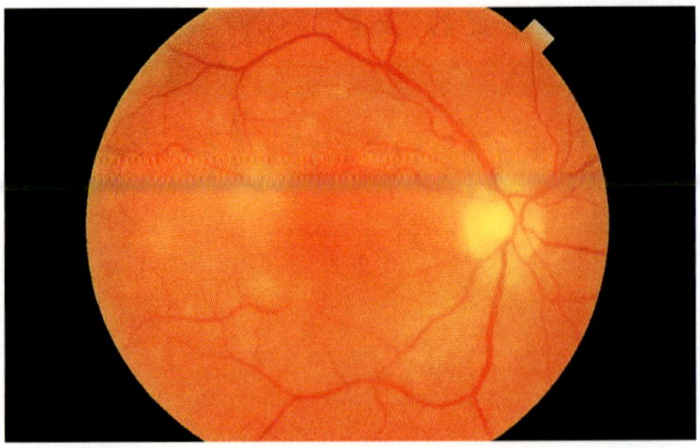

Figure 9-1 Primary central nervous system lymphoma. Fundus photograph of multifocal, subretinal pigment epithelial lesions. *(Courtesy of E. Mitchel Opremcak, MD.)*

Other neurologic signs include hemiparesis, cerebellar signs, epileptic seizures, and cranial nerve palsies. Cerebrospinal fluid seeding of lymphoma cells occurs in 42% of patients with PCNSL.

Diagnostic testing

Ultrasonography may indicate vitreous debris, elevated chorioretinal lesions, and serous retinal detachment. Fluorescein angiography may show hypofluorescent areas due to blockage from a sub-RPE tumor mass or from RPE clumping. Hyperfluorescent window defects may also be caused by RPE atrophy from resolved RPE infiltration. An unusual leopard-spot pattern of alternating hyperfluorescence and hypofluorescence may also be noted.

With CNS involvement, magnetic resonance imaging (MRI) studies of the brain show isointense lesions on T1-weighted images and isointense to hyperintense lesions on T2-weighted images; computed tomography (CT) without use of contrast shows multiple diffuse periventricular lesions. If intravenous contrast is used with CT, these periventricular lesions may be enhanced. Cerebrospinal fluid analysis reveals lymphoma cells in one-third of patients.

The presence of vitreous cells in cases of uveitis that do not respond to therapy necessitates a vitreous biopsy. Ideally, at least 1 mL of undiluted vitreous sample should be obtained. A retinal biopsy, an aspirate of sub-RPE material, or both, may be considered when previous vitreous biopsy results have been negative. Prior to surgery, communication with an experienced pathologist for instructions on the proper and prompt handling of the specimens is necessary to avoid degeneration of the typically friable cells that may occur with delay. Examination by an experienced pathologist is crucial, as the diagnosis may be difficult to establish because of the frequently sparse cellularity of the specimens. Portions of the specimen are typically prepared for both cytologic examination and cell surface marker determination by flow cytometry. As many as one-third of vitreous biopsies incur a false-negative result; thus, a second biopsy of the vitreous should be performed if the clinical picture warrants.

Cytokine analysis of vitreous samples can be helpful in supporting the diagnosis of intraocular lymphoma. Interleukin-10 (IL-10) levels are elevated in the vitreous of patients with lymphoma. In contrast, high levels of IL-6 are found in the vitreous of patients with inflammatory uveitis. Thus, the ratio of IL-10 to IL-6 is often elevated in intraocular lymphoma and supports the diagnosis.

If diagnosis by vitreous aspiration or subretinal aspiration cannot be established, either internal or external chorioretinal biopsy techniques may be used to aid in the diagnosis of PCNSL.

Histology

Cytologic specimens obtained from the vitreous or subretinal space often show pleomorphic cells with scanty cytoplasm, hyperchromatic nuclei with multiple irregular nucleoli, and an elevated nuclear-to-cytoplasm ratio (Fig 9-2). Monoclonality of cells is likely to be present in PCNSL. This can be established through immunophenotyping by immunohistochemistry or flow cytometry to demonstrate the clonality of B lymphocytes by the presence of abnormal immunoglobulin κ or λ light chain predominance, specific B-lymphocyte markers (CD19, CD20, and CD22), and/or gene or oncogene translocations or gene rearrangements. Abnormal lymphocytes may be isolated manually or by laser capture and polymerase chain reaction (PCR)–based assays performed to improve the diagnostic yield of paucicellular samples.

Treatment

Treatment regimens vary among experts. If only 1 eye is affected and there is no CNS involvement, intravitreal methotrexate or rituximab may be considered, although long-term survival studies are not available. This modality does work for some eyes, but given the high rate of eventual CNS involvement, caution is indicated. If both eyes are involved, intraocular treatment alone is even more controversial. In patients with CNS involvement, systemic therapy is indicated. High-dose methotrexate has been used; it may be delivered intravenously, with or without intrathecal administration, and alone or in combination with brain radiation therapy and other chemotherapeutic drugs. Because of the neurotoxicity of radiation, many experts do not use whole-brain radiation, especially in elderly patients. Approximately one-half of patients with ocular involvement eventually develop CNS involvement, prompting some specialists to use prophylactic treatment of the CNS even in cases of seemingly isolated ocular disease.

Itty S, Pulido JS. Rituximab for intraocular lymphoma. *Retina.* 2009;29(2):129–132.

Prognosis

The prognosis for survival depends on whether there is CNS involvement. Despite the availability of multiple treatment modalities and regimens, the long-term prognosis for

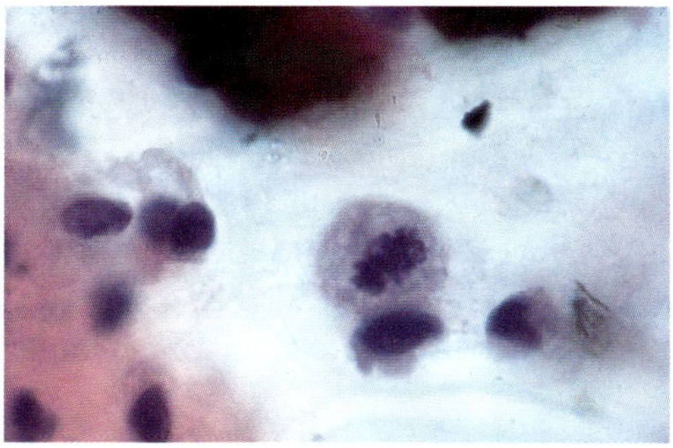

Figure 9-2 Vitreous aspirate showing mitotic figure and cellular atypia in large cell lymphoma. *(Courtesy of E. Mitchel Opremcak, MD.)*

patients with PCNSL remains poor; the median survival with supportive care alone is 2–3 months, and with surgery alone, median survival is in the range of 1–5 months. The longest median survival in various reports approaches 40 months with treatment. Factors that negatively influence outcome include advanced age, worse neurologic functional classification level, multiple rather than single lesions present in the CNS, and deep nuclei/periventricular lesions rather than superficial cerebral and cerebellar hemispheric lesions.

Chan CC, Rubenstein JL, Coupland SE, et al. Primary vitreoretinal lymphoma: a report from an international primary central nervous system lymphoma collaborative group symposium. *Oncologist.* 2011;16(11):1589–1599.

Raparia K, Chang CC, Chévez-Barrios P. Intraocular lymphoma: diagnostic approach and immunophenotypic findings in vitrectomy specimens. *Arch Pathol Lab Med.* 2009; 133(8):1233–1237.

Read RW, Zamir E, Rao NA. Neoplastic masquerade syndromes. *Surv Ophthalmol.* 2002; 47(2):81–124.

Rothova A, Ooijman F, Kerkhoff F, Van der Lelij A, Lokhorst HM. Uveitis masquerade syndromes. *Ophthalmology.* 2001;108(2):386–399.

Sen HN, Bodaghi B, Hoang PL, Nussenblatt R. Primary intraocular lymphoma: diagnosis and differential diagnosis. *Ocul Immunol Inflamm.* 2009;17(3):133–141.

Zaldivar RA, Martin DF, Holden JT, Grossniklaus HE. Primary intraocular lymphoma: clinical, cytologic, and flow cytometric analysis. *Ophthalmology.* 2004;111(9):1762–1767.

Neoplastic Masquerade Syndromes Secondary to Systemic Lymphoma

Though rare, systemic lymphomas can spread hematogenously to the choroid, the subretinal space, the vitreous, and the anterior chamber. These entities can present with a pseudohypopyon, vitritis, creamy subretinal infiltrates, retinal vasculitis, necrotizing retinitis, and diffuse choroiditis or uveal masses. All T-lymphocyte lymphomas can present in this fashion.

Neoplastic Masquerade Syndromes Secondary to Leukemia

Patients with leukemia may have retinal findings, including intraretinal hemorrhages, cotton-wool spots, white-centered hemorrhages, microaneurysms, and peripheral neovascularization. In rare instances, leukemic cells may invade the vitreous cavity. If the choroid is involved, exudative retinal detachment may be present and is angiographically similar to Vogt-Koyanagi-Harada (VKH) syndrome. Leukemia may also present with a hypopyon or hyphema, iris heterochromia, or a pseudohypopyon, which can be gray-yellow.

Neoplastic Masquerade Syndromes Secondary to Uveal Lymphoid Proliferations

The uveal tract may be a site for benign reactive uveal lymphoid hyperplasia that can mimic chronic uveitis. Presenting symptoms may include vision loss that is gradual, painless, and unilateral or bilateral. Early-stage disease shows multifocal creamy choroidal lesions that may mimic sarcoid uveitis or birdshot uveitis. Cystoid macular edema (CME) may be present. Anterior uveitis with acute symptoms of pain, redness, and photophobia may also be present. Glaucoma and elevated intraocular pressure (IOP) are common. Angle structures may be infiltrated by lymphocytes, resulting in elevation of IOP. There may be overlap in presentation with posterior scleritis and uveal effusion syndrome.

Fleshy episcleral or conjunctival masses that may appear salmon-pink may be present. Unlike subconjunctival lymphomas, these masses are not mobile and are attached firmly to the sclera. Biopsy specimens demonstrate mature lymphocytes and plasma cells, quite different from the appearance of specimens with PCNSL.

Therapy using corticosteroids, radiation, or both has been used with variable results. Systemic and periocular corticosteroid therapy can lead to rapid regression of the lesions, as can external-beam radiation.

Nonlymphoid Malignancies

Uveal melanoma

Approximately 5% of patients with uveal melanoma present with signs of ocular inflammation, including episcleritis, anterior or posterior uveitis, or panuveitis. Most tumors that present in this fashion are epithelioid-cell or mixed-cell choroidal melanomas. Ultrasonography is useful in diagnosing atypical cases because of the characteristically low internal reflectivity of these lesions. Management of uveal melanomas is discussed in BCSC Section 4, *Ophthalmic Pathology and Intraocular Tumors.*

Retinoblastoma

Approximately 1%–3% of retinoblastomas may present with the appearance of inflammation, caused primarily by the relatively rare variant of diffuse infiltrating retinoblastoma. Patients are usually between age 4 and 6 years at presentation. These cases can be diagnostically confusing because of the limited visibility of the fundus and the lack of calcification on radiography or ultrasonography. Patients may have conjunctival chemosis, pseudohypopyon, and vitritis. The pseudohypopyon typically shifts with changes in head position and is usually white as opposed to the yellowish color of inflammatory hypopyon.

Juvenile xanthogranuloma

Juvenile xanthogranuloma is the result of a histiocytic process affecting mainly the skin and eyes, and, in rare instances, viscera. Patients usually present before the age of 1 year with characteristic reddish-yellow skin lesions. Histologic investigation shows large histiocytes with foamy cytoplasm and Touton giant cells. Ocular lesions can involve the iris and result in a spontaneous hyphema. Iris biopsy samples show fewer foamy histiocytes and fewer Touton giant cells than do skin biopsy specimens. Other ocular structures may rarely be involved. If the skin of the eyelids is involved, the globe is usually spared. Intraocular lesions may respond to topical, periocular, or systemic corticosteroid therapy. Resistant cases may require local resection, radiation, or immunomodulatory therapy.

Zamir E, Wang RC, Krishnakumar S, Aiello Leverant A, Dugel PU, Rao NA. Juvenile xanthogranuloma masquerading as pediatric chronic uveitis: a clinicopathologic study. *Surv Ophthalmol.* 2001;46(2):164–171.

Metastatic Tumors

Most intraocular malignancies in adults are metastatic tumors. The most common primary cancers include lung and breast. Choroidal metastasis may be marked by vitritis, serous retinal detachment, and, occasionally, CME. These lesions are often bilateral and multifocal.

Anterior uveal metastasis may present with cells in the aqueous humor, iris nodules, rubeosis iridis, and elevated IOP. Anterior chamber paracentesis may help confirm the diagnosis. Retinal metastases are extremely rare. Primary cancers metastatic to the retina include cutaneous melanoma (the most common), followed by lung, gastrointestinal, and breast cancer. Metastatic melanoma often produces brown spherules in the retina, whereas other metastatic cancers appear white to yellow and may result in perivascular sheathing, simulating a retinal vasculitis or necrotizing retinitis.

Bilateral Diffuse Uveal Melanocytic Proliferation

Bilateral diffuse uveal melanocytic tumors have been associated with systemic malignancy. Such tumors can be accompanied by rapid vision loss, cataracts, multiple pigmented and nonpigmented placoid iris and choroidal nodules, and serous retinal detachments. This condition can mimic VKH syndrome. Histologic investigation shows diffuse infiltration of the uveal tract by benign nevoid or spindle-shaped cells. Necrosis within the tumors may be present, and scleral involvement is common. The cause of this entity is unknown. Treatment should be directed at finding and treating the underlying primary lesion.

Nonneoplastic Masquerade Syndromes

Retinitis Pigmentosa

Patients with retinitis pigmentosa (RP) often have variable numbers of vitreous and anterior chamber cells and can develop CME. Features of RP that differentiate it from uveitis include nyctalopia, positive family history, and on fundus examination, waxy disc pallor, attenuation of arterioles, and a bone-spicule pattern of pigmentary changes in the midperiphery. Electroretinographic responses of patients with RP often appear severely depressed or extinguished, even early in the disease. However, these findings can be found in late posterior uveitis, making differentiation between the entities very difficult in some cases. See BCSC Section 12, *Retina and Vitreous,* for additional information.

Ocular Ischemic Syndrome

Ocular ischemic syndrome results from hypoperfusion of the entire eye and sometimes the orbit, usually because of carotid artery obstruction. Patients with ocular ischemic syndrome are typically men aged 65 years or older. Patients present with decreased vision and mild ocular pain. Examination findings may include corneal edema, anterior chamber cells, and moderate flare, the latter often greater than and out of proportion to the number of cells. Anterior segment neovascularization may be present. IOP may be low from decreased aqueous production due to ischemia or high due to neovascular glaucoma. A cataract may be more prominent on the involved side. The vitreous is usually clear. Dilated fundus examination may show mild disc edema associated with dilated tortuous retinal venules, narrowed artcriolcs, and medium to large intraretinal scattered blot hemorrhages in the midperiphery and far periphery of the retina. Neovascularization may be present on the disc or elsewhere in the retina.

Fluorescein angiography shows delayed arteriolar filling, diffuse leakage in the posterior pole as well as from the optic disc, and signs of capillary nonperfusion. Retinal vascular staining may be present in the absence of any physical vascular sheathing on examination.

Diagnostic studies include carotid Doppler ultrasonography; ipsilateral carotid stenosis greater than 90% supports the diagnosis of ocular ischemic syndrome.

Definitive treatment involves carotid endarterectomy. Local treatment consists of topical corticosteroids and cycloplegics, as well as panretinal photocoagulation, especially if rubeosis or retinal neovascularization is present. Intraocular injection of vascular endothelial growth factor (VEGF) inhibitors may also be considered. The 5-year mortality rate of patients with ocular ischemic syndrome is 40%, primarily from cardiovascular disease and myocardial infarction. The visual prognosis is guarded, and many patients improve transiently with treatment but eventually worsen.

Mendrinos E, Machinis TG, Pournaras CJ. Ocular ischemic syndrome. *Surv Ophthalmol.* 2010;55(1):2–34.

Chronic Peripheral Rhegmatogenous Retinal Detachment

Chronic peripheral rhegmatogenous retinal detachment can be associated with anterior segment cell and flare and vitreous inflammatory and pigment cells. Patients often have good vision that can sometimes deteriorate because of CME. Careful dilated fundus examination with scleral depression is of paramount importance in establishing the diagnosis. Findings may include peripheral pigment demarcation lines, subretinal fluid, retinal breaks, subretinal fibrosis, and peripheral retinal cysts. Photoreceptor outer segments liberated from the subretinal space may be present in the anterior chamber, simulating inflammatory cells. In such situations, IOP may be elevated, as these photoreceptor outer segments are phagocytosed by the endothelial cells in the trabecular meshwork, resulting in secondary open-angle glaucoma. This condition is called *Schwartz syndrome.*

Schwartz A. Chronic open-angle glaucoma secondary to rhegmatogenous retinal detachment. *Am J Ophthalmol.* 1973;75(2):205–211.

Intraocular Foreign Bodies

Retained intraocular foreign bodies may produce chronic intraocular inflammation as the result of mechanical, chemical, toxic, or inflammatory irritation of uveal tissues (particularly the ciliary body). A high index of suspicion followed by a careful history; clinical examination; and ancillary testing, including gonioscopy, ultrasonography, and CT of the eye and orbits, are essential. If this condition is suspected and recognized quickly, identification and removal of the foreign body often results in a cure. If the diagnosis is delayed, ocular complications such as proliferative vitreoretinopathy and endophthalmitis result in a poorer visual prognosis.

Pigment Dispersion Syndrome

Pigment dispersion syndrome is characterized by pigment granules that have been released from the iris, ciliary body, or both and are floating in the anterior chamber; these granules may be confused with the cells of anterior uveitis. Refer to BCSC Section 10, *Glaucoma,* for a complete discussion.

Other Syndromes

Certain infectious uveitic entities may also be mistaken for immunologic uveitis. Thus, nonneoplastic masquerade syndromes can also include bacterial uveitis caused by infection with *Nocardia* species or *Tropheryma whipplei* (Whipple disease), as well as fungal endophthalmitis due to infection with *Candida* species, *Aspergillus* species, or *Coccidioides immitis.* These entities are discussed in Chapter 7 and Chapter 8.

CHAPTER 10

Complications of Uveitis

This chapter includes a related video, which can be accessed by scanning the QR code provided in the text or going to www.aao.org/bcscvideo_section09.

Calcific Band Keratopathy

Patients with chronic uveitis, especially children, may develop calcium deposition along the epithelial basement membrane and the Bowman layer, a condition termed *band keratopathy.* This complication may arise within months of onset of the uveitis. These calcium deposits are usually located in the interpalpebral zone. Calcific band keratopathy may become visually significant when it extends into the visual axis, or it may cause symptoms of foreign body sensation; in such cases, removal may be required. The calcium deposits are located beneath the corneal epithelium; thus, their removal requires epithelial debridement followed by chelation with disodium ethylenediaminetetraacetic acid (EDTA). Recurrences may require repeat EDTA treatments. Photorefractive keratotomy can also be considered.

Cataracts

Any eye with chronic or recurrent uveitis may develop cataract as a result of the inflammation or the corticosteroids used for treatment. Indications for cataract surgery in uveitic eyes are the same as for all cataracts: when the cataract causes functional impairment that interferes with activities of daily living; when the cataract is responsible for at least a portion of that visual decrease; and when functional improvement is likely to occur after cataract extraction (a particularly important consideration in children who may develop amblyopia). Additional considerations for cataract surgery in uveitic eyes are whether a cataract precludes the clinician from obtaining an adequate view of the fundus—thereby inhibiting appropriate monitoring of posterior segment disease or health—and the degree to which the uveitis has been controlled.

As mentioned previously, careful preoperative evaluation is necessary to ascertain whether the cataract is actually contributing to visual dysfunction. Vision loss in uveitis may stem from a variety of other ocular complications of uveitis, including corneal or vitreous opacity, cystoid macular edema, macular scarring, and glaucoma.

Studies have shown that phacoemulsification with posterior chamber (in-the-bag) intraocular lens (IOL) implantation effectively improves vision and is well tolerated in many eyes with uveitis, even over long periods. Excellent surgical and visual results have been reported for eyes with Fuchs heterochromic uveitis. Cataract surgery in other types of uveitis—including uveitis associated with sarcoidosis, herpes simplex virus, herpes zoster, syphilis, toxoplasmosis, spondyloarthropathies, and juvenile idiopathic arthritis (JIA); idiopathic uveitis; and pars planitis—can be more problematic, although such surgery may also yield very good results.

Management

Uveitic eyes are at greater risk for postoperative complications than nonuveitic eyes. Thus, careful planning for surgery, including preoperative medical management and the timing of the procedure, is of utmost importance. The key to a successful visual outcome is meticulous long-term control of inflammation before proceeding with surgery. Common advice is to achieve the best control possible without flare-ups for at least 3 months prior to cataract surgery. The rationale is to ensure the eye is stable on the current medical regimen and the tissues are allowed to recover from prior inflammation before the eye is challenged with a surgical procedure that can lead to a profound postoperative inflammatory response. The recommendation for maintenance of maximum control for at least 3 months before surgery is based on retrospective clinical case series and clinical experience; no prospective or controlled trials provide definitive data. As such, exceptions may be made when the considered opinion of the treating physician is that a delay in surgery is not indicated, for example, in eyes with mild uveitis without sequelae, in disorders that have a good surgical prognosis (eg, Fuchs heterochromic uveitis), or under special circumstances such as lens-induced uveitis or the need to view the posterior segment (eg, to repair a rhegmatogenous retinal detachment). It should be noted that the "best control possible" is not achieved by incomplete control with corticosteroids alone. The clinician must utilize all appropriate means for control, including immunosuppression if needed. If the clinician is uncomfortable with such means of treatment, then referral to a specialist with that experience is required before proceeding with cataract surgery.

Once appropriate control is achieved, preoperative pulsing with oral corticosteroids (0.5–1.0 mg/kg/day, usually for 3 days—although opinions vary as to dose and duration) and/or intensive topical corticosteroid treatment should be considered. Dosages may be tapered over weeks to months after surgery, based on the severity of the underlying uveitis before surgery and the postoperative inflammatory response. Postoperative use of nonsteroidal anti-inflammatory drugs (NSAIDs) has not been studied in eyes with uveitis but is frequently employed in nonuveitic eyes that are undergoing cataract surgery, with the goal of preventing cystoid macular edema (CME). Corneal toxicity from topical NSAIDs used concurrently with topical corticosteroids is a concern. Patients with certain infectious uveitides (eg, uveitis caused by *Toxoplasma gondii* infection and herpetic uveitis) may require perioperative prophylactic antimicrobial therapy to prevent surgically induced recurrence; in such situations, preoperative oral corticosteroids are usually not given.

Cataract surgery in uveitic eyes is generally more complex than in nonuveitic eyes because of the potential presence of sequelae of uveitis, including posterior synechiae, pupillary membranes, corneal edema or opacity, and hypotony. Entrance into the eye using a clear corneal approach is often used and may be particularly desirable in cases of scleritis that may be prone to postoperative scleral necrosis. Posterior synechiae and pupillary miosis may require mechanical or viscoelastic pupil stretching, sphincterotomies, or the use of flexible iris retractors (Video 10-1).

VIDEO 10-1 Synechiolysis, placement of iris dilator, and capsular staining in a uveitic cataract (07:15).
Courtesy of Russell W. Read, MD, PhD.
Scan the QR code or access the video at www.aao.org/bcscvideo_section09.

A continuous curvilinear capsulorrhexis is preferred, as it appears to reduce posterior synechiae formation, reduces the risk of posterior capsular tear, and facilitates placement of IOL haptics in the capsular bag. A fibrotic anterior capsule may be more difficult to open with a capsulorrhexis. Zonular insufficiency may be present, which may make phacoemulsification and lens implantation challenging or impossible. In such cases, there may be few alternatives, and the surgeon's preference may be to perform pars plana lensectomy and vitrectomy and avoid placing an IOL because of the lack of capsular support or zonular dehiscence. Fortunately, this scenario is rare. Meticulous cortical cleanup is important to avoid leaving behind potentially proinflammatory material in the eye. For intraocular lens choice, many surgeons prefer hydrophobic acrylic posterior chamber IOLs placed in the capsular bag. The possibility of future vitreoretinal surgery with silicone oil should be considered when deciding whether to use silicone IOLs. At the conclusion of the surgery, periocular or intravitreal corticosteroids may be administered. Postoperatively, immunomodulation is continued and supplemented with liberal use of topical corticosteroids, which are slowly tapered.

Phacoemulsification with IOL implantation can also be done in conjunction with pars plana vitrectomy if clinical or ultrasonographic findings suggest the presence of substantial vision-limiting vitreous debris or macular pathology such as epiretinal membranes. When there has been significant structural damage from inflammation, or in cases in which the surgical prognosis is more guarded—for example, in JIA-associated uveitis—vitrectomy and aphakia may be the best course. Relative contraindications for IOL implantation include the prior development of rubeosis, a history of extensive membrane formation, and hypotony, although even in these circumstances, an IOL may be used in select cases. There is controversy regarding IOL placement in children with JIA-associated uveitic cataracts. Avoiding aphakia in children is desirable but may not always be in the best interest of the patient. Choosing the proper IOL power, especially in children under the age of 10 years, is difficult because of normal ocular/orbital growth. Regardless, the most important step in the treatment of these children is stringent control of preoperative and postoperative intraocular inflammation using corticosteroids and immunomodulatory therapy (IMT). If IOLs are used, in-the-bag implantation of acrylic IOLs and primary posterior capsulorrhexis are preferred in children. Some surgeons may also perform a core anterior vitrectomy through the posterior capsulorrhexis prior to IOL placement. Administration of intraocular corticosteroids at the end of the procedure is extremely useful for controlling postoperative inflammation and CME. Using these methods, 75% of patients will obtain a visual acuity of better than 20/40.

Complications

Close monitoring with immediate attention to any postoperative increase in inflammation or complications is imperative. Visual compromise following phacoemulsification with posterior chamber lens implantation in patients with uveitis is usually attributed to posterior segment abnormalities, most commonly CME. Postoperative CME rates may be reduced through the use of perioperative corticosteroids and with delay of surgery until the uveitis has been controlled for at least 3 months. The postoperative course may also be complicated by the recurrence or exacerbation of uveitis. The incidence of posterior capsule opacification is higher in uveitic than nonuveitic eyes, leading to earlier use of Nd:YAG laser capsulotomy. In some uveitic conditions such as pars planitis, inflammatory debris may accumulate and membranes may form on the surface of the IOL. Strict control of inflammation remains paramount to reducing the chance of these deposits. Long-term administration of topical corticosteroids may be necessary. Despite aggressive use of IMT, inflammatory cocooning of the IOL–lens capsule complex and uncontrolled inflammation may necessitate IOL explantation in 5%–10% of patients. Frequent follow-up, a high index of suspicion, and aggressive IMT can optimize short- and long-term visual results.

Adán A, Gris O, Pelegrin L, Torras J, Corretger X. Explantation of intraocular lenses in children with juvenile idiopathic arthritis–associated uveitis. *J Cataract Refract Surg.* 2009; 35(3):603–605.

Bélair ML, Kim SJ, Thorne JE, et al. Incidence of cystoid macular edema after cataract surgery in patients with and without uveitis using optical coherence tomography. *Am J Ophthalmol.* 2009;148(1):128–135.

Jancevski M, Foster CS. Cataracts and uveitis. *Curr Opin Ophthalmol.* 2010;21(1):10–14.

Nemet AY, Raz J, Sachs D, et al. Primary intraocular lens implantation in pediatric uveitis: a comparison of 2 populations. *Arch Ophthalmol.* 2007;125(3):354–360.

Quiñones K, Cervantes-Castañeda RA, Hynes AY, Daoud YJ, Foster CS. Outcomes of cataract surgery in children with chronic uveitis. *J Cataract Refract Surg.* 2009;35(4):725–731.

Glaucoma

Elevated intraocular pressure (IOP) in uveitic eyes may be acute, chronic, or recurrent. In eyes with long-term ciliary body inflammation, the IOP may fluctuate between abnormally high and low values. Numerous morphologic, cellular, and biochemical alterations occur in the uveitic eye that cause uveitic glaucoma and ocular hypertension. Successful management of uveitic glaucoma and ocular hypertension requires the identification and treatment of each of these contributing factors.

Elevation of IOP to levels above 24 mm Hg increases the risk of glaucoma. Most practitioners tend to treat eyes with IOP greater than 30 mm Hg, even without evidence of glaucomatous optic nerve damage. Assessment of patients with uveitis and elevated IOP should include the same measures taken as for any case of ocular hypertension: slit-lamp and dilated fundus examination, gonioscopy, evaluation of the optic nerve head with disc photographs and optical coherence tomography (OCT), and serial automated visual fields.

Uveitic Ocular Hypertension

Unilateral uveitis of sudden onset with open angles and increased IOP may be of infectious origin, particularly from viral causes but also toxoplasma. Thus, in the presence of active inflammation early in the course of uveitis, clinicians should resist the urge to prematurely taper corticosteroids because of a fear of corticosteroid-induced ocular hypertension. Corticosteroid-induced ocular hypertension rarely occurs before 3 weeks after the initiation of corticosteroid therapy. Early IOP elevations with active inflammation are almost always caused by inflammation that requires aggressive anti-inflammatory treatment.

Uveitic Glaucoma

Uveitic glaucoma often results from a combination of mechanisms. Glaucoma associated with uveitis is best classified by morphologic changes in angle structure; thus, uveitic glaucoma may be divided into secondary angle-closure and secondary open-angle glaucoma. These entities may be further subdivided into acute and chronic types. In addition, corticosteroid-induced ocular hypertension and glaucoma are other components that must be addressed in cases of chronic uveitic glaucoma. Gonioscopic evaluation of the peripheral angle, optic nerve evaluation with disc photographs, imaging to evaluate the nerve fiber layer, and automated visual fields are essential in the evaluation of patients with uveitic glaucoma. See also BCSC Section 10, *Glaucoma*.

Secondary angle-closure glaucoma

Acute Acute secondary angle-closure glaucoma may occur when choroidal inflammation results in forward rotation of the ciliary body and lens–iris diaphragm. It can be the presenting sign of Vogt-Koyanagi-Harada (VKH) syndrome or sympathetic ophthalmia. Patients present with pain, elevated IOP, and no posterior synechiae. Ultrasound biomicroscopy (UBM) or ultrasound evaluation showing choroidal thickening and anterior rotation of the ciliary body is diagnostic. Treatment is with aggressive corticosteroid therapy, aqueous suppressants, and cycloplegia to induce a posterior rotation of the ciliary body. As the inflammation subsides, the chamber deepens and the IOP normalizes. Peripheral iridotomy or iridectomy is not useful in these acute cases because the underlying cause is not pupillary block.

Subacute Chronic or acute recurrent anterior segment inflammation may result in the formation of circumferential posterior synechiae with pupillary block due to seclusion of the pupil and resultant iris bombé, producing secondary peripheral angle closure. Whereas synechiae formation usually occurs over time, the development of iris bombé may be an acute event. Peripheral laser iridotomy or surgical iridectomy results in resolution of the bombé and angle closure if performed before permanent peripheral anterior synechiae form. Iridotomies should be multiple, created as large as possible. Exacerbation of inflammation can be anticipated after laser iridotomy in these eyes, making the iridotomies prone to close and requiring re-treatment or surgical iridectomy. Intensive topical corticosteroid and cycloplegic therapy is given following the procedure. In patients with brown irides, pretreatment of the iris with an argon laser before using the Nd:YAG laser may lessen the chance of bleeding and facilitate a wider opening. If laser iridotomy is not successful, surgical iridectomy is required. The procedure may be supplemented with goniosynechialysis if peripheral anterior synechiae have started to develop, but this approach is controversial.

Chronic In addition to posterior synechiae, chronic intraocular inflammation may result in peripheral anterior synechiae and chronic secondary angle-closure glaucoma. Eyes with these complications often have chronic secondary open-angle glaucoma and corticosteroid-induced glaucoma superimposed. Topical aqueous suppressants may be inadequate to prevent progression of optic nerve head damage. These eyes may require goniosynechialysis and trabeculectomy with mitomycin C or placement of a glaucoma drainage device.

Secondary open-angle glaucoma

Acute Inflammatory open-angle glaucoma occurs when the trabecular meshwork is inflamed (trabeculitis), as commonly occurs with infectious causes of uveitis such as toxoplasma retinochoroiditis, necrotizing herpetic retinitis, herpes simplex and varicella-zoster anterior uveitis, cytomegalovirus anterior uveitis (including the Posner-Schlossman type), sarcoid uveitis, and Fuchs heterochromic uveitis (rubella-associated) or when inflammatory debris clogs the angle. This type of glaucoma usually responds to specific treatment of the infectious agent supplemented by topical cycloplegics and corticosteroids.

Chronic Chronic outflow obstruction is caused by direct damage to the trabecular meshwork. The management of chronic secondary open-angle glaucoma is similar to that of primary open-angle glaucoma (see BCSC Section 10, *Glaucoma*), with the added complexity of maintaining strict control of intraocular inflammation through the use of IMT.

Combined-mechanism uveitic glaucoma

Multiple mechanisms may be responsible for elevated pressure in uveitic eyes. Treatment should be aimed at controlling the inflammation and IOP through a multimodal approach, including both medical and surgical therapy aimed at the responsible mechanisms.

Corticosteroid-Induced Ocular Hypertension and Glaucoma

Elevated IOP in the setting of uveitis should prompt consideration of whether the cause is one of the aforementioned angle issues or is corticosteroid induced. Corticosteroids in any formulation—topical, periocular, intraocular (injection and sustained release), or oral—may induce an elevation of IOP that may be difficult to distinguish from other causes of ocular hypertension in uveitis. Use of the fluocinolone intraocular implant is associated with an eventual need for glaucoma surgery in approximately 40% of eyes. Difluprednate used topically also appears to be associated with severe and sometimes rapid increases in IOP. This IOP rise may be avoided by use of a less-potent topical corticosteroid preparation, a less-frequent administration schedule, or both. Fluorometholone, loteprednol, and rimexolone may be less likely to induce an IOP elevation but are also less effective in controlling intraocular inflammation.

Management

Medical management of uveitic glaucoma requires aggressive control of both intraocular inflammation and IOP as well as prevention of glaucomatous optic nerve damage and visual field loss (see BCSC Section 10, *Glaucoma*). Aqueous suppressants are generally the first-line agents. Prostaglandin analogues may be used to treat uveitic glaucoma and generally do not exacerbate intraocular inflammation, especially when used concomitantly with IMT and corticosteroids. However, caution should be used in eyes with herpetic uveitis. Use of pilocarpine should be avoided in uveitis, as the smaller fixed pupil may be at risk for worsening of posterior synechiae, and pilocarpine causes breakdown of the blood–aqueous barrier.

When medical management fails, glaucoma filtering surgery is indicated. Standard trabeculectomy has a greater risk of failure in these eyes. Results may be improved by using mitomycin C with intensive topical corticosteroids. However, intense and recurrent postoperative inflammation can often lead to failure of filtering surgery in uveitic eyes. Up to 90% of patients 1 year after surgery and approximately 62% 5 years after surgery achieve IOP control with 1 or 0 medications. Surgical complications include cataract formation, bleb leakage (early and late) that could lead to endophthalmitis, and choroidal effusions. Because peripheral iridectomy is performed with trabeculectomy, the excised trabecular block and iris should be submitted for pathologic evaluation.

Alternatives to classic trabeculectomy are numerous and have been used with some short-term success in uveitic glaucoma. Nonpenetrating deep sclerectomy with or without a drainage implant has been shown effective in controlling IOP in up to 90% of uveitic eyes for 1 year after surgery. Among pediatric uveitis patients, goniotomy has up to a 75% chance of reducing IOP to 21 mm Hg or less after 2 surgeries. This procedure may be complicated by transient hyphema and worsening of the preexisting cataract. Trabeculodialysis and laser sclerostomy have high rates of failure because of recurrent postoperative inflammation. Viscocanalostomy has shown higher success rates in a limited number of studies.

Most cases of uveitic glaucoma, especially in pseudophakic or aphakic eyes, require aqueous drainage devices. These devices may be tunneled into the anterior chamber or placed through the pars plana directly into the vitreous cavity. A unidirectional valve design (valve implant) can prevent postoperative hypotony. These implants are more likely than trabeculectomy to successfully control IOP in the long term; results indicate up to a 75% reduction of IOP from preoperative levels and that nearly 75% of patients achieve target IOP levels with use of 0 or 1 topical antiglaucoma medication after 4 years. Complications of glaucoma-drainage-device surgery (10%/patient-year) include shallow anterior chamber, hypotony, suprachoroidal hemorrhage, and blockage of the drainage device by blood, fibrin, or iris. Long-term complications include device erosion through the conjunctiva, valve migration, corneal decompensation, drainage device–cornea touch, and retinal detachment. Unlike trabeculectomy, these drainage devices have proven to be robust and continue to function despite chronic, recurrent inflammation; they provide excellent long-term IOP control in eyes with uveitic glaucoma.

Cyclodestructive procedures may worsen ocular inflammation and lead to hypotony and phthisis bulbi. Laser trabeculoplasty is generally considered ineffective in eyes with uveitis.

As with all surgeries in uveitic eyes, tight and meticulous control of perioperative inflammation—including the use of preoperative regimens similar to those used before cataract surgery as well as of immunomodulators and corticosteroids—not only improves the success of glaucoma surgery but also improves visual acuity outcomes by limiting sight-threatening complications such as CME and hypotony. Additional details and information on newer surgical procedures for uveitic glaucoma are described in BCSC Section 10, *Glaucoma.*

Fortuna E, Cervantes-Castañeda RA, Bhat P, Doctor P, Foster CS. Flare-up rates with bimatoprost therapy in uveitic glaucoma. *Am J Ophthalmol.* 2008;146(6):876–882.

Heinz C, Koch JM, Heiligenhaus A. Transscleral diode laser cyclophotocoagulation as primary surgical treatment for secondary glaucoma in juvenile idiopathic arthritis: high failure rate after short term follow up. *Br J Ophthalmol.* 2006;90(6):737–740.

Kafkala C, Hynes A, Choi J, Topalkara A, Foster CS. Ahmed valve implantation for uncontrolled pediatric uveitic glaucoma. *J AAPOS.* 2005;9(4):336–340.

Markomichelakis NN, Kostakou A, Halkiadakis I, Chalkidou S, Papakonstantinou D, Georgopoulos G. Efficacy and safety of latanoprost in eyes with uveitic glaucoma. *Graefes Arch Clin Exp Ophthalmol.* 2009;247(6):775–780.

Moorthy RS, Mermoud A, Baerveldt G, Minckler DS, Lee PP, Rao NA. Glaucoma associated with uveitis. *Surv Ophthalmol.* 1997;41(5):361–394.

Noble J, Derzko-Dzulynsky L, Rabinovitch T, Birt C. Outcome of trabeculectomy with intraoperative mitomycin C for uveitic glaucoma. *Can J Ophthalmol.* 2007;42(1):89–94.

Papadaki TG, Zacharopoulos IP, Pasquale LR, Christen WB, Netland PA, Foster CS. Long-term results of Ahmed glaucoma valve implantation for uveitic glaucoma. *Am J Ophthalmol.* 2007;144(1):62–69.

Hypotony

Acute inflammation of the ciliary body may cause aqueous hyposecretion and low IOP. This reduction in IOP is reversible with control of intraocular inflammation. In contrast, chronic inflammation may lead to ciliary body damage and atrophy of the ciliary processes, resulting in permanent hypotony. Serous choroidal detachment often accompanies hypotony and complicates management. Prolonged choroidal effusions may require surgical drainage. Chronic hypotony in long-standing uveitis may be helped by surgery if there is ciliary body traction from a cyclitic membrane that can be released and if the ciliary processes are preserved (as shown on UBM). If ciliary processes are atrophic, vitrectomy with intraocular silicone oil or viscoelastic may help maintain ocular anatomy and increase IOP. In some of these cases, visual improvement after surgery can be significant; these gains may, however, be transient. Hypotony recurs in nearly one-half of eyes, requiring reinjection of silicone oil between 1 and 3 times over 1 year.

de Smet MD, Gunning F, Feenstra R. The surgical management of chronic hypotony due to uveitis. *Eye (Lond).* 2005;19(1):60–64.

Kapur R, Birnbaum AD, Goldstein DA, et al. Treating uveitis-associated hypotony with pars plana vitrectomy and silicone oil injection. *Retina.* 2010;30(1):140–145.

Tosi GM, Schiff W, Barile G, Yoshida N, Chang S. Management of severe hypotony with intravitreal injection of viscoelastic. *Am J Ophthalmol.* 2005;140(5):952–954.

Cystoid Macular Edema

Cystoid macular edema is a common cause of vision loss in eyes with uveitis. CME is usually caused by active intraocular inflammation and appears to be mediated by the pro-inflammatory cytokines vascular endothelial growth factor (VEGF) and interleukin-6, which cause retinal vascular leakage and retinal pigment endothelium dysfunction. Less commonly, CME may be caused by mechanical vitreomacular traction; the distinction can be differentiated by OCT. CME can also be quantitatively evaluated and monitored by serial spectral-domain OCT and fluorescein angiography studies. The severity of CME does not necessarily correspond to the level of inflammatory disease activity. CME is often slow to respond and clear and frequently remains even after visible, active inflammation has resolved. Smoking appears to be associated with a greater prevalence of CME, especially in patients with intermediate uveitis and panuveitis.

Treatment of CME must first be directed toward control of intraocular inflammation. If CME persists despite control of inflammation, therapy directed specifically toward the CME is required. This treatment may be regional or systemic. Periocular injections of corticosteroid may be used; a superotemporal posterior sub-Tenon injection of 20–40 mg of triamcinolone acetonide is preferred. Theoretically, this technique delivers juxtascleral corticosteroid closest to the macula. The injections may be repeated monthly. If CME persists, then 2–4 mg of intravitreal preservative-free triamcinolone may be considered. Intravitreal triamcinolone can be highly effective in reducing CME, particularly in non-vitrectomized eyes, but its effect is time limited; the drug is eliminated more quickly from the vitreous cavity of vitrectomized eyes. Maximum visual improvement and reduction of CME after intravitreal triamcinolone injection occurs within 4 weeks. Eyes with a longer duration of uveitic CME and worse vision on presentation tend to show the least amount of visual improvement after treatment with intravitreal triamcinolone. Corticosteroid-induced elevation of IOP may occur in up to 40% of patients, especially in those younger than 40 years. Sustained delivery of corticosteroid to the vitreous cavity through the use of implants is also effective. Currently available implants in the United States include the fluocinolone acetonide implant and an intravitreal sustained-release drug-delivery system for dexamethasone (700 μg). The risk of ocular hypertension is lower for the dexamethasone delivery system than for the fluocinolone implant. Anti-VEGF therapies can also reduce inflammatory CME, but the action is of short duration and repeat injections are required. Intravitreal methotrexate (400 μg/0.1 mL) has been shown to be effective in reducing uveitic CME in a limited number of patients and is under active investigation. Additional information on the use of corticosteroids in the treatment of uveitis including CME can be found in Chapter 5.

Topical NSAIDs can be beneficial in treating pseudophakic CME, but their effectiveness in the treatment of uveitic CME has not been well established. Oral acetazolamide, 500 mg once or twice daily, has also been effective in reducing uveitic CME, particularly in patients whose inflammation is well controlled. Systemic interferon therapy has shown efficacy in resolving recalcitrant CME, with complete control in 62.5% of patients in one study. Common adverse effects include flulike symptoms.

Surgical therapy for uveitic CME is still controversial. Pars plana vitrectomy for uveitic CME in the presence of hyaloidal traction on the macula (as demonstrated on OCT imaging) may be visually and anatomically beneficial. In the absence of vitreomacular traction, however, the efficacy of pars plana vitrectomy in treating CME is not well understood. There is some suggestion that vitrectomy may be beneficial in managing recalcitrant uveitic CME, but this application requires further investigation.

Androudi S, Letko E, Meniconi M, Papadaki T, Ahmed M, Foster CS. Safety and efficacy of intravitreal triamcinolone acetonide for uveitic macular edema. *Ocul Immunol Inflamm.* 2005;13(2–3):205–212.

Angunawela RI, Heatley CJ, Williamson TH, et al. Intravitreal triamcinalone acetonide for refractory uveitic cystoid macular oedema: longterm management and outcome. *Acta Ophthalmol Scand.* 2005;83(5):595–599.

Becker M, Davis J. Vitrectomy in the treatment of uveitis. *Am J Ophthalmol.* 2005;140(6): 1096–1105.

Deuter CM, Kötter I, Günaydin I, Stübiger N, Doycheva DG, Zierhut M. Efficacy and tolerability of interferon alpha treatment in patients with chronic cystoid macular oedema due to non-infectious uveitis. *Br J Ophthalmol.* 2009;93(7):906–913.

Jennings T, Rusin MM, Tessler HH, Cunha-Vaz JG. Posterior sub-Tenon's injections of corticosteroids in uveitis patients with cystoid macular edema. *Jpn J Ophthalmol.* 1988; 32(4):385–391.

Kok H, Lau C, Maycock N, McCluskey P, Lightman S. Outcome of intravitreal triamcinolone in uveitis. *Ophthalmology.* 2005;112(11):1916.e1–e7.

Lin P, Loh AR, Margolis TP, Acharya NR. Cigarette smoking as a risk factor for uveitis. *Ophthalmology.* 2010;117(3):585–590.

Rothova A. Inflammatory cystoid macular edema. *Curr Opin Ophthalmol.* 2007;18(6): 487–492.

Schilling H, Heiligenhaus A, Laube T, Bornfeld N, Jurklies B. Long-term effect of acetazolamide treatment of patients with uveitic chronic cystoid macular edema is limited by persisting inflammation. *Retina.* 2005;25(2):182–188.

Taylor SR, Habot-Wilner Z, Pacheco P, Lightman SL. Intraocular methotrexate in the treatment of uveitis and uveitic cystoid macular edema. *Ophthalmology.* 2009;116(4): 797–801.

Tran TH, de Smet MD, Bodaghi B, Fardeau C, Cassoux N, Lehoang P. Uveitic macular oedema: correlation between optical coherence tomography patterns with visual acuity and fluorescein angiography. *Br J Ophthalmol.* 2008;92(7):922–927.

Vitreous Opacification and Vitritis

Vitreous opacification to a degree that vision is affected may occur in uveitis. Vitrectomy may improve visual acuity in these cases, with one review of studies on pars plana vitrectomy in uveitis showing visual acuity improved in 68%. A standard small (25- or 23-gauge) 3-port pars plana vitrectomy is the preferred technique, with a few minor variations. See BCSC Section 12, *Retina and Vitreous.*

Becker M, Davis J. Vitrectomy in the treatment of uveitis. *Am J Ophthalmol.* 2005;140(6): 1096–1105.

Davis JL, Miller DM, Ruiz P. Diagnostic testing of vitrectomy specimens. *Am J Ophthalmol.* 2005;140(5):822–829.

Manku H, McCluskey P. Diagnostic vitreous biopsy in patients with uveitis: a useful investigation? *Clin Experiment Ophthalmol.* 2005;33(6):604–610.

Rhegmatogenous Retinal Detachment

Rhegmatogenous retinal detachment (RRD) occurs in 3% of patients with uveitis. The high prevalence of RRD means that uveitis itself may be an independent risk factor for the condition. Panuveitis and infectious uveitis are the entities most frequently associated with RRD, although pars planitis and posterior uveitis can also be associated with rhegmatogenous or tractional retinal detachments. Uveitis is often still active in eyes that present with RRD. Up to 30% of patients with uveitis and RRD may have proliferative vitreoretinopathy (PVR) at presentation; this percentage is significantly higher than in primary RRD in patients without uveitis. Repair is often complicated by preexisting PVR, vitreous membranes, and poor visualization. Scleral buckling may still be useful in cases of retinal detachment associated with pars planitis. Acute retinal necrosis and cytomegalovirus retinitis frequently lead to retinal detachments that are difficult to repair because of multiple large posterior retinal breaks. Prophylactic laser treatment applied as soon as adequate visualization is possible may be desirable, but the rate of detachment is still high. Pars plana vitrectomy and endolaser treatment with internal silicone oil tamponade are required to repair the detachment. When PVR is present, combined scleral buckling and pars plana vitrectomy is often required to reattach the retina.

Kerkhoff FT, Lamberts QJ, van den Biesen PR, Rothova A. Rhegmatogenous retinal detachment and uveitis. *Ophthalmology.* 2003(2);110:427–431.

Nussenblatt RB, Whitcup SM. *Uveitis: Fundamentals and Clinical Practice.* 4th ed. Philadelphia, PA: Mosby; 2010.

Retinal and Choroidal Neovascularization

Retinal neovascularization is most often associated with pars planitis, sarcoid panuveitis, and retinal vasculitis of various causes, including Eales disease. Retinal neovascularization results from chronic inflammation or capillary nonperfusion. Treatment is directed toward the underlying etiology. The presence of uveitic retinal neovascularization does not always require panretinal photocoagulation. Some cases of sarcoid panuveitis, for example, may present with neovascularization of the disc that resolves completely with immunomodulatory and corticosteroid therapy alone. Thus, treatment must first be directed toward reduction of inflammation. If ischemia is angiographically extensive, as in retinal vasculitis or Eales disease, scatter laser photocoagulation in the ischemic areas is therapeutic. Dramatic regression of neovascularization of the disc and elsewhere in various inflammatory disorders typically occurs after 1 or 2 intravitreal injections of a VEGF inhibitor. This treatment may be used as an adjunct to IMT and scatter laser photocoagulation.

Choroidal neovascularization (CNV) can develop in uveitis as a result of a disruption of the Bruch membrane from choroidal inflammation and the presence of inflammatory cytokines that promote angiogenesis. The prevalence of CNV varies among different entities; for example, it can occur in up to 10% of patients with VKH syndrome. Patients present with metamorphopsia and scotoma, and diagnosis is based on clinical and angiographic findings. Treatment should be directed toward reducing inflammation as well as anatomical ablation of the CNV. Focal laser photocoagulation of peripapillary, extrafoveal, and juxtafoveal CNV may be performed. Treatment of subfoveal CNV is accomplished with VEGF inhibitors; results of one study showed that 2–3 intravitreal injections improved vision and reduced the size of subfoveal CNV in nearly all patients. Photodynamic therapy with verteporfin may also be a useful adjunct in some cases. Control of inflammation in these cases may reduce the risk of recurrence of CNV and the need for repeated intravitreal injections.

Doctor PP, Bhat P, Sayed R, Foster CS. Intravitreal bevacizumab for uveitic choroidal neovascularization. *Ocul Immunol Inflamm.* 2009;17(2):118–126.

Lott MN, Schiffman JC, Davis JL. Bevacizumab in inflammatory eye disease. *Am J Ophthalmol.* 2009;148(5):711–717.

Mansour AM, Arevalo JF, Ziemssen F, et al. Long-term visual outcomes of intravitreal bevacizumab in inflammatory ocular neovascularization. *Am J Ophthalmol.* 2009; 148(2):310–316.

O'Toole L, Tufail A, Pavesio C. Management of choroidal neovascularization in uveitis. *Int Ophthalmol Clin.* 2005;45(2):157–177.

Vision Rehabilitation

Despite optimal treatment, inflammatory disorders of the eye can lead to decreased vision. Worldwide, inflammatory disease is a significant cause of blindness and low vision. In the United States, 10% of all blindness is attributed to inadequately treated uveitis. Clinicians can assist their patients by inquiring if vision loss secondary to inflammation is affecting day-to-day functions, such as reading or enjoying leisure activities, and by advising patients about vision rehabilitation resources. Referral to vision rehabilitation is recommended for patients with visual acuity less than 20/40 in the better eye, reduced contrast sensitivity, disabling glare, or central or peripheral visual field loss (see BCSC Section 3, *Clinical Optics*). The SmartSight patient handout on the American Academy of Ophthalmology website (http://one.aao.org/smart-sight-low-vision) outlines how patients can identify vision rehabilitation resources in their community.

It is particularly important for clinicians to provide parents of children with uveitis information about rehabilitation to optimize functioning at school and in other activities. A useful guide for teachers and parents can be found at www.uveitis.org/patients/education/patient-guides.

American Academy of Ophthalmology Vision Rehabilitation Committee. Preferred Practice Pattern Guidelines. *Vision Rehabilitation.* San Francisco: American Academy of Ophthalmology; 2013. Available at: www.aao.org/ppp.

CHAPTER 11

Ocular Involvement in AIDS

Acquired immunodeficiency syndrome (AIDS) is caused by the human immunodeficiency virus (HIV), which infects and results in the depletion of $CD4^+$ helper T lymphocytes. This loss of $CD4^+$ T lymphocytes causes profound immune deficiency with subsequent opportunistic infections. Refer to BCSC Section 1, *Update on General Medicine,* for a full discussion of HIV infection and AIDS.

Ophthalmic Manifestations

Ophthalmic manifestations may be the first sign of disseminated systemic HIV infection and have been reported in up to 70% of infected people. These manifestations include

- HIV-related microangiopathy of the retina
- opportunistic viral, bacterial, and fungal infections
- Kaposi sarcoma of the eyelid and conjunctiva
- lymphomas involving the retina (primary intraocular lymphoma), adnexal structures, and orbit
- squamous cell carcinoma of the conjunctiva

Reports also suggest that HIV infection itself may cause anterior or intermediate uveitis that is not responsive to corticosteroids but improves with antiretroviral therapy.

HIV retinopathy is the most common ocular finding in patients infected with HIV. It is characterized by retinal hemorrhages, microaneurysms, and cotton-wool spots (Fig 11-1). HIV has been isolated from the human retina, and its antigen has been detected in retinal endothelial cells. It is thought that HIV endothelial infection and/or rheologic abnormalities may play a role in the development of cotton-wool spots and other vascular alterations. It has also been suggested that accelerated aging may be a part of HIV-associated eye disease, with earlier onset of macular degeneration and cataracts.

Other infectious agents that can affect the eye in HIV-infected patients include cytomegalovirus (CMV), herpes zoster virus, *Toxoplasma gondii, Mycobacterium tuberculosis, Mycobacterium avium-intracellulare, Cryptococcus neoformans, Pneumocystis jirovecii, Histoplasma capsulatum, Candida* species, molluscum contagiosum virus, microsporidia, and others. These pathogens can infect the ocular adnexa, anterior segment, or posterior segment. Visual morbidity, however, occurs primarily with posterior segment involvement, particularly retinitis caused by CMV, herpes zoster virus, or *T gondii.*

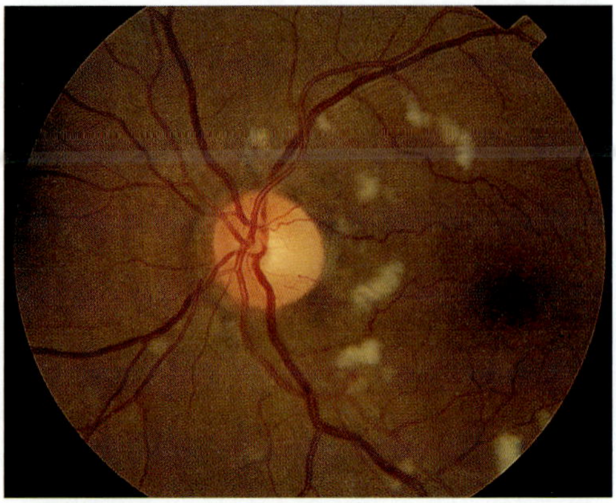

Figure 11-1 Fundus photograph of human immunodeficiency virus (HIV) retinopathy with numerous cotton-wool spots. *(Reprinted with permission from Cunningham ET Jr, Belfort R Jr.* HIV/AIDS and the Eye: A Global Perspective. Ophthalmology Monograph 15. *San Francisco, CA: American Academy of Ophthalmology; 2002:55.)*

Dadgostar H, Holland GN, Huang X, et al. Hemorheologic abnormalities associated with HIV infection: in vivo assessment of retinal microvascular blood flow. *Invest Ophthalmol Vis Sci.* 2006;47(9):3933–3938.

Kalyani PS, Fawzi AA, Gangaputra S, et al; Studies of the Ocular Complications of AIDS Research Group. Retinal vessel caliber among people with acquired immunodeficiency syndrome: relationships with visual function. *Am J Ophthalmol.* 2012;153(3):428–433.

Cytomegalovirus Retinitis

Before the availability of potent antiretroviral treatment regimens, disseminated CMV infection was the most common opportunistic infection in people with AIDS, and retinal infection was its most clinically important manifestation, occurring in up to 40% of patients with AIDS. CMV retinitis is found mostly in the eyes of individuals with $CD4^+$ counts of 50 cells/μL or less; it is now uncommon in areas where potent combination antiretroviral therapy is available. Even so, it remains the most common opportunistic ocular infection in patients with AIDS and occasionally is the first AIDS-defining infection found in an individual. Although CMV retinitis has become rare in regions where potent antiretroviral treatment is available, it is an increasing problem in the resource-limited world, particularly in Southeast Asia. See Chapter 7 for a full discussion of CMV retinitis.

Ford N, Shubber Z, Saranchuk P, et. al. Burden of HIV-related cytomegalovirus retinitis in resource-limited settings: a systematic review. *Clin Infect Dis.* 2013;57(9):1351–1361.

Immune recovery uveitis

Immune recovery uveitis (IRU) may occur in patients with previous CMV retinitis whose immune status improves with combination antiretroviral therapy. IRU occurs only in eyes infected with CMV and manifests as anterior or intermediate uveitis; the risk of developing IRU appears to be proportional to the surface area of retina involved.

A prospective study recorded IRU in 10% of patients with previous CMV retinitis. Immune recovery was defined as an increase in the $CD4^+$ T-lymphocyte count of at least 50 cells/μL to at least 100 cells/μL. IRU was associated with a CMV retinitis surface area of 25% or more. The likelihood of developing IRU was greater (odds ratio, 10.6) in patients who had ever been treated with cidofovir.

Eyes with IRU were more likely to have macular edema or epiretinal membrane. The macular edema can be resistant to treatment with sub-Tenon injections of depot corticosteroids, although such injections do not seem to cause reactivation of CMV infection. In contrast, intravitreal injections of corticosteroids must be avoided. IRU has been associated with moderate vision loss in the eyes in which it occurs but has not been linked to active replication of CMV or with the continuation or discontinuation of anti-CMV medication.

Retinal detachment

Retinal detachment occurs in up to 50% of patients with CMV retinitis. It may occur during active disease or after successful treatment. With potent antiretroviral regimens available, the rate of retinal detachment has been reduced to 0.06 per patient-year. Risk factors for developing retinal detachment include involvement of all 3 retinal zones, lower $CD4^+$ T-lymphocyte count, and more extensive retinitis. The retinal detachments in patients with CMV retinitis may be difficult to repair because of extensive retinal necrosis and multiple, often posterior, hole formation. Most of these detachments require pars plana vitrectomy with long-term silicone oil tamponade. Anatomical reattachment can be achieved in 90% of patients.

El-Bradey MH, Cheng L, Song MK, Torriani FJ, Freeman WR. Long-term results of treatment of macular complications in eyes with immune recovery uveitis using a graded treatment approach. *Retina.* 2004;24(3):376–382.

Holland GN, Vaudaux JD, Shiramizu KM, et al; Southern California HIV/Eye Consortium. Characteristics of untreated AIDS-related cytomegalovirus retinitis. II. Findings in the era of highly active antiretroviral therapy (1997 to 2000). *Am J Ophthalmol.* 2008;145(1):12–22.

Jabs DA, Van Natta ML, Thorne JE, et al; Studies of Ocular Complications of AIDS Research Group. Course of cytomegalovirus retinitis in the era of highly active antiretroviral therapy: 1. Retinitis progression. *Ophthalmology.* 2004;111(12):2224–2231.

Jabs DA, Van Natta ML, Thorne JE, et al; Studies of Ocular Complications of AIDS Research Group. Course of cytomegalovirus retinitis in the era of highly active antiretroviral therapy: 2. Second eye involvement and retinal detachment. *Ophthalmology.* 2004; 111(12):2232–2239.

Kempen JH, Min YI, Freeman WR, et al; Studies of Ocular Complications of AIDS Research Group. Risk of immune recovery uveitis in patients with AIDS and cytomegalovirus retinitis. *Ophthalmology.* 2006;113(4):684–694.

Schrier RD, Song MK, Smith IL, et al. Intraocular viral and immune pathogenesis of immune recovery uveitis in patients with healed cytomegalovirus retinitis. *Retina.* 2006;26(2):165–169.

Necrotizing Herpetic Retinitis

Patients with AIDS may develop necrotizing herpetic retinitis, which appears to manifest as a spectrum of disease; the severity is directly proportional to the level of immunologic compromise.

Progressive outer retinal necrosis (PORN)—a rare variant of necrotizing herpetic retinitis—may be caused by varicella-zoster virus or herpes simplex virus infections (Fig 11-2). It may occur in the absence of, at the same time as, or subsequent to a cutaneous varicella-zoster infection. (See also Chapter 7.)

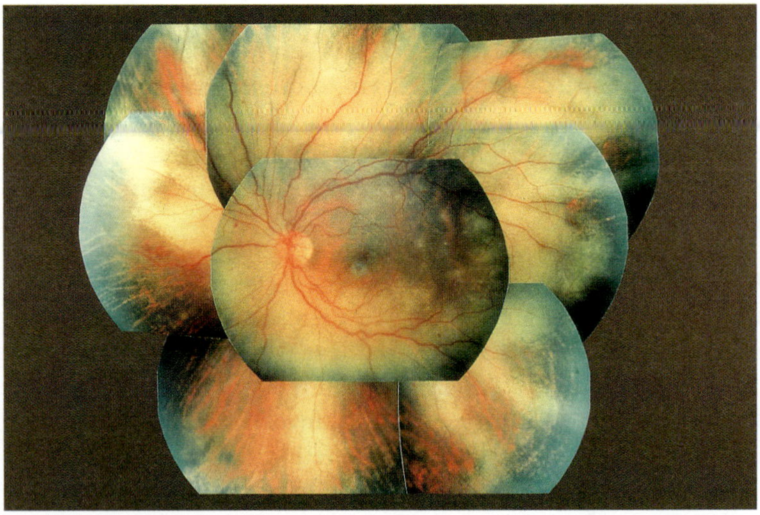

Figure 11-2 Fundus photomontage of retinal necrosis with preservation of vessels in a patient with progressive outer retinal necrosis (PORN). *(Courtesy of Narsing A. Rao, MD.)*

In its early stages, PORN may be difficult to differentiate from peripheral CMV retinitis. However, PORN's characteristically rapid progression and relative absence of vitreous inflammation usually allow this entity to be distinguished from CMV retinitis and acute retinal necrosis (ARN). PORN is associated with a high incidence of retinal detachment, and bilateral involvement is common. Treatment with intravitreous ganciclovir, foscarnet, or acyclovir as well as combination antiretroviral therapy has been reported to preserve vision.

Engstrom RE Jr, Holland GN, Margolis TP, et al. The progressive outer retinal necrosis syndrome. A variant of necrotizing herpetic retinopathy in patients with AIDS. *Ophthalmology.* 1994;101(9):1488–1502.

Kim SJ, Equi R, Belair ML, Fine HF, Dunn JP. Long-term preservation of vision in progressive outer retinal necrosis treated with combination antiviral drugs and highly active antiretroviral therapy. *Ocul Immunol Inflamm.* 2007;15(6):425–427.

Toxoplasma Retinochoroiditis

Toxoplasmosis in patients with AIDS differs from toxoplasmosis in immunocompetent patients. In general, the lesions are larger in people with AIDS, and up to 40% of cases have bilateral disease. Solitary, multifocal, and miliary patterns of retinitis have been observed (Fig 11-3). A vitreous inflammatory reaction usually appears overlying the area of active retinochoroiditis, but the degree of vitreous reaction may be less than that observed in immunocompetent patients. (See also Chapter 7.)

The diagnosis of ocular toxoplasmosis may also be more difficult in patients with AIDS. Preexisting scars are rare (present in 6% of patients at most). Newly acquired *T gondii* infections or dissemination from nonocular sites are the most likely causes among patients with AIDS, although reactivation of quiescent toxoplasmosis also occurs. Ocular toxoplasmosis in patients with AIDS may be difficult to distinguish from ARN,

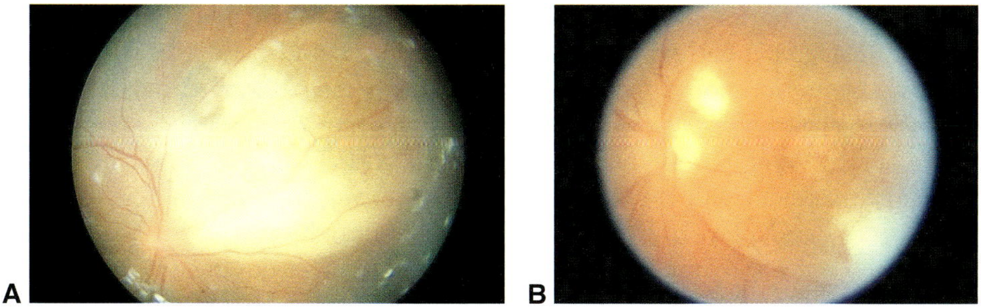

Figure 11-3 **A,** Fundus photograph showing a large area of macular toxoplasmic retinochoroiditis in a patient infected with HIV. **B,** Fundus photograph of multifocal toxoplasmic retinochoroiditis in another HIV-infected patient. *(Courtesy of Emmett T. Cunningham, Jr, MD.)*

necrotizing herpetic retinitis, or syphilitic retinitis. Diagnosis may require aqueous and vitreous samples for culture and polymerase chain reaction techniques.

In general, the inflammatory reaction in the choroid, retina, and vitreous is less prominent than in patients with an intact immune system. Trophozoites and cysts can be observed in greater numbers within areas of retinitis, and *T gondii* organisms can occasionally be noted invading the choroid, a finding not present in immunocompetent patients.

The prompt diagnosis of ocular toxoplasmosis is especially important in patients who are immunocompromised because the condition inevitably progresses if left untreated, in contrast to the self-limiting disease in immunocompetent patients. In addition, ocular toxoplasmosis in immunocompromised patients may be associated with cerebral or disseminated toxoplasmosis, an important cause of morbidity and mortality in patients with AIDS. For HIV-infected patients with active ocular toxoplasmosis, magnetic resonance imaging (MRI) of the brain and consultation with specialists in infectious diseases should be pursued to rule out central nervous system (CNS) involvement.

Antitoxoplasmic therapy with various combinations of pyrimethamine, sulfadiazine, azithromycin, atovaquone, or clindamycin is required. Corticosteroids should be used with caution and only in the presence of appropriate antimicrobial cover because of the risk of further immunosuppression in this population. In selecting the therapeutic regimen, the physician should consider the possibility of coexisting cerebral or disseminated toxoplasmosis as well as the toxic effects of pyrimethamine and sulfadiazine on bone marrow. Continued maintenance therapy may be necessary for patients with poor immune status that is not improving.

Moshfeghi DM, Dodds EM, Couto CA, et al. Diagnostic approaches to severe, atypical toxoplasmosis mimicking acute retinal necrosis. *Ophthalmology.* 2004;111(4):716–725.

Syphilitic Chorioretinitis

The clinical presentations of ocular syphilitic chorioretinitis include uveitis, optic neuritis, and nonnecrotizing retinitis. Patients may also experience dermatologic and CNS symptoms. A classic manifestation of syphilis in patients with AIDS is unilateral or bilateral, pale-yellow, placoid retinal lesions that preferentially involve the macula (syphilitic posterior placoid chorioretinitis). Exudative retinal detachment may also be present. Some HIV-infected patients with syphilis may present with dense vitritis without clinical evidence of chorioretinitis. In these patients, vitritis can be the first manifestation of syphilis. (See also Chapter 7.)

The course of syphilis may be more aggressive in HIV-infected patients. These patients require treatment with 18–24 million units of intravenous penicillin G administered daily for 10–14 days, followed by 2.4 million units of intramuscular benzathine penicillin G administered weekly for 3 weeks. Monitoring of results from the quantitative rapid plasma reagin (RPR) test is recommended, as symptomatic disease can recur.

Browning DJ. Posterior segment manifestations of active ocular syphilis, their response to a neurosyphilis regimen of penicillin therapy, and the influence of human immunodeficiency virus status on response. *Ophthalmology.* 2000;107(11):2015–2023.

Pneumocystis jirovecii Choroiditis

Patients with AIDS are at much greater risk for *Pneumocystis jirovecii* pneumonia. In rare cases, this infection can result in choroidal infiltrates that contain the microorganisms.

Fundus changes that are characteristic of *P jirovecii* choroiditis consist of slightly elevated, plaquelike, yellow-white lesions located in the choroid, with minimal vitritis (Fig 11-4). On fluorescein angiography, these lesions tend to be hypofluorescent in the early phase and hyperfluorescent in the later phases. If disseminated *P jirovecii* infection is suspected, an extensive examination is required by an infectious diseases specialist.

Treatment of *P jirovecii* choroiditis involves a 3-week regimen of intravenous trimethoprim (20 mg/kg/day) and sulfamethoxazole (100 mg/kg/day) or pentamidine (4 mg/kg/day). Within 3–12 weeks, most of the yellow-white lesions disappear, leaving mild overlying pigmentary changes. Vision is usually not affected.

Cryptococcus neoformans Choroiditis

The dissemination of *Cryptococcus neoformans* in patients with AIDS may result in a multifocal choroiditis. Some patients with *C neoformans* choroiditis show choroidal lesions before clinical evidence of dissemination develops. More typically, *C neoformans* infection involves the cerebrospinal fluid, and there is secondary optic nerve edema as a result of increased intracranial pressure that can slowly lead to optic atrophy. Direct invasion of the

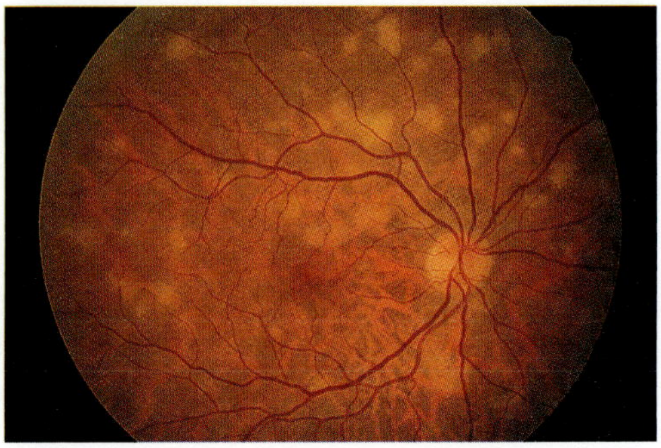

Figure 11-4 Fundus photograph of *Pneumocystis jirovecii* choroiditis. The fellow eye revealed similar findings. *(Reprinted with permission from Cunningham ET Jr, Belfort R Jr.* HIV/AIDS and the Eye: A Global Perspective. *Ophthalmology Monograph 15. San Francisco, CA: American Academy of Ophthalmology; 2002:67.)*

optic nerve by organisms is also possible and can lead to more rapid vision loss. Treatment may include amphotericin and flucytosine.

Kestelyn P, Taelman H, Bogaerts J, et al. Ophthalmic manifestations of infections with *Cryptococcus neoformans* in patients with the acquired immunodeficiency syndrome. *Am J Ophthalmol.* 1993;116(6):721–727.

Multifocal Choroiditis and Systemic Dissemination

Multifocal choroidal lesions from a variety of infectious agents are found in up to 10% of patients with AIDS. Most of these lesions are caused by *C neoformans, P jirovecii, M tuberculosis,* or atypical mycobacteria. Because of the profound immunosuppression, multiple infectious agents may cause simultaneous infectious multifocal choroiditis.

The choroid is often a site of opportunistic disseminated infections and thus needs to be carefully examined in patients with AIDS. Multifocal choroiditis should prompt an exhaustive workup because it frequently is a sign of disseminated infection.

External Eye Manifestations

Other ophthalmic manifestations of AIDS include Kaposi sarcoma; molluscum contagiosum; herpes zoster ophthalmicus; and keratitis caused by various viruses, protozoa, conjunctival infections, and microvascular abnormalities. All of these conditions affect mainly the anterior segment of the globe and the ocular adnexa. These conditions are also discussed in BCSC Section 8, *External Disease and Cornea.*

Ocular Adnexal Kaposi Sarcoma

Human herpesvirus 8 is associated with Kaposi sarcoma. Two aggressive variants of this tumor have been described: an endemic variety especially prevalent in Kenya and Nigeria and a second variant, epidemic Kaposi sarcoma, which was first noted in renal transplant recipients and in patients with AIDS. AIDS-associated Kaposi sarcoma may be found in visceral organs (the gastrointestinal tract, lung, and liver) in up to 50% of patients. Before the availability of potent antiretroviral therapy, ocular adnexal involvement occurred in approximately 20% of patients with AIDS-associated systemic Kaposi sarcoma (Fig 11-5). Histologic investigation shows spindle cells mixed with vascular structures. Treatment

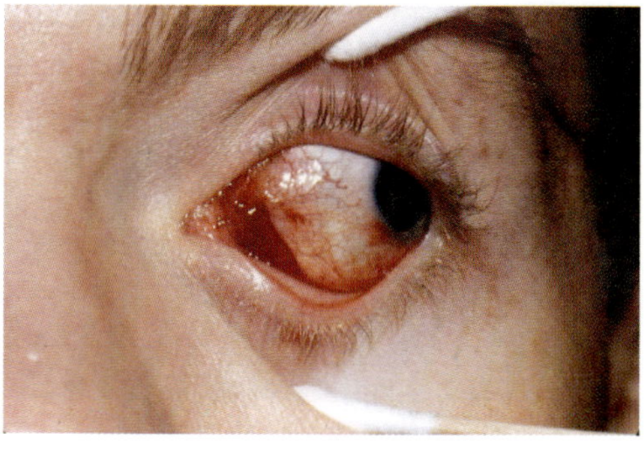

Figure 11-5 Conjunctival involvement in Kaposi sarcoma; hemorrhagic conjunctival tumor. *(Courtesy of Elaine Chuang, MD.)*

of Kaposi sarcoma consists of excision, cryotherapy, radiation, or a combination of these methods and is based on the clinical stage of the tumor as well as its location and the presence or absence of disseminated lesions.

Molluscum Contagiosum

Molluscum contagiosum is caused by a DNA virus of the poxvirus family. The characteristic skin lesions show a small elevation with central umbilication. Molluscum contagiosum lesions in immunocompetent individuals are few, unilateral, and involve the eyelids. In patients with AIDS, however, these lesions may be numerous and bilateral. If molluscum contagiosum lesions in patients with AIDS are symptomatic or cause conjunctivitis, surgical excision may be necessary.

Herpes Zoster

People younger than 50 years of age who present with herpes zoster lesions of the face or eyelids should be considered for HIV testing. Corneal involvement can cause a persistent, chronic epithelial keratitis. Treatment consists of intravenous and topical acyclovir. These patients should receive periodic monitoring with retinal examinations to ensure that posterior segment involvement does not occur.

Other Infections

HIV infection does not appear to predispose patients to bacterial keratitis, although bacterial and fungal keratitis can occur in patients with AIDS who have no obvious predisposing factors such as trauma or topical corticosteroid use. Infections appear to be more severe and are more likely to cause corneal perforation in patients with AIDS than in immunocompetent patients. Similarly, herpes simplex keratitis does not appear to have a higher incidence in patients with AIDS, but it may have a prolonged course or multiple recurrences and involve the limbus. Microsporidia have been shown to cause a coarse, punctate epithelial keratitis with minimal conjunctival reaction in patients with AIDS (Fig 11-6). Electron microscopy of epithelial scrapings has revealed the organism, which is an obligate, intracellular, protozoal parasite.

Solitary granulomatous conjunctivitis caused by cryptococcal or mycotic infections or by tuberculosis can occur in HIV-infected persons. The possibility of dissemination

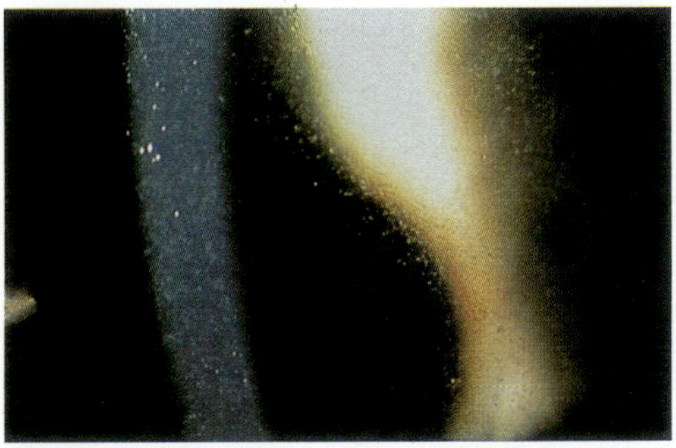

Figure 11-6 Slit-lamp photograph of cornea showing punctate epithelial keratitis caused by microsporidia.

must be aggressively investigated, and, if present, treated. Both orbital and intraocular lymphomas have been described in patients with AIDS. These neoplasms are mostly large B-cell lymphomas. Conjunctival squamous cell carcinomas have been reported, and in some patients, these neoplasms show spindle cells with frequent abnormal mitotic figures.

HIV Infection in Resource-Limited Regions of the World

HIV infection remains a major global health problem despite the fact that effective antiretroviral therapy and education have greatly improved outcomes and decreased the rate of ocular complications in resource-rich nations. In 2013 it was estimated that more than 35 million people are living with HIV/AIDS, including 2.1 million adolescents (ages 10–19 years). The World Health Organization estimates that 3.34 million children are HIV infected. Up to 95% of new HIV infections occur in individuals living in low- and middle-income countries. Economic and social factors limit access to care; in addition, genetic differences and differences in the prevalence of opportunistic infections such as tuberculosis result in a different spectrum of HIV-related ocular complications than that seen in higher-income countries. Hopes are that the impact of HIV infection will be ameliorated worldwide by efforts at education and prevention, increasing the availability of antiretroviral medication, training paramedical personnel, and the use of telemedicine and other methods for remote screening for CMV retinitis, tuberculosis, syphilis, squamous cell carcinoma of the conjunctiva, herpes zoster infections, and other ocular complications of HIV/AIDS.

Precautions in the Health Care Setting

Universal precautions as advocated in the United States by the Centers for Disease Control and Prevention (CDC) and other governmental agencies, including the Occupational Safety and Health Administration (OSHA), should always be followed.

Precautions in Ophthalmic Practice

There are no published reports of HIV transmission in ophthalmic health care settings. Regardless, the American Academy of Ophthalmology advocates that ophthalmic health care practitioners take precautionary measures against exposure to infectious agents. Hands should be washed or a hand sterilizer solution used between tests on an individual and between patients. Tonometers, diagnostic contact lenses, and contact lens trial sets should be appropriately disinfected according to the manufacturers' guidelines. BCSC Section 10, *Glaucoma,* gives more specific instructions for infection control in tonometry.

Minimizing transmission of bloodborne pathogens and surface infectious agents in ophthalmic offices and operating rooms. Information Statement. San Francisco, CA: American Academy of Ophthalmology; 2002.

APPENDIX

Diagnostic Survey for Uveitis

FAMILY HISTORY

These questions refer to your grandparents, parents, aunts, uncles, brothers and sisters, children, or grandchildren.

To your knowledge, has anyone in your family ever had any of the following?

Arthritis or rheumatism	Yes	No
Syphilis	Yes	No
Tuberculosis	Yes	No
Sickle cell disease or trait	Yes	No
Lyme disease	Yes	No
Uveitis, or inflammation in the eye?	Yes	No

SOCIAL HISTORY

Your age (years):		
Your current job:		
Have you ever traveled outside of the United States?	Yes	No
If yes, where and when?		
Have you ever owned a dog or cat?	Yes	No
Have you ever eaten raw meat or uncooked sausage?	Yes	No
Have you ever had unpasteurized milk or cheese?	Yes	No
Have you ever been exposed to sick animals?	Yes	No
Do you drink untreated stream, well, or lake water, or have you gone hunting or camping?	Yes	No
Do you smoke cigarettes?	Yes	No
Have you ever used recreational intravenous drugs?	Yes	No
Have you ever had sexual relations with a person of the same sex or with a person who engages in same-sex relations?	Yes	No

PERSONAL MEDICAL HISTORY

Are you allergic to any medications?	Yes	No
If yes, which medications?		

Please list the medications that you are currently taking, including nonprescription or over-the-counter drugs, nutritional supplements, and herbal or other alternative remedies:

______

______

Please list all the eye surgeries you have had (including laser surgery) and the dates of the surgeries:

______

______

______

______

Please list all the operations besides on the eye you have had and the dates of the surgeries:

____

____

____

Have you ever been told by a medical doctor that you have the following conditions?

Anemia (low blood count)	Yes	No
Cancer	Yes	No
Diabetes mellitus	Yes	No
Hepatitis	Yes	No
High blood pressure	Yes	No
Pleurisy	Yes	No
Pneumonia	Yes	No
Ulcers	Yes	No
Herpes (sores in or on the mouth or genitals)	Yes	No
Chickenpox	Yes	No
Shingles (zoster)	Yes	No
German measles (rubella)	Yes	No
Measles (rubeola)	Yes	No
Mumps	Yes	No
Chlamydia or trachoma	Yes	No
Syphilis	Yes	No
Gonorrhea	Yes	No
Any other sexually transmitted disease	Yes	No
Tuberculosis	Yes	No
Leprosy	Yes	No
Leptospirosis	Yes	No
Lyme disease	Yes	No
Histoplasmosis	Yes	No
Candida infection or moniliasis	Yes	No
Coccidioidomycosis	Yes	No
Sporotrichosis	Yes	No
Toxoplasmosis	Yes	No
Toxocariasis	Yes	No
Cysticercosis	Yes	No
Trichinosis	Yes	No
Whipple disease	Yes	No
HIV infection or AIDS	Yes	No
Hay fever	Yes	No
Allergies	Yes	No
Vasculitis	Yes	No
Arthritis	Yes	No
Rheumatoid arthritis	Yes	No
Lupus (systemic lupus erythematosus)	Yes	No
Scleroderma	Yes	No
Reactive arthritis	Yes	No
Colitis (Crohn disease, ulcerative colitis)	Yes	No
Behçet disease	Yes	No

Sarcoidosis	Yes	No
Ankylosing spondylitis	Yes	No
Erythema nodosa	Yes	No
Temporal arteritis	Yes	No
Multiple sclerosis	Yes	No

Have you ever had any of the following symptoms?

GENERAL HEALTH

Chills	Yes	No
Fever (persistent or recurrent)	Yes	No
Painful or swollen glands	Yes	No
Night sweats	Yes	No
Fatigue (tire easily)	Yes	No
Poor appetite	Yes	No
Unexplained weight loss	Yes	No
Do you feel sick?	Yes	No

HEAD

Headaches	Yes	No
Fainting	Yes	No
Numbness or tingling in your body	Yes	No
Paralysis in parts of your body	Yes	No
Seizures or convulsions	Yes	No

EARS

Hard of hearing or deafness	Yes	No
Ringing or noise in your ears	Yes	No
Frequent or severe ear infections	Yes	No
Painful or swollen ear lobes	Yes	No

NOSE AND THROAT

Sores in your nose or mouth	Yes	No
Severe or recurrent nosebleeds	Yes	No
Frequent sneezing	Yes	No
Sinus trouble	Yes	No
Persistent hoarseness	Yes	No
Tooth or gum infections	Yes	No

SKIN

Rashes	Yes	No
Skin sores	Yes	No
Sunburn easily (photosensitivity)	Yes	No
White patches of skin or hair	Yes	No
Loss of hair	Yes	No
Tick or insect bites	Yes	No
Painfully cold fingers	Yes	No
Severe itching	Yes	No

RESPIRATORY

Severe or frequent colds	Yes	No
Constant coughing	Yes	No

Coughing up blood	Yes	No
Recent flu or viral infection	Yes	No
Wheezing or asthma attacks	Yes	No
Difficulty breathing	Yes	No

CARDIOVASCULAR

Chest pain	Yes	No
Shortness of breath	Yes	No
Swelling of your legs	Yes	No

BLOOD

Frequent or easy bruising	Yes	No
Frequent or easy bleeding	Yes	No
Have you received blood transfusions?	Yes	No

GASTROINTESTINAL

Trouble swallowing	Yes	No
Diarrhea	Yes	No
Bloody stools	Yes	No
Stomach ulcers	Yes	No
Jaundice or yellow skin	Yes	No

BONES AND JOINTS

Stiff joints	Yes	No
Stiff lower back	Yes	No
Back pain while sleeping or awakening	Yes	No
Muscle aches	Yes	No

GENITOURINARY

Kidney problems	Yes	No
Bladder trouble	Yes	No
Blood in your urine	Yes	No
Urinary discharge	Yes	No
Genital sores or ulcers	Yes	No
Prostatitis	Yes	No
Testicular pain	Yes	No
Are you pregnant?	Yes	No
Do you plan to be pregnant in the future?	Yes	No

Adapted with permission from Foster CS, Vitale AT. *Diagnosis and Treatment of Uveitis*. 2nd ed. Jaypee Brothers Medical Publishers, New Delhi, India; 2012:123–128.

Basic Texts

Intraocular Inflammation and Uveitis

Albert DM, Miller JW, Azar DT, Blodi BA, eds. *Albert & Jakobiec's Principles and Practice of Ophthalmology.* 3rd ed. Philadelphia: Saunders; 2008.

Delves PJ, Martin SJ, Burton DR, Roitt IM. *Roitt's Essential Immunology.* 12th ed. Hoboken, NJ: Wiley-Blackwell; 2011.

Dick AD, Okada AA, Forrester JV. *Practical Manual of Intraocular Inflammation.* New York: Informa Healthcare USA; 2008.

Foster CS, Vitale AT, eds. *Diagnosis & Treatment of Uveitis.* 2nd ed. New Dehli, India: Jaypee Brothers Medical Publishers; 2013.

Giles CL. Uveitis in childhood. In: Tasman W, Jaeger EA, eds. *Duane's Clinical Ophthalmology.* Philadelphia: Lippincott Williams & Wilkins; 2005.

Kanski JJ, Bowling B. *Clinical Ophthalmology: A Systematic Approach.* 7th ed. London: Elsevier; 2011.

Michelson JB. *Color Atlas of Uveitis.* 2nd ed. St Louis: Mosby; 1992.

Nussenblatt RB, Whitcup SM. *Uveitis: Fundamentals and Clinical Practice.* 4th ed. St Louis: Mosby; 2010.

Pepose JS, Holland GN, Wilhelmus KR, eds. *Ocular Infection and Immunity.* St Louis: Mosby; 1996.

Rao NA, section ed. Part 7: Uveitis and other intraocular inflammations. In: Yanoff M, Duker JS, eds. *Ophthalmology.* 3rd ed. St Louis: Mosby; 2009.

Related Academy Materials

The Academy is dedicated to providing a wealth of high-quality clinical education resources for ophthalmologists.

Print Publications and Electronic Products

For a complete listing of Academy products related to topics covered in this BCSC Section, visit our online store at http://store.aao.org/clinical-education/topic/uveitis.html. Or call Customer Service at 866-561-8558 (toll free, US only) or +1 415-561-8540, Monday through Friday, between 8:00 AM and 5:00 PM (PST).

Online Resources

Visit the Ophthalmic News and Education (ONE®) Network at www.aao.org/clinical-education to find relevant videos, online courses, journal articles, practice guidelines, self-assessment quizzes, images, and more. The ONE Network is a free Academy-member benefit.

Access free, trusted articles and content with the Academy's collaborative online encyclopedia, EyeWiki, at www.aao.org/eyewiki.

Requesting Continuing Medical Education Credit

The American Academy of Ophthalmology is accredited by the Accreditation Council for Continuing Medical Education to provide continuing medical education for physicians.

The American Academy of Ophthalmology designates this enduring material for a maximum of 10 *AMA PRA Category 1 Credits*™. Physicians should claim only the credit commensurate with the extent of their participation in the activity.

The American Medical Association requires that all learners participating in activities involving enduring materials complete a formal assessment before claiming continuing medical education (CME) credit. To assess your achievement in this activity and ensure that a specified level of knowledge has been reached, a posttest for this Section of the Basic and Clinical Science Course is provided online. A minimum score of 80% must be obtained to pass the test and claim CME credit.

To take the posttest and request CME credit online:

1. Go to www.aao.org/cme-central and log in.
2. Click on "Claim CME Credit and View My CME Transcript" and then "Report AAO Credits."
3. Select the appropriate Academy activity. You will be directed to the posttest.
4. Once you have passed the test with a score of 80% or higher, you will be directed to your transcript. *If you are not an Academy member, you will be able to print out a certificate of participation once you have passed the test.*

CME expiration date: June 1, 2018. *AMA PRA Category 1 Credits*™ may be claimed only once between June 1, 2015, and the expiration date.

For assistance, contact the Academy's Customer Service department at 866-561-8558 (US only) or +1 415-561-8540 between 8:00 AM and 5:00 PM (PST), Monday through Friday, or send an e-mail to customer_service@aao.org.

Study Questions

Please note that these questions are *not* part of your CME reporting process. They are provided here for your own educational use and identification of any professional practice gaps. The required CME posttest is available online (see "Requesting CME Credit"). Following the questions are a blank answer sheet and answers with discussions. Although a concerted effort has been made to avoid ambiguity and redundancy in these questions, the authors recognize that differences of opinion may occur regarding the "best" answer. The discussions are provided to demonstrate the rationale used to derive the answer. They may also be helpful in confirming that your approach to the problem was correct or, if necessary, in fixing the principle in your memory. The Section 9 faculty thanks the Self-Assessment Committee for reviewing the self-assessment questions.

1. What inflammatory cell type dominates the infiltrate in acute bacterial infections?
   a. eosinophils
   b. neutrophils
   c. macrophages
   d. mast cells

2. The initial recognition, transport, and presentation of antigenic substances to the adaptive immune system constitute what phase of the immune response arc?
   a. afferent
   b. memory
   c. processing
   d. effector

3. Mast cells bind which immunoglobulin (Ig) type to their cell surfaces?
   a. IgM
   b. IgG
   c. IgE
   d. IgA

4. Regional immunity refers to
   a. the idea that many organs and tissues possess modifications to the classic immune response
   b. variations in immune responses that occur in different geographic areas of the world
   c. the different zones present in draining lymph nodes
   d. the isolation and tolerance of antigens present in the various structures within the eye

5. AIRE (autoimmune regulator)-deficient mice develop spontaneous uveitis because
   a. autoreactive T cells escape deletion
   b. retinal antigens are overexpressed in regional lymph nodes
   c. complement regulatory molecules are absent in the eyes of these animals
   d. the CD4:CD8 T helper cell ratio is reversed compared with that in wild type mice

6. The fluocinolone acetonide implant releases therapeutic levels of corticosteroids to the vitreous cavity for approximately how long?
   a. 10 months
   b. 20 months
   c. 30 months
   d. 40 months

7. What inhibitor of tumor necrosis factor α is least effective for uveitis?
   a. infliximab
   b. adalimumab
   c. golimumab
   d. etanercept

8. What mechanism of action produces the anti-inflammatory effects of methotrexate?
   a. inhibition of folate metabolism
   b. nucleotide crosslinking during DNA replication
   c. inhibition of calcineurin
   d. extracellular release of adenosine

9. What is the most common noninfectious systemic disease associated with scleritis?
   a. granulomatosis with polyangiitis (formerly, Wegener granulomatosis)
   b. multiple sclerosis
   c. rheumatoid arthritis
   d. systemic lupus erythematosus

10. The white dot lesions of which disease are least apparent on fluorescein angiography?
    a. serpiginous choroiditis
    b. punctate inner choroiditis
    c. acute posterior multifocal placoid pigment epitheliopathy
    d. birdshot uveitis

11. What finding can suggest the diagnosis of multiple evanescent white dot syndrome after the white dots have disappeared?
    a. granular pigment changes in the fovea
    b. punched-out lesions in the retinal periphery
    c. perivascular pigment alterations
    d. peripapillary scarring

12. What entity can present with marked visual symptoms but minimal findings on clinical examination?
    a. serpiginous choroiditis
    b. Vogt-Koyanagi-Harada syndrome
    c. acute zonal occult outer retinopathy
    d. punctate inner choroiditis

13. A patient with necrotizing scleritis is found to have antibodies directed against proteinase 3. What disease is most likely to be associated with this finding?
    a. polyarteritis nodosa
    b. microscopic polyangiitis
    c. granulomatosis with polyangiitis
    d. Churg-Strauss syndrome

14. What stage of Vogt-Koyanagi-Harada syndrome is most likely to be associated with exudative retinal detachments?
    a. prodromal
    b. acute uveitic
    c. convalescent
    d. chronic recurrent

15. What factor is associated with vision loss in patients with ocular sarcoidosis?
    a. need for systemic immunomodulatory therapy (IMT)
    b. delay of more than 1 year in presentation to a uveitis specialist
    c. anterior uveitis associated with nummular corneal infiltrates
    d. presence of "string-of-pearls" condensations within the vitreous

16. What test is useful in the diagnosis of tubular interstitial nephritis and uveitis?
    a. urine β2-microglobulin level
    b. antinuclear antibody (ANA) level
    c. erythrocyte sedimentation rate
    d. angiotensin-converting enzyme level

17. What class of infectious organisms has been associated with glaucomatocyclitic crisis (also known as *Posner-Schlossman syndrome*)?
    a. viruses such as cytomegalovirus (CMV)
    b. fungi such as *Candida* species
    c. bacteria such as *Mycobacterium tuberculosis*
    d. helminths such as *Toxocara* species

18. Lyme disease–associated intermediate uveitis occurs most commonly in what stage of the disease?
    a. stage 1, local disease
    b. stage 2, disseminated disease
    c. stage 3, persistent disease
    d. recurrent disease

19. What is the US Centers for Disease Control and Prevention (CDC)–recommended testing protocol for suspected Lyme disease in a patient with intermediate uveitis and a history of a recent tick bite?
    a. polymerase chain reaction (PCR) testing for Lyme (ie, *Borrelia burgdorferi*) DNA in aqueous humor
    b. PCR testing for Lyme DNA in vitreous humor
    c. enzyme-linked immunosorbent assay for Lyme IgM and IgG antibodies followed by Western immunoblot testing
    d. determinations of Lyme IgM and IgG titers in aqueous humor

20. The term *pars planitis* describes
    a. any type of intermediate uveitis; can be used interchangeably
    b. any form of infectious or noninfectious intermediate uveitis in which pars plana exudates are noted
    c. intermediate uveitis in children only
    d. idiopathic intermediate uveitis with snowbank or snowball formation (in the absence of an associated infection or systemic disease)

21. Juvenile idiopathic arthritis (JIA)–associated uveitis occurs most commonly in oligoarticular-onset JIA, and a subset typically affects girls who test positive for ANA. What should the treatment strategy include?
    a. short-term treatment with topical corticosteroids to eliminate inflammation in the eye; early consideration of systemic IMT such as with methotrexate
    b. long-term therapy with oral corticosteroids to control inflammation as the mainstay of therapy
    c. topical corticosteroids and cycloplegics only, at whatever dose is required for as long as required, avoiding systemic IMT in children
    d. intravitreal corticosteroids repeated periodically based on the level of disease activity

22. You suspect your patient has intraocular inflammation related to toxoplasmosis and wish to perform a Goldmann-Witmer test. What 2 tissue samples are needed to perform this test?
    a. aqueous and serum
    b. aqueous and vitreous
    c. aqueous and urine
    d. aqueous and saliva

23. A 65-year-old man is found to have unilateral decline in vision as well as occlusive arteritis, vitritis, and a multifocal yellow-white peripheral retinitis. What is the best therapy for this case?
    a. prednisolone acetate drops
    b. trifluridine drops
    c. systemic prednisone
    d. systemic acyclovir

24. What endogenous fungal infection is the most common cause of endophthalmitis?
    a. *Cryptococcus*
    b. *Blastomyces*
    c. *Aspergillus*
    d. *Candida*

25. A 70-year-old woman underwent cataract surgery. What organism aside from *Propionibacterium acnes* should be suspected if a chronic, indolent, intraocular inflammation develops?
    a. *Candida parapsilosis*
    b. *Streptococcus pneumoniae*
    c. *Staphylococcus aureus*
    d. *Pseudomonas aeruginosa*

26. A 70-year-old woman has chronic anterior uveitis that is poorly responsive to treatment with topical prednisolone acetate, 1%. On examination, there is no view to the posterior segment because of fibrin formation and posterior synechiae. On gonioscopy, there appears to be a pigmented mass in the angle from 10 to 1 o'clock. What is the next step?
    a. obtain a B scan
    b. inject intravitreal corticosteroids
    c. initiate oral corticosteroids
    d. obtain a vitreous biopsy

27. What is the treatment for visually significant calcific band keratopathy?
    a. epithelial debridement and chelation with ethylenediaminetetraacetic acid (EDTA)
    b. intense treatment with topical steroids
    c. corneal transplantation
    d. corneal crosslinking

28. A patient with sarcoid anterior and intermediate uveitis exhibits less than ½+ anterior chamber cells, minimal vitreous haze, and no macular edema on mycophenolate and infliximab treatment. Before treatment, the patient exhibited 3+ anterior chamber cells, mutton-fat keratic precipitates, extensive posterior synechiae without iris bombé, and 2+ vitreous haze in both eyes. She now needs cataract surgery in order to drive. What is the most appropriate approach to cataract surgery in this patient?
    a. Wait until her level of inflammation is stable on this regimen for at least 3 months and then perform cataract surgery.
    b. Perform cataract surgery now.
    c. Insert a fluocinolone implant and then perform cataract surgery as soon as possible.
    d. Increase the infliximab dosage until there are absolutely no anterior chamber cells for 6 months.

29. What intraocular infection is most commonly associated with immune recovery uveitis in a patient with AIDS whose immune function has improved with antiretroviral therapy?
    a. CMV retinitis
    b. toxoplasmosis
    c. Kaposi sarcoma (caused by human herpesvirus 8)
    d. syphilitic uveitis

Answer Sheet for Section 9 Study Questions

Question	Answer	Question	Answer
1	a b c d	16	a b c d
2	a b c d	17	a b c d
3	a b c d	18	a b c d
4	a b c d	19	a b c d
5	a b c d	20	a b c d
6	a b c d	21	a b c d
7	a b c d	22	a b c d
8	a b c d	23	a b c d
9	a b c d	24	a b c d
10	a b c d	25	a b c d
11	a b c d	26	a b c d
12	a b c d	27	a b c d
13	a b c d	28	a b c d
14	a b c d	29	a b c d
15	a b c d		

Answers

1. **b.** Neutrophils are efficient phagocytes that readily clear tissues and degrade ingested material. They act as important effector cells through the release of granule products and cytokines. Neutrophils dominate the infiltrate in experimental models and clinical examples of active bacterial infections of the conjunctiva (conjunctivitis), sclera (scleritis), cornea (keratitis), and vitreous (endophthalmitis).
2. **a.** Following ingestion of antigen, antigen-presenting cells (APCs) migrate via afferent lymphatics to lymph nodes. In the APCs, enzymatic digestion of proteins within endocytic vesicles produces short amino acid chains of 7–11 amino acids: the antigenic epitopic fragments. Each antigenic fragment is combined with a groove-shaped HLA peptide residing on the APC surface, and this surface complex forms a unique epitope. The combination of peptide and HLA protein is recognized by the T-lymphocyte receptors CD4 and CD8.
3. **c.** Immunoglobulin E (IgE) binds to the surface of mast cells and participates in allergic reactions. IgM and IgG are involved in the initial and memory responses of the immune arc, respectively. IgA is primarily involved in mucosal immunity.
4. **a.** The concept that many organs and tissue sites possess modifications to the classic immune response arc is termed *regional immunity.* Regional immunity can affect all 3 phases of the response arc—afferent, processing, and effector. Regional differences in immune response occur because of differences in the immunologic microenvironments of various tissue sites; these regional differences can occur down to the level of specific locations within and around the eye.
5. **a.** AIRE (autoimmune regulator) is a transcription factor used by the thymus in the process of establishing thymic tolerance. Early in life, the thymus expresses many cell-type–specific proteins; T-cell clones reactive to these proteins are deleted. This mechanism is important in the development of self-tolerance. Mice deficient in AIRE do not express these proteins during development; thus, autoreactive T cells escape deletion, and the mice spontaneously develop a posterior uveitis.
6. **c.** Multicenter, controlled clinical studies have shown that the 0.59-mg fluocinolone implant is effective for a median of 30 months. The sustained-release implant was approved by the US Food and Drug Administration (FDA) in 2005 for the treatment of chronic noninfectious uveitis affecting the posterior segment. The implant is inserted through a small pars plana incision and sutured to the sclera.
7. **d.** Etanercept, a tumor necrosis factor α (TNF-α) decoy receptor, has proved effective in controlling joint inflammation in polyarticular juvenile idiopathic arthritis (JIA) and adult rheumatoid arthritis. It is generally less effective than infliximab and adalimumab for uveitis and is not a preferred biologic for uveitis treatment. There are also some reports of paradoxical inflammation with etanercept. Golimumab is a new TNF agonist that is a monoclonal antibody similar to infliximab and adalimumab, but data on its usefulness in uveitis are lacking at present.
8. **d.** Methotrexate, a folic acid analogue and inhibitor of dihydrofolate reductase, inhibits DNA replication, but its anti-inflammatory effects result from extracellular release of adenosine.

9. **c.** Approximately 40% of scleritis cases are associated with systemic disease, most commonly rheumatoid arthritis. Granulomatosis with polyangiitis (formerly, Wegener granulomatosis) and systemic lupus erythematosus are also associated with scleritis, but much less frequently. Multiple sclerosis is not associated with scleritis but rather with intermediate uveitis and pars planitis.
10. **d.** Fluorescein angiography (FA) in birdshot uveitis reveals inconsistent findings depending on the age of the lesions and the phase of the study. Early birdshot uveitis lesions may show initial hypofluorescence with subtle late staining. In general, however, FA does not typically highlight the lesions themselves but rather is useful in identifying more subtle types of active inflammation such as retinal vasculitis, cystoid macular edema, and optic nerve head leakage. In contrast, in patients with acute posterior multifocal placoid pigment epitheliopathy (APMPPE), FA shows characteristic early blockage with late staining of the lesions, and in patients with punctate inner choroiditis (PIC), it reveals early hyperfluorescence with late staining of the lesions. In patients with serpiginous choroiditis, FA reveals blockage of the choroidal flush in the early stage of the study and staining of the active edge of the lesion in the later stage. Early hyperfluorescence with late leakage is indicative of choroidal neovascular membranes, which are observed frequently in patients with PIC and less often in those with serpiginous choroiditis or birdshot uveitis.
11. **a.** Subtle granular pigment changes in the fovea are present after the acute stage of multiple evanescent white dot syndrome (MEWDS), and they are considered pathognomonic for the disease. The finding can be very useful in making the diagnosis in patients who present with symptoms after the white dots have faded. MEWDS patients do not typically develop peripheral punched-out lesions or peripapillary scarring, as can be present in ocular histoplasmosis syndrome and multifocal choroiditis. Perivascular pigment alterations can be present in retinal vasculitis but not in MEWDS.
12. **c.** Acute zonal occult outer retinopathy (AZOOR) can present with numerous visual complaints but very minimal funduscopic changes; patients may, however, have marked abnormalities on electroretinography (ERG), multifocal ERG, and visual field testing. The condition may even be misdiagnosed as functional vision loss if no additional testing is performed. Fundus pigment changes often appear in the later stages of the disease and may be more apparent on fluorescein angiography or fundus autofluorescence. Serpiginous choroiditis and PIC present with characteristic scars and foci of localized inflammation. Although the prodromal phase of Vogt-Koyanagi-Harada syndrome may have minimal ocular findings, patients have typical systemic symptoms, and by the time they present with vision loss, they have panuveitis and exudative retinal detachments.
13. **c.** Testing for antineutrophil cytoplasmic antibodies (ANCA) involves 2 techniques: (1) immunofluorescent testing, which evaluates for the presence of cytoplasmic or perinuclear immunofluorescence patterns (c-ANCA and p-ANCA, respectively), and (2) testing for the specific antibodies that cause each immunofluorescent pattern. Antibodies to proteinase 3 (PR3-ANCA) are associated with c-ANCA, and antibodies to myeloperoxidase (MPO-ANCA) are associated with p-ANCA. Tests for PR3-ANCA and c-ANCA are sensitive and specific for granulomatosis with polyangiitis. Positivity for MPO-ANCA and p-ANCA is more commonly associated with microscopic polyangiitis. Approximately 50% of patients with Churg-Strauss syndrome test positive for ANCA; they are typically, but not uniformly, MPO-ANCA positive. In a patient with antibodies to proteinase 3, the most likely associated disease will be granulomatosis with polyangiitis.

14. **b.** The acute uveitic stage is typically associated with exudative retinal detachments. By definition, the prodromal stage is characterized by systemic symptoms, such as a flulike syndrome and headaches, prior to the development of clinically apparent ophthalmic disease. The convalescent stage occurs weeks to months after the exudative retinal detachments have resolved; patients can develop gradual depigmentation in the fundus and findings such as vitiligo, alopecia, and poliosis. The chronic recurrent stage is associated with repeated bouts of anterior uveitis that can lead to significant structural damage, but it is not commonly associated with recurrence of the exudative retinal detachments.
15. **b.** Referral to a uveitis specialist should be strongly considered for patients who have ocular sarcoidosis that is difficult to control. The need for immunomodulatory therapy (IMT) is not necessarily associated with vision loss; patients receiving such treatment may eventually fare better than patients who receive intermittent treatment for flare-ups. Findings such as anterior uveitis, nummular corneal infiltrates, and "string of pearls" cells in the vitreous occur in ocular sarcoidosis, but they are not specifically associated with an increased risk of vision loss.
16. **a.** An increased urine level of β2-microglobulin is a useful marker for tubular interstitial nephritis and uveitis (TINU). Patients with TINU may also test positive for antinuclear antibody and have an elevated sedimentation rate, but these findings are not always present and are not specific. Elevated angiotensin-converting enzyme level has not been reported with TINU. Patients with TINU may also have hematuria and proteinuria along with elevated serum creatinine level, eosinophilia, and slightly abnormal results on liver function tests.
17. **a.** Glaucomatocyclitic crisis has been associated with cytomegalovirus (CMV) infection, and the virus has been isolated from the eyes of patients with this disease. Topical corticosteroids and aqueous suppressants are utilized to treat the episodes of acute anterior uveitis and intraocular pressure elevation in these patients. Presenting intraocular pressure may be very high (>40 mm Hg) during these episodes. The inflammation responds readily to topical corticosteroids.
18. **b.** The most common ocular manifestation of early stage 1 Lyme disease (LD) is follicular conjunctivitis. LD-associated uveitis occurs most commonly in stage 2 disease and less commonly in stage 3 disease. It can manifest as anterior, intermediate, or posterior uveitis or as panuveitis; intermediate uveitis is the most common form. Granulomatous anterior chamber reaction, severe vitritis, papillitis, retinal vasculitis, neuroretinitis, and choroiditis with exudative retinal detachment may also occur.
19. **c.** Lyme disease is diagnosed on the basis of clinical signs, symptoms, and a history of possible exposure. The US Centers for Disease Control and Prevention (CDC) currently recommends a 2-step approach to testing for Lyme antibodies. The first step is an enzyme-linked immunosorbent assay (or rarely, an indirect immunofluorescence assay), and the second step is an immunoblot (in this case, a Western blot). Both steps can be done using the same blood specimen. If the first step's result is negative, no further testing is necessary. Results are considered positive only if both steps test positive. Skipping the enzyme immunoassay and performing only the Western blot analysis can increase the false-positive rate. Polymerase chain reaction–based assays can be used to amplify *Borrelia burgdorferi* DNA found in ocular fluids; however, this assay is rarely performed at present.

20. **d.** The diagnostic term *pars planitis* should be used only for the subset of idiopathic intermediate uveitis with snowbank or snowball formation in the absence of associated infection or systemic disease. For example, if the patient has multiple sclerosis as an underlying etiology, the term *intermediate uveitis* should be used.

21. **a.** The main goals of therapy in the treatment of JIA-associated uveitis are the elimination of active intraocular inflammation, preservation of vision, and prevention of new structural complications such as posterior synechiae, cataract formation, and development of macular edema. Because the long-term use of both oral and topical corticosteroids typically leads to significant complications in children, it is important to consider systemic IMT early in the disease course.

22. **a.** The Goldmann-Witmer (GW) coefficient for a specific pathogen is calculated by dividing the amount of IgG reactive to a specific pathogen (xIgG) in aqueous by the total amount of IgG in the aqueous, and then dividing that ratio by a ratio created by dividing the amount of the same specific antigen IgG (xIgG) in serum by the total amount of IgG in serum:

    GW = (xIgG in aqueous/total IgG in aqueous)/(xIgG in serum/total IgG in serum)

23. **d.** Patients with acute retinal necrosis usually present with acute unilateral loss of vision, photophobia, floaters, and pain. Panuveitis is observed, beginning with significant anterior segment inflammation with keratic precipitates, posterior synechiae, and elevated intraocular pressure, together with heavy vitreous cellular infiltration. Within 2 weeks, the classic triad of occlusive retinal arteriolitis, vitritis, and a multifocal yellow-white peripheral retinitis has evolved. Widespread necrosis of the midperipheral retina, multiple posterior retinal breaks, and proliferative vitreoretinopathy predispose to combined tractional–rhegmatogenous retinal detachments in 75% of patients. Timely diagnosis and prompt antiviral therapy are essential given the rapidity of disease progression, the frequency of retinal detachment, and the guarded visual prognosis. Intravenous acyclovir, 10 mg/kg every 8 hours for 10–14 days, is effective against herpes simplex virus and varicella-zoster virus. After 24–48 hours of antiviral therapy, systemic corticosteroids (prednisone, 1 mg/kg/day) are introduced to treat active inflammation and subsequently tapered over several weeks. Aspirin and other anticoagulants have been used to treat an associated hypercoagulable state and prevent vascular occlusions, but the results have been inconclusive. More recently, oral valacyclovir at doses of up to 2 g, 3 times daily, has been used successfully as an alternative to intravenous acyclovir as induction therapy. Additionally, intravitreal ganciclovir (0.2–2.0 mg/0.1 mL) and foscarnet (1.2–2.4 mg/0.1 mL) have been used to achieve a rapid induction in combination with both intravenous and oral antivirals as first-line therapy or in patients who fail to respond to systemic acyclovir.

24. **d.** *Candida* species are the most common fungal cause of endogenous endophthalmitis.

25. **a.** Although all of the organisms listed can cause endophthalmitis, only *Candida parapsilosis* causes an indolent chronic inflammation similar to that which occurs with *Propionibacterium acnes.*

26. **a.** Melanomas can be associated with an impressive inflammatory response, and ciliary body melanomas can break through to the anterior segment. In any case, the differential diagnosis includes infections, chronic retinal detachment, and metastatic tumors. In the absence of a posterior segment view, B scan ultrasonography and, when available, ultrasound biomicroscopy or anterior segment optical coherence tomography can be very helpful.

27. **a.** Not all band keratopathy needs to be treated, but if it is symptomatic or visually significant, the treatment is epithelial debridement followed by chelation with ethylenediaminetetraacetic acid (EDTA).
28. **a.** Ensuring that the current regimen is effective in controlling inflammation for at least 3 months and allowing the ocular tissues to recover from recent inflammation are both highly desirable. In some cases, it may not be necessary to wait 3 months; examples include a very mild uveitis that was easily controlled and is without sequelae as well as Fuchs heterochromic uveitis, which has a good surgical prognosis. The fluocinolone implant is not necessary in this case, as the patient is already being treated systemically, her disease is well controlled, and there is no macular edema. Reduction of anterior chamber cells to zero for 6 months is not necessary.
29. **a.** Immune recovery uveitis is observed in patients with previous CMV retinitis and recovered immune systems, most often in patients with AIDS who have received antiretroviral therapy. CMV retinitis is usually associated with a minimal inflammatory response in AIDS patients; the inflammation of immune recovery uveitis is presumably the reconstituted immune system's response to CMV antigens.

Index

(*f* = figure; *t* = table)